T0226409

Equine Genetic Diseases

Editor

CARRIE J. FINNO

VETERINARY CLINICS OF NORTH AMERICA: EQUINE PRACTICE

www.vetequine.theclinics.com

Consulting Editor
THOMAS J. DIVERS

August 2020 • Volume 36 • Number 2

ELSEVIER

1600 John F. Kennedy Boulevard ● Suite 1800 ● Philadelphia, Pennsylvania, 19103-2899

http://www.vetequine.theclinics.com

VETERINARY CLINICS OF NORTH AMERICA: EQUINE PRACTICE Volume 36, Number 2
August 2020 ISSN 0749-0739, ISBN-13: 978-0-323-70859-3

Editor: Katerina Heidhausen
Developmental Editor: Donald Mumford

Veterinary Clinics of North America: Equine Practice (ISSN 0749-0739) is published in April, August, and December by Elsevier Inc., 360 Park Avenue South, New York, NY 10010-1710. Business and Editorial Offices: 1600 John F. Kennedy Blvd., Suite 1800, Philadelphia, PA 19103-2899. Subscription prices are $290.00 per year (domestic individuals), $585.00 per year (domestic institutions), $100.00 per year (domestic students/residents), $334.00 per year (Canadian individuals), $737.00 per year (Canadian institutions), $365.00 per year (international individuals), $737.00 per year (international institutions), $100.00 per year (Canadian students/residents), and $180.00 per year (international students/residents). To receive student/resident rate, orders must be accompanied by name of affiliated institution, date of term, and the signature of program/residency coordinator on institution letterhead. Orders will be billed at individual rate until proof of status is received. Foreign air speed delivery is included in all *Clinics* subscription prices. All prices are subject to change without notice. **POSTMASTER:** Send address changes to *Veterinary Clinics of North America: Equine Practice*, 3251 Riverport Lane, Maryland Heights, MO 63043. Customer Service (orders, claims, online, change of address): Elsevier Health Sciences Division, Subscription **Customer Service, 3251 Riverport Lane, Maryland Heights, MO 63043. Tel: 1-800-654-2452 (U.S. and Canada); 314-447-8871 (outside U.S. and Canada). Fax: 314-447-8029. E-mail: journalscustomerservice-usa@elsevier.com (for print support);** E-mail: **journalsonlinesupport-usa@ elsevier.com (for online support).**

Reprints. For copies of 100 or more of articles in this publication, please contact the Commercial Reprints Department, Elsevier Inc., 360 Park Avenue South, New York, NY 10010-1710. Tel.: 212-633-3874; Fax: 212-633-3820; E-mail: reprints@elsevier.com.

Veterinary Clinics of North America: Equine Practice is covered in *MEDLINE/PubMed (Index Medicus)*, *Excerpta Medica*, *Current Contents/Agriculture, Biology and Environmental Sciences*, and *ISI*.

Contributors

CONSULTING EDITOR

THOMAS J. DIVERS, DVM
Diplomate, American College of Veterinary Internal Medicine; Diplomate, American College of Veterinary Emergency and Critical Care; Steffen Professor of Veterinary Medicine, Department of Clinical Sciences, Section of Large Animal Medicine, College of Veterinary Medicine, Cornell University, Ithaca, New York, USA

EDITOR

CARRIE J. FINNO, DVM, PhD
Diplomate, American College of Veterinary Internal Medicine (LA), Associate Professor and Gregory L. Ferraro Endowed Chair of the Center for Equine Health, Department of Population Health and Reproduction, School of Veterinary Medicine, University of California, Davis, Davis, California, USA

AUTHORS

DOUGLAS F. ANTCZAK, VMD, PhD
Dorothy Havemeyer McConville Professor of Equine Medicine, Baker Institute for Animal Health, College of Veterinary Medicine, Cornell University, Ithaca, New York, USA

FELIPE AVILA, PhD
Research Geneticist, Veterinary Genetics Laboratory, School of Veterinary Medicine, University of California, Davis, Davis, California, USA

REBECCA R. BELLONE, PhD
Adjunct Professor, Department of Population Health and Reproduction, Director, Veterinary Genetics Laboratory, School of Veterinary Medicine, University of California, Davis, Davis, California, USA

MARIA JULIA BEVILAQUA FELIPPE, MV, MS, PhD
Diplomate, American College of Veterinary Internal Medicine; Professor of Medicine, Department of Clinical Sciences, College of Veterinary Medicine, Cornell University, Ithaca, New York, USA

SAMANTHA A. BROOKS, PhD
Department of Animal Sciences, UF Genetics Institute, University of Florida, Gainesville, Florida, USA

STEPHEN J. COLEMAN, MS, PhD
Assistant Professor, Department of Animal Sciences, Colorado State University, Fort Collins, Colorado, USA

OTTMAR DISTL, Dr. med. vet., Dr. habil
Institute for Animal Breeding and Genetics, University of Veterinary Medicine Hannover, Hannover, Germany

LISA EDWARDS, DVM
Department of Veterinary Population Health and Reproduction, School of Veterinary Medicine, University of California, Davis, Davis, California, USA

CARRIE J. FINNO, DVM, PhD
Diplomate, American College of Veterinary Internal Medicine (LA), Associate Professor and Gregory L. Ferraro Endowed Chair of the Center for Equine Health, Department of Population Health and Reproduction, School of Veterinary Medicine, University of California, Davis, Davis, California, USA

SAMANTHA L. FOUSSE
Stern Comparative Cardiac Genetics Laboratory, Department of Medicine and Epidemiology, School of Veterinary Medicine, University of California, Davis, Davis, California, USA

REBECKA FREY, DVM
AniCura Norsholms Djursjukhus, Norsholm, Sweden

HANNAH GALANTINO-HOMER, VMD, PHD
Diplomate, American College of Theriogenologists; Department of Clinical Studies, New Bolton Center, School of Veterinary Medicine, University of Pennsylvania, Kennett Square, Pennsylvania, USA

VINZENZ GERBER, Professor, Dr. med. vet., PhD
Diplomate, American College of Veterinary Internal Medicine; Diplomate European College of Veterinary Internal Medicine; Department of Clinical Veterinary Medicine, Vetsuisse Faculty, Professor, Swiss Institute of Equine Medicine (ISME), University of Bern, Agroscope, Berne, Switzerland

THEODORE S. KALBFLEISCH, PhD
Associate Professor, Department of Veterinary Science, Gluck Equine Research Center, University of Kentucky, Lexington, Kentucky, USA

GABRIELLA LINDGREN, PhD
Department of Animal Breeding and Genetics, Swedish University of Agricultural Sciences, Uppsala, Sweden; Livestock Genetics, Department of Biosystems, KU Leuven Leuven, Leuven, Belgium

JAMES N. MACLEOD, VMD, PhD
Professor, John S. and Elizabeth A. Knight Chair, Department of Veterinary Science, Gluck Equine Research Center, University of Kentucky, Lexington, Kentucky, USA

MOLLY E. McCUE, DVM, MS, PhD
Diplomate, American College of Veterinary Internal Medicine, Large Animal; Faculty and Associate Dean of Research, Veterinary Population Medicine Department, University of Minnesota, St Paul, Minnesota, USA

JULIA METZGER, Dr. med. vet., Dr. habil
Institute for Animal Breeding and Genetics, University of Veterinary Medicine Hannover, Hannover, Germany

RAKAN NABOULSI, PhD
Department of Animal Breeding and Genetics, Swedish University of Agricultural Sciences, Uppsala, Sweden

ELAINE NORTON, DVM, MS, PhD
Diplomate, American College of Veterinary Internal Medicine, Large Animal; Veterinary Population Medicine Department, University of Minnesota, St Paul, Minnesota, USA

JESSICA L. PETERSEN, MS, PhD
Assistant Professor, Department of Animal Science, University of Nebraska-Lincoln, Lincoln, Nebraska, USA

TERJE RAUDSEPP, PhD
Professor and Director of Molecular Cytogenetic Laboratory, Department of Veterinary Integrative Biosciences, Molecular Cytogenetics laboratory, Texas A&M University, College of Veterinary Medicine and Biomedical Sciences, College Station, Texas, USA

ROBERT J. SCHAEFER, PhD
Department of Veterinary Population Medicine, College of Veterinary Medicine, University of Minnesota, St Paul, Minnesota, USA

MARINA SOLÉ, PhD
Department of Animal Breeding and Genetics, Swedish University of Agricultural Sciences, Uppsala, Sweden

JOSHUA A. STERN, DVM, PhD
Diplomate, American College of Veterinary Internal Medicine (Cardiology); Associate Professor and Chief of Service, Stern Comparative Cardiac Genetics Laboratory, Department of Medicine and Epidemiology, School of Veterinary Medicine, University of California, Davis, Davis, California, USA

REBECCA L. TALLMADGE, PhD
Research Support Specialist, Animal Health Diagnostic Center, College of Veterinary Medicine, Cornell University, Ithaca, New York, USA

STEPHANIE J. VALBERG, DVM, PhD
Diplomate, American College of Veterinary Internal Medicine; American College of Veterinary Sports Medicine and Rehabilitation; Endowed Professor, Mary Anne McPhail Dressage Chair, Equine Sports Medicine, Department of Large Animal Clinical Sciences, College of Veterinary Medicine, Michigan State University, East Lansing, Michigan, USA

CARISSA WICKENS, PHD
Department of Animal Sciences, University of Florida, Gainesville, Florida, USA

Contents

James N. MacLeod and Theodore S. Kalbfleisch

The first equine reference genome was completed in 2007 and published in 2009. This major accomplishment has enabled equine science to advance in ways that broadly parallel the transformative impact that genomics has had on many animal species including humans. A conceptual overview of reference genomes, genome annotation, and the major implications for equine science is presented. The relationship between genomic sequencing and the accelerating application of precision P4 medicine is discussed in the context of human and equine patients. Emergent technologies built on the foundation of genomic sequencing and rapidly gaining traction in research and clinical settings are introduced.

Robert J. Schaefer and Molly E. McCue

High-quality genomic tools have been integral in understanding genomic architecture and function in the modern-day horse. The equine genetics community has a long tradition of pooling resources to develop genomic tools. Since the equine genome was sequenced in 2006, several iterations of high throughput genotyping arrays have been developed and released, enabling rapid and cost-effective genotyping. This review highlights the design considerations of each iteration, focusing on data available during development and outlining considerations in selecting the genetic variants included on each array. Additionally, we outline recent applications of equine genotyping arrays as well as future prospects and applications.

Jessica L. Petersen and Stephen J. Coleman

The sequencing and assembly of a reference genome for the horse has been revolutionary for investigation of horse health and performance. Next-generation sequencing (NGS) methods represent a second revolution in equine genomics. Researchers can align and compare DNA and RNA sequencing data to the reference genome to explore variation that may contribute or be attributed to disease. NGS has also facilitated the translation of research discovery to clinically relevant applications. This article discusses the history and development of NGS, details some of the available sequencing platforms, and describes currently available applications in the context of both discovery and clinical settings.

Genetic testing in horses began in the 1960s, when parentage testing using blood group markers became the standard. In the 1990s, parentage testing shifted from evaluating blood groups to DNA testing. The development of genetics and genomics in both human and veterinarian medicine, along with continued technological advances in the last 2 decades, has helped unravel the causal variants for many horse traits. Genetic testing is also now possible for a variety of phenotypic and disease traits and is used to assist in breeding and clinical management decisions. This article describes the genetic tests that are currently available for horses.

There have been some advances in understanding the genetic contribution to ventricular septal defects in Arabians, sudden death in racehorses, and atrial fibrillation in racehorses. No genetic analyses have been published for aortic rupture in Friesians or atrioventricular block in donkeys despite strong evidence for a genetic cause. To date, no genetic mutation has been identified for any equid cardiac disease. With the advancement of genetic tools and resources, we are moving closer to discoveries that may explain the heritable basis of inherited equid cardiac disease.

Genetic factors influence the development of guttural pouch tympany, recurrent laryngeal neuropathy, severe equine asthma, exercise-induced pulmonary hemorrhage, and possibly also some malformations and infectious diseases of the respiratory tract. The current data suggest that most of these diseases are complex, resulting from the interaction between several genes and environmental factors. To date, no specific genes or causative mutations have been identified that would allow the development of practical genetic tests. In the future, genetic profiling panels, based on multiple genetic markers and environmental risk factors, may allow identification of individuals with an increased genetic risk.

Neurologic disease in horses can be particularly challenging to diagnose and treat. These diseases can result in economic losses, emotional distress to owners, and injury to the horse or handlers. To date, there are five neurologic diseases caused by known genetic mutations and several more are suspected to be heritable: lethal white foal syndrome (LWFS), lavender foal syndrome (LFS), cerebellar abiotrophy (CA), occipitoatlantoaxial malformation (OAAM), and Friesian hydrocephalus. Genetic testing allows owners, breeders, and veterinarians to make informed decisions when selecting dams and sires for breeding or deciding the treatment or prognosis of a neurologic animal.

Host defenses against infection by viruses, bacteria, fungi, and parasites are critical to survival. It has been estimated that upwards of 7% of the coding genes of mammals function in immunity and inflammation. This high level of genomic investment in defense has resulted in an immune system characterized by extraordinary complexity and many levels of redundancy. Because so many genes are involved with immunity, there are many opportunities for mutations to arise that have negative effects. However, redundancy in the mammalian defense system and the adaptive nature of key immune mechanisms buffer the untoward outcomes of many such deleterious mutations.

Orthopedic diseases are a common cause for limited exercise capacity in the horse. They often underlie genetic risk factors, which can affect bone, articular cartilage, tendons, ligaments, and adnexal structures among others. The genetic effects can directly interfere with tissue development and skeletal growth or can trigger degenerative or inflammatory processes. Many of these diseases of the locomotor system like osteochondrosis are complex and can be affected by multifactorial influences. For this reason, it is important for those performing diagnostic procedures to have a comprehensive knowledge of orthopedic diseases, their prevalence within breeds, and genetic background.

Horses perform in a variety of disciplines that are visually demanding, and any disease impacting the eye has the potential to threaten vision and thus the utility of the horse. Advances in equine genetics have enabled the understanding of some inherited ocular disorders and ocular manifestations and are enabling cross-species comparisons. Genetic testing for multiple congenital ocular anomalies, congenital stationary night blindness, equine recurrent uveitis, and squamous cell carcinoma can identify horses with or at risk for disease and thus can assist in clinical management and breeding decisions. This article describes the current knowledge of inherited ocular disorders.

Equine skin diseases are common, causing increased costs and reduced welfare of affected horses.Genetic testing, if available, can complement early detection, disease diagnosis, and clinical treatment and offers horse breeders the possibility to rule out carrier status. The mechanisms of complex disease can be investigated by using the latest state-of-the-art genomic technologies. Genome-based strategies may also serve as an efficient and cost-effective strategy for the management of the disease

The only available genetic test for stallion subfertility is based on a suscep-tibility gene FKBP6. The ongoing progress in equine genomics will improve the status of genetic testing. However, because subfertile phenotypes do not facilitate collection of large numbers of samples or pedigrees, and clin-ical causes of many cases remain unknown, further progress requires constructive cross-talk between geneticists, clinicians, breeders, and owners.

Carissa Wickens and Samantha A. Brooks

Behavior is a valuable quantitative trait in the horse because of its impact on performance, work, recreation, and prerequisite close interactions with humans. This article reviews what is known about the genetics of behavior in horses with an emphasis on the genetic basis for temperament traits, neuroendocrine function, and stereotypic behavior. The importance of us-ing modern molecular genetic techniques to the study of equine behavior and recommendations for future research are also discussed. Ultimately, these studies enhance the understanding of the biology of behavior in the horse, improve handler and rider safety, and benefit horse welfare.

VETERINARY CLINICS OF NORTH AMERICA: EQUINE PRACTICE

RELATED SERIES

Veterinary Clinics of North America: Food Animal Practice

THE CLINICS ARE NOW AVAILABLE ONLINE!
Access your subscription at:
www.theclinics.com

Preface

Equine Genetic Diseases

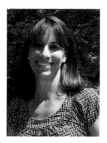

Carrie J. Finno, DVM, PhD
Editor

The publication of a reference genome sequence of a single domestic horse in 2009 resulted in unprecedented advancements in the field of equine genetics. Subsequent technologies, including the development of high-density single nucleotide polymorphism arrays and affordable next-generation sequencing, provided the tools necessary to fully explore the genetic contribution to equine traits and diseases. Of the 46 equine traits for which a genetic test is available to date, 29 were discovered from 2009 to 2019. This issue of *Veterinary Clinics of North America: Equine Practice* highlights these recent discoveries. A new version of the equine genome, EquCab3.0, became available in 2018, and functional annotation of the equine genome, aimed at defining regulatory marks associated with tissue-specific promoters, enhancers, insulators, repressive marks, and open chromatin, was initiated in 2016. These advances will serve to integrate genetics into many facets of equine medicine, while providing exciting insight into new disease mechanisms.

Carrie J. Finno, DVM, PhD
Veterinary Genetics
Department of Population Health
and Reproduction
UC Davis School of Veterinary Medicine
Room 4206 Vet Med 3A
One Shields Avenue
Davis, CA 95616, USA

E-mail address:
cjfinno@ucdavis.edu

Genetics, Genomics, and Emergent Precision Medicine 12 Years After the Equine Reference Genome Was Published

James N. MacLeod, VMD, PhD*, Theodore S. Kalbfleisch, PhD

KEYWORDS

- Equine • Reference genome • EquCab2 • EquCab3 • Genomics
- Precision medicine • Genome sequencing

KEY POINTS

- Historically, the equine reference genome represents one of the most important achievements in equine science. It has enabled fundamental new discoveries and knowledge in multiple disciplines.
- Applied aspects of genomics are coming to fruition in many areas of equine science and veterinary medicine. This includes the emergence of equine precision P4 medicine: predictive, preventive, personalized, and participatory.
- Future use of genomic knowledge, resources, and strategies will continue to expand in biomedical and animal husbandry aspects of equine science.

By the mid-1990s, a small community of scientists from around the world with a shared interested in equine genetics had already recognized the huge impact that genomics was going to have on animal biology. The human genome project was underway, but widely considered such a massive undertaking that it simply was not going to be logistically feasible for most other mammalian species. Yet just 10 years later, blood samples were drawn from a small gray filly of Thoroughbred descent living at Cornell University in Ithaca, New York and named Twilight. The blood samples were needed to isolate the filly's genomic DNA and formally launch the sequencing effort for the equine genome project.

Generating the first whole-genomic DNA sequence of the horse in 2006 to 2007, followed by assembly of the primary Sanger reads into the equine reference genome,

Department of Veterinary Science, Gluck Equine Research Center, University of Kentucky, Lexington, KY 40546-0099, USA
* Corresponding author.
E-mail address: jnmacleod@uky.edu

Vet Clin Equine 36 (2020) 173–181
https://doi.org/10.1016/j.cveq.2020.04.002
0749-0739/20/© 2020 Elsevier Inc. All rights reserved.

qualifies as one of equine science's greatest achievements.[1] Much of the actual technical and computational work was completed by scientists at the Broad Institute in Boston and funded by the National Human Genome Research Institute. Yet the equine-specific intellectual and scientific resources that provided a foundation for this achievement, and substantial improvements to the structural and functional annotation of the reference genome over the last 12 years have been international in scope and highly collaborative. The current 2.41-Gb reference, EquCab 3, has a contig N50 of 4.5 Mb and near chromosome-limited scaffold contiguity.[2]

With regard to the understanding of horse biology, the impact of the equine reference genome, together with the related genomic, molecular, and computational resources that have been developed, has been profound (**Fig. 1**). As demonstrated by more than 600 citations of the equine reference genome paper in the scientific literature and detailed elsewhere in this issue of *Veterinary Clinics of North America*, biologic and biomedical knowledge is being advanced in every body system, from individuals to populations, from evolution to epidemiology, and from the most basic cell biology questions to clinical medicine. Most importantly, however, translational applications are increasingly coming to fruition. This is the dawn of P4 medicine: predictive, preventive, personalized, and participatory. Fortunately for horses and the people who care about them, equine science and equine veterinary medicine are well-positioned to participate.

Precision medicine, earlier referred to as personalized medicine, is now an established concept that has become a major driver for transformative changes underway in health care and biomedical research. Each individual patient, as opposed to a large group or population of patients, is the focus. This is true for human and veterinary patients, including prophylactic, diagnostic, therapeutic, and patient monitoring applications. DNA sequencing has been the primary enabling technology, with logistical challenges being addressed as sequencing costs continue to fall, computational

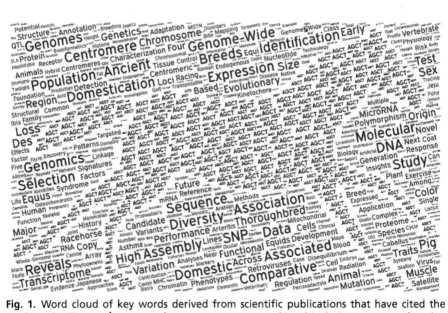

Fig. 1. Word cloud of key words derived from scientific publications that have cited the Wade and colleagues[1] equine reference genome paper. (Graphic design courtesy of Jordan R. Smith, University of Kentucky.)

methods improve, and structural and functional genome annotation advances. In effect, DNA sequencing and genomics have added a fourth leg to the stool of medical practice (**Fig. 2**).

Delivery of precision medicine is developing on multiple levels, both molecular and cellular. Targeted and genomic DNA sequencing applications are increasingly being used not only as diagnostic tests for a suspected condition in diseased patients, but also as broad diagnostic screens, assessments of disease susceptibility, and to identify patients for specific therapies. For certain conditions in human medicine, affordable costs coupled with improved clinical outcomes are compelling enough to motivate the establishment of sponsored testing partnerships. In these programs, the full cost of genetic testing is paid by a biopharmaceutical company working to identify patients who might benefit from a specific therapy. The physician, patient, genetic testing company, and biopharmaceutical company are working collaboratively to deliver personalized and more progressive health care to each individual. Most recently, improvements in DNA and RNA editing technologies, such as CRISPR, are rapidly advancing precise nucleotide sequence manipulations. Patient applications are nascent at present, but the compelling potential on multiple levels is clear for direct and cell-based therapies.

Four broad areas of personalized medicine are advanced through a detailed understanding of the genome: (1) prophylactics, (2) diagnostics, (3) therapeutics, and (4) patient assessment.

Shifting the emphasis of health care from treating disease (reaction) to maintaining health (prevention), or at least balancing these relationships, is a foundation of the changes underway. Inherited mutations or other genetic determinants can either be the direct cause of an inherited disease or alter a patient's susceptibility for specific acquired conditions. Understanding these relationships enables compensatory methods that alter environmental variables to lower disease risk and customize disease prevention strategies.

DNA diagnostic tests are already standard of care for several conditions and the list continues to expand as underlying molecular mechanisms for additional diseases are defined. Multiple analyses in human medicine have demonstrated medical and

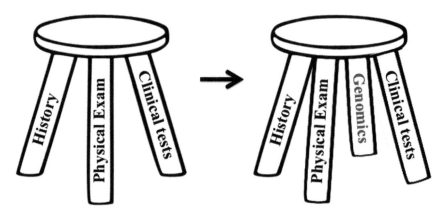

Fig. 2. Genomics has become an important variable in many aspects of health care. In caring for individual patients, this is depicted as a new, but now fundamental fourth leg of the doctor's decision-making stool.

economic benefits of genetic testing and screens. Specific examples include noninvasive prenatal testing during pregnancy,[3] neonatal genomic sequencing,[4] childhood epilepsy,[5] and cancer.[6] Closely related molecular tests, DNA and RNA, are used for patient monitoring and assessment of therapy.

Personalized prophylactic and diagnostic parameters tie directly into precision therapies. There are a couple of general considerations. First, therapeutic intervention earlier in the pathogenesis of a disease, often before clinical signs develop, usually has a higher efficacy with an improved prognosis. Second, drug resistance, absence of efficacy, or an unacceptable side effect is interpreted not as a drug failure, but rather as a failure of accurate patient selection. Optimally, drug selection is customized to maximize the net positive outcome for each individual patient and therapeutic target. The prospective pairing of specific drugs to individual patients based on genomic testing of either patients or infectious pathogens is accelerating. From 2008 to 2020, the number of Food and Drug Administration–approved personalized therapies on the market in the United States has risen from 5 to 170.[7] Personalized therapies not only include the consideration of individual drugs in the context of DNA-based tests of the patient, but also additional areas, such as small interfering RNA molecules. In the future, the list will undoubtedly include molecular and cellular therapies personalized using CRISPR and related nucleotide-editing technologies.[8]

Applications of precision medicine in equine patients are currently centered on DNA-based diagnostic tests. Knowledge obtained not only informs therapeutic options, but also managerial decisions such as breeding considerations, optimization of nutrition, and modifications to training programs. Areas of active research include molecular profiling of biopsy, microbial, and parasitic samples. Because many health and welfare decisions involving horses are based on the care of individual animals rather than herd health, the development and adoption of these new prospective personalized medical practices will continue and undoubtedly accelerate in ways that broadly parallel advances in human health care.

WHAT IS A REFERENCE GENOME?

What exactly is a reference genome, and how does having one benefit your horse? A horse has 31 pairs of autosomal chromosomes. One-half of that pair is inherited from the sire, the other half is inherited from the dam. There is also what is called the sex chromosome (chromosome X) where, for a female, the sire and dam pass on their version of that chromosome, and for a male, the dam passes an X chromosome, and the sire passes on a Y chromosome. These chromosomes are large molecules, big enough that they can be seen and analyzed under the lens of a microscope. The picture shown in **Fig. 3** is termed a karyotype and shows the maternal and paternal copies of equine chromosomes grouped with one another and ordered by size. To make things easier, they have been assigned names based on their size and type. The big pair in the upper left-hand corner are named chromosome 1. Each of these is a single molecule, comprised of approximately 190 million molecular subunits called nucleotides. These subunits adenine, thymine, cytosine, and guanine, referred to as A, T, C, and G, respectively, are arranged in an order that has been honed by the trial and error process of evolution for many millions of years. The genomes of any two horses are going to be nearly identical to one another, but the differences that do exist (occurring at an overall rate of about 1 in every 1000 nucleotides) are primarily responsible for the many, and substantial differences between any two individuals.

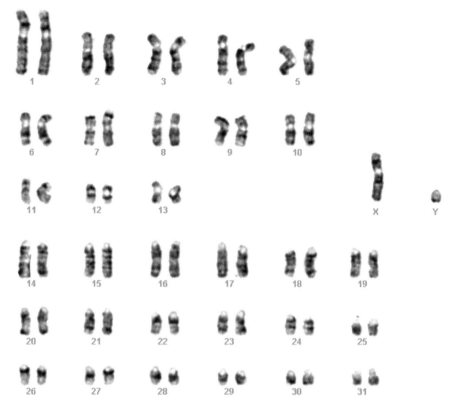

Fig. 3. A karyotype of a horse produced by Dr. Teri Lear. The pairs of chromosomes are ordered by size and type. The metacentric chromosomes are those with the centromere in the center of the chromosome, and they are arranged first, chromosomes 1 through 13. Chromosomes 14 through 31 are acrocentric because their centromeres are physically located near the end of the chromosome. The sex chromosomes, X and Y for a male, and X and X for a female, are typically positioned separately from the autosomal (nonsex) chromosomes.

A reference genome for a species is the ordering of these nucleotides to generate a single representation of each chromosome. We make several compromises when building reference genomes. The first among them is the aforementioned single representation of each chromosome. All horses are diploid, that is, each animal has a maternal and paternal copy of each autosomal chromosome. When we build a reference, we isolate several million physical copies of each of these chromosomes when we sample the chosen reference animal, and randomly break the genome into between hundreds of thousands to tens of millions of pieces depending on the approach. These pieces, originating from different maternal and paternal copies of the same chromosomes (eg, chromosome 1), when compared partially overlap one another, and this nucleotide level identity allows us to position them in consecutive order to form a consensus sequence that includes the overlapped region plus the bits from each sequence that extend beyond the overlap. We look for these overlaps over and over again until, if fortunate, we are able to tile the entire length of a chromosome. It is important to remember that the maternal and paternal versions of the chromosomes are nearly identical, but not completely. Typically, we do not have any notion as to whether a fragment is maternal or paternal in origin. So, when we come to a place where the two differ, the choice regarding which version of the region to include in the reference is made more or less at random.

The second notable compromise is that we use one animal as a representative for the entire species: all horses in the current case. From work done in other species, namely human, we know that there are substantial pieces of the human genome content that were simply missed because they did not exist in the few individuals sampled for the reference genome construction. In one case, there were segments as large as 5 million bases missing from the human reference that could be accurately identified in an individual with a different ethnic origin than those sampled for the reference.[9] In fact, the sequence missing from the original reference contained protein-coding genes, which would have been effectively invisible in any genome-wide studies conducted using this reference as a basis. Nevertheless, these compromises have proven themselves worthy because our efforts have provided a faithful representation of the equine genome.[1,2]

The reference genome, even with the compromises, has given us a perspective that we never had before in biomedical science. We can inexpensively sequence the genome of an animal (current 2020 cost for sequencing to a useful depth for research is ~$1000) and know quickly how this specific animal differs from others. This is powerful in research, because we can sequence a cohort of healthy animals and compare them with a cohort of animals with a condition that seems to be heritable. In many cases, copies or variants of genes common to those with the condition and missing from those without the condition emerge as potentially important genetic determinants and become the basis for research aimed at understanding the cause, and perhaps methods to prevent or treat the condition.

WHAT IS ANNOTATION?

As seen in subsequent articles, scientists sequence different sample types to gain a functional understanding of the genome. Whole-genome shotgun sequencing is done to identify sequence variants in an individual. RNA sequencing (RNA-Seq) is performed to catalog and quantify the RNA transcripts that are produced in a given cell type or tissue. There are also various types of epigenetic sequencing projects done to identify regions within the genome that regulate what genes are transcribed and at what level. The reference genome is used to place all of this information in a single unified context (**Fig. 4**).

We can, for example, identify a genetic variant in an animal and, leveraging what is known about gene structures from the RNA-Seq data (intron-exon boundaries, coding sequence start and end positions), predict an impact for this variant based on its position in that larger context. In an extreme example, we may see a variant allele present in an individual that is positioned in the coding sequence of a gene. Based on its position in a codon, it changes the amino acid normally present in the protein of horses to a stop codon. If near the beginning of the gene's coding sequence, this would dramatically truncate the encoded protein and likely prove to be deleterious. There are other questions we could ask. Is the variant common in horses? Does it exist in healthy animals? If the answer to either or both of these questions is yes, then the variant is likely not as impactful as we might have predicted. Otherwise, it is an obvious candidate to study as a potential causative variant. To be clear, as tantalizing as this variant may seem to be, it is still just one of several million found in that animal, all of which merit consideration.

Historically, in the pregenome era, measurements would have been performed and recorded, often by hand, in laboratory notebooks. This approach is simply impossible

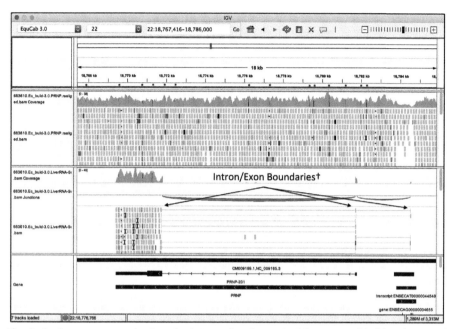

Fig. 4. An image prepared using the Integrative Genomics Viewer provided by the Broad Institute. These sequence data were produced as part of the Equine FAANG project and described in Burns and colleagues.[10] The data shown in the *top panel* are whole-genome shotgun sequence data. The positions indicated with an *asterisk* are positions where the animal has an allele that differs from the reference sequence. The animal is heterozygous (indicated by the *vertical bars* comprised of *two colors*) meaning that one chromosome contains the reference allele, and the other contains a nonreference allele. RNA-Seq for the same animal's liver is shown in the *middle panel*. The data when mapped indicate what portion of the genomic sequence was transcribed to the mRNA (the exons) and what was omitted (the introns). The physical annotation known for this region of the horse genome at the time of this publication is shown in the *bottom panel*. What is most interesting about this is that the RNA-Seq data suggest an exon 5′ (to the right in this rendering) of the current 5′ most annotated exon. This new information will likely be incorporated into the next version of the annotation.

in the postgenome era. Software has been written that will use as foundational knowledge the equine reference genome and structural annotation for comparison to the information garnered from the animals being studied. Using the power of now readily accessible high-performance computers, these large datasets are analyzed to remove such things as common variants, or transcripts whose expression levels are not statistically different from those of the population. This winnowing process will take us from tens of thousands or even millions of pieces of data and result in tens to hundreds of pieces of individual information that can be studied further. The ability to aggregate all of these disparate data sources has proven essential in contemporary biomedical disciplines, and has, as a result, turned the life sciences into a data science.

PARADIGM SHIFT IN RESEARCH

One of the most profound impacts of next-generation sequencing is that the results produced are unbiased in the sense that we are not testing a sample to quantify any single transcript or probe any single locus of a genetic sequence. In fact, the data produced will contain representative sequence data sampled from the entirety of the RNA or DNA present. This will include every cell type present in the sample of the animal being tested, and even every bacteria or virus present in that same sample, or inadvertently swept along during sample collection or sample preparation.

This new perspective has introduced a transformative paradigm shift in life science research. Before the advent of high throughput arrays and sequencing, a researcher was required to limit the scope of their query to one or only a few transcripts, using polymerase chain reaction and agarose gels to quantify expression levels. These targeted transcripts would have typically been within a pathway central to the researcher's established interest. In contrast, next-generation sequencing is completely unbiased. Specifically for whole-genome shotgun sequencing or RNA-Seq experiments, the sequence data are captured from everything in the sample. That is, all of the genomic DNA or transcribed RNA in the sample is characterized and quantified. Our knowledge of exactly how cells work and the specific identity of active transcriptional components have been improved greatly by the new sequencing technologies and data-driven approaches, greatly enabled by the fact that we have an equine reference genome to put all of the nucleotide sequences into a genomic context.

New high throughput RNA-Seq datasets, when mapped to the reference genome, not only provide sufficient data to quantify transcripts, but also allow structural assessments of those same transcripts (ie, exon-intron boundaries). This enables comparison of the transcript structure in the experimental sample to the current known structures for the gene and transcribed RNAs from that locus. Perhaps the biggest benefit is that any sequences that do not map to known genes or RNA structures represent novel transcripts that expand knowledge of the functional elements in the genome. This is a vastly broader perspective than we had before and provides the opportunity for a new research paradigm that shifts from hypothesis testing to one of hypothesis generation. Simply put, for a given condition, collect some number of samples that have been unchallenged and collect another set of samples that have been challenged, perform RNA-Seq, and see just what transcripts are differentially expressed. Again, this is not hypothesis-based testing, but an opportunity to determine how a cell responds when challenged with a disease, a drug, an environmental change, or with a genetic mutation known to alter the function of a certain gene or protein. This, in turn, will lead the researcher to an understanding of what is dysregulated and will often enable the development of hypotheses that can be tested in the traditional manner.

CRYSTAL BALL GAZING

The first version of the human reference genome was published at the start of the new millennium in 2000. This monumental scientific achievement took approximately 10 years, engaged hundreds of scientists, and reflected a global investment totaling several billions of dollars to complete. In the two decades since, from the year 2000 to 2020, the landscape has changed to an extent that few would have predicted. For roughly $20,000 and less than 2 weeks of computational time, an expert in the field can generate genome sequences representing all pairs of chromosomes for a mammal, completely phased, and gap free.[11] With costs continuing to fall, what exactly does this change? Instead of looking at an animal's genomic content in the context of Twilight, equine scientists and veterinarians will soon be able to fully sequence and assemble the genomes of horses in research and clinical settings. All of the efforts that have been directed at the infrastructure necessary to build genomic references are now rapidly being redirected toward the task of annotating the genome of individual subjects, complete with assessment of known and predicted risk alleles. This is powerful on multiple levels. As our computer models become more sophisticated and our functional understanding of the genome becomes more complete, we will ultimately be able to comprehensively predict the physical and chemical behavior of a diploid genome in much the same way a cell experiences it. This is no longer science fiction. A decade or two from now, we will likely be able to predict simple and complex phenotypes that may take years to manifest themselves, while adjusting management and other environmental variables to minimize the impact of disease susceptibilities or avoid potential pathologies altogether. It is an exciting time to be biologist.

DISCLOSURE

The authors have nothing to disclose.

REFERENCES

1. Wade CM, Giulotto E, Sigurdsson S, et al. Genome sequence, comparative analysis, and population genetics of the domestic horse. Science 2009;326:865–7.
2. Kalbfleisch TS, Rice RS, DePriest MS Jr, et al. EquCab3: improved reference genome for the domestic horse increases assembly contiguity and composition. Nat Commun Biol 2018;16(1):197.
3. Benachi A, Caffrey J, Calda P, et al. Understanding attitudes and behaviors towards cell-free DNA-based noninvasive prenatal testing (NIPT): a survey of European health-care providers. Eur J Med Genet 2020;63(1):103616.
4. Ceyhan-Birsoy O, Murry JB, Machini K, et al, BabySeq Project Team. Interpretation of genomic sequencing results in healthy and ill newborns: results from the BabySeq Project. Am J Hum Genet 2019;104(1):76–93.
5. Truty R, Patil N, Sankar R, et al. Possible precision medicine implications from genetic testing using combined detection of sequence and intragenic copy number variants in a large cohort with childhood epilepsy. Epilepsia Open 2019;4(3):397–408.
6. Brown NA, Elenitoba-Johnson KSJ. Enabling precision oncology through precision diagnostics. Annu Rev Pathol 2020;15:97–121.
7. Personalized Medicine Coalition, Strategic Plan, 2020. Available at: http://www.personalizedmedicinecoalition.org/Userfiles/PMC-Corporate/file/PMC_Strategic_Plan_20202.pdf.
8. Zipkin M. "CRISPR's "magnificent moment" in the clinic". Nat Biotechnol 2019. https://doi.org/10.1038/d41587-019-00035-2.
9. Li R, Li Y, Zheng H, et al. Building the sequence map of the human pan-genome. Nat Biotechnol 2010;28(1):57–63.
10. Burns EN, Bordbari M, Mienaltowski MJ, et al. Generation of an equine functional annotation of animal genomes biobank. Anim Genet 2018. https://doi.org/10.1111/age.12717.
11. Rice ES, Koren S, Rhie A, et al. Continuous chromosome-scale haplotypes assembled from a single interspecies F1 hybrid of yak and cattle. Gigascience 2020;9(4):giaa029.

Equine Genotyping Arrays

Robert J. Schaefer, PhD*, Molly E. McCue, DVM, MS, PhD

KEYWORDS

- SNP • Genotyping array • Equine • GWAS • Population genomics • Imputation

KEY POINTS

- High-quality single nucleotide polymorphism genotyping arrays have in the horse have been crucial for mapping equine diseases and characterizing equid populations.
- In the past decade, several iterations of commercially available single nucleotide polymorphism genotyping arrays with varying densities and technical capabilities have been available.
- Equine single nucleotide polymorphism chips have been used in association mapping, population genomics, and imputation.
- Genotype imputation has become a crucial component of improving accuracy and combining datasets from varying equine single nucleotide polymorphism arrays.

INTRODUCTION

High-quality genomic tools have been integral in understanding genomic architecture and function in the modern-day horse. The equine genetics community has had a long tradition of pooling resources to communally develop genomic tools. Since the equine genome was first sequenced, several iterations of high-throughput genotyping arrays (commonly called "single nucleotide polymorphism [SNP] chips") have been developed and released, enabling rapid and cost-effective genotyping. The first generation genotyping array (Illumina EquineSNP50 BeadChip; Illumina, San Diego, CA) with 54,602 SNPs was developed using SNPs discovered by limited Sanger sequencing in a small cohort of 7 horses.[1] Soon after, a slightly higher density array (Illumina EqineSNP70 BeadChip) with 65,157 SNPs was released. Most recently, both the SNP50 and SNP70 BeadChips have been superseded by the MNEc670 K array, which surveys 670,805 sites throughout the equine genome using SNPs identified from whole genome sequencing of a cohort of 153 horses.[2] This review highlights the design of each generation of equine SNP genotyping array, focusing on the data that were available during development and outlining the efforts and considerations

Department of Veterinary Population Medicine, College of Veterinary Medicine, University of Minnesota, 1365 Gortner Avenue, St Paul, MN 55108, USA
* Corresponding author.
E-mail address: schae234@umn.edu
Twitter: @CSciBio (R.J.S.); @Molly_McCue_DVM (M.E.M.)

Vet Clin Equine 36 (2020) 183–193
https://doi.org/10.1016/j.cveq.2020.03.001
0749-0739/20/© 2020 Elsevier Inc. All rights reserved.

in selecting the SNPs chosen for each array. We also outline relevant applications of equine genotyping arrays along with future prospects and applications.

DESIGN AND IMPLEMENTATION OF EQUINE GENOTYPING ARRAYS

The development of each generation of equine SNP genotyping array has required a multistep process involving SNP discovery, prioritization based on the feasibility of probe design, balancing the marker informativeness among breeds of interest, and, finally, downstream validation and characterization in a cohort of diverse individuals. Since the equine reference genome was sequenced, 2 major SNP discovery efforts have resulted in 4 equine genotyping arrays being developed. The development process for each generation of arrays was slightly different, influenced largely by the genotyping technology available at the time of development, as well as the wealth of data the equine genetics community was able to collectively pool together.

Equine SNP50 BeadChip Design

Development of the first-generation EquineSNP50 array (54,602 SNPs) occurred shortly after the whole genome sequencing of Twilight in 2006 (a female Thoroughbred), funded by the National Human Genome Research Institute and led by the Broad Institute. This massive Sanger sequencing project also incorporated an SNP discovery effort that resequenced 7 individuals at very low coverage, each representing different breeds (Akhal-Teke, Andalusian, Arabian, Icelandic, Quarter Horse, Standardbred, and Thoroughbred). These efforts resulted in a pool of approximately 750,000 SNPs discovered from Twilight in addition to approximately 400,000 SNPs discovered from the low coverage sequencing of the 7 additional horses. The SNP selection criteria for inclusion on the array was performed as a single step process that largely involved assigning scores to each SNP based on their ability to be converted to a reliable oligonucleotide probe for the Illumina Infinium II assay. From the pool of approximately 1.1 million candidate SNPs from Twilight and the 7 additional horses, approximately 60,000 SNPs were suitable for array design based on their ability to be converted to oligonucleotide probes.

Subsequently, McCue and associates[1] evaluated the design performance on a cohort of diverse horse breeds based on across breed informativeness, as well as overall genome coverage. The initial panel of 60,000 SNP probes were assessed in 354 horses representing 14 breeds (Andalusian, Arabian, Belgian, Franches-Montanges, French Trotter, Hanoverian, Icelandic, Mongolian, Norwegian Fjord, Quarter Horse, Saddlebred, Standardbred, Swiss Warmblood, and Thoroughbred), yielding 54,602 probes that reliably produced consistent genotypes (91% conversion rate). The average spacing between SNPs across the autosomes was 43.1 kb, with only 12 regions larger than 500 kb. Among the breeds, approximately one-half (26,473) of the SNPs were polymorphic across all breeds, and between 43,287 and 52,085 SNPs were polymorphic within each breed. The number of informative SNPS (minor allele frequency of >5%) varied between 37,053 and 47,669, with 17,428 SNPs that were informative in all 14 sampled breeds. Because the SNP discovery cohort was heavily biased to the breed of the reference genome (Thoroughbred), the SNP selection process included a breed balancing step that prioritized SNPs that were observed to be polymorphic in 1 of the 7 additional breeds.[3,4] More than two-thirds of SNPs were identified exclusively in 1 of the 7 alternative breeds, and the remaining SNPs were present in at least 1 alternative breed as well as Twilight.[1]

Equine SNP70 BeadChip Design

Shortly after the initial design of the Equine SNP50 BeadChip, the commercial provider of the assay replaced the technology with an updated array containing 65,157 SNP markers. The design of this array represented an extension to the larger, first-generation design with an opportunity to address some of the gaps in coverage, although without the massive SNP discovery stage. In addition to approximately 45,000 informative markers from the SNP50 BeadChip with a minor allele frequency of greater than 0.005 in the 354 horses used for validation of the SNP50 chip, an additional approximately 20,000 SNPs were needed to reach 65,000. Because there were insufficient SNPs discovered from the original 7 discovery breeds suitable for array design,[5] an additional approximately 3900 SNPs discovered from Twilight alone were included as well as approximately 2800 SNPs from RNASeq data[6] were included. Despite a limited SNP discovery stage, this incremental update yielded an average of one SNPs per 35-kb window, substantially increasing the density of the array, especially in places with known gaps in the previous design as well as the equine major histocompatibility region and X chromosome.

Equine MNEc2M and MNEc670K Axiom Array Design

An increased number of available short-read based whole genome sequences (WGS), coupled with advances in chip based genotyping technologies, prompted a massive SNP chip redesign in February 2017 that produced 2 new arrays, the MNEc2M and MNEc670k arrays. Despite changes in genotyping platform technologies, from Illumina-based Infinium to Affymetrix-based Axiom (Affymetrix, Santa Clara, CA), the MNEc2M and MNEc670k Axiom arrays overall followed a similar design process as previous generation arrays, with several major exceptions. The eventual selection of 670,805 SNPs to be included on the commercially available MNEc670 K array followed a 6-stage filtering process.[2] Within this selection process, a limited edition test array containing 2,001,826 SNPs (MNEc2M) genotyped on a test cohort of 332 horses was used to inform the design of the commercially available MNEc670k array. This multistage design process allowed for a finer tuned SNP selection process and an overall higher quality final product because the SNP conversion rates, breed representation, and imputation accuracy from the MNEc2M test array were informative for selection SNPs selected for the MNEc670k array.[2]

SNP discovery was significantly expanded, including WGS from 154 individuals representing 24 distinct breeds.[2] In total, approximately 23 million SNPs were discovered from WGS, of which approximately 10 million were candidates for array design based on the ability to reliably design an oligonucleotide probe. A set of approximately 5 million SNPs selected for probe design were identified based on backward compatibility with the approximately 74,000 SNPs on the legacy (54,000/65,000) arrays, even genome distribution, informativeness among the 24 discovery breeds, and low linkage disequilibrium (LD). This set of 5 million SNPs was evaluated and scored by Affymetrix (now Thermo-Fisher Scientific) for probe design feasibility. A set of 2,001,826 SNPs were then filtered based on their recommendation as well as a greedy selection algorithm targeting approximately 37 SNPs per 50-kb window. Furthermore, all SNPs within the equine major histocompatibility were automatically included. These filtering steps resulted in the 2 million SNPs used to build the MNEc2M test array.[2]

A cohort of 347 horses were genotyped on the MNEc2M test array to validate SNP conversion and provide information for selecting the final set of SNPs used on the more affordable MNEc670k array. After quality control of SNP probe clustering quality, 1,846,988 SNPs remained. As previously seen during the design of the 54,000

BeadChip, SNPs that were discovered in more than 1 breed group were more likely to produce high-quality genotypes. Genotypes at the approximately 1.8 million SNP sites from the 347 genotyped horses were combined with WGS genotypes to identify tagging SNPs, thus allowing for efficient reconstruction of genomic haplotypes (imputation) both within and across breeds. In total, 355,903 tag SNPs were included that tagged haplotypes across breeds as well as 206,822 tag SNPs that were informative in 5 or more of the 15 tagging breeds. Finally, 7394 SNPs within the major histocompatibility region were included, 16,398 SNPs were added to increase SNP density in 50-kb windows with fewer than 8 SNPs, and 70,295 SNPs were included owing to backward compatibility with previous SNP50 and SNP70 arrays. In total, these 670,805 SNPs represent the MNEc670k commercial array.

USEFULNESS IN ASSOCIATION MAPPING

One of the main applications of SNP chips is rapid genotyping of large cohorts of individuals to map a trait of interest. Each generation of genotyping assay has increased the number of available SNPs as well as the number of breeds where SNPs have been evaluated for informativeness. Genome-wide LD analysis of both the SNP50 array as well as the MNEc2M array have demonstrated general as well as breed-specific utility for genome wide association mapping.[1,2] **Fig. 1** shows a composite plot, summarizing the LD decay for the SNP50 chip and the MNEc2M chip as reported by McCue and colleagues[1] and Schaefer and colleagues,[2] respectively. In general, for both chips, the initial LD decays rapidly across all breeds dropping to approximately 0.2 within 50 kb; however, breed-specific patterns of LD show higher r^2 values up to a megabase away.

To date, the SNP50 Chip has been used to map many different traits, often times focused on specific breeds. Studies have included: osteochondrosis in Norwegian Standardbred[7]; palmar/plantar osteochondral fragments in Norwegian Standardbred Trotters[8]; hoof wall separation disease in Connemara Ponies[9]; "splashed white" and other coat color phenotypes Quarter Horses[10]; sprinting ability and racing Stamina,[11] optimum racing distance,[12] osteochondrosis,[13] and impaired acrosomal reaction of sperm[14] in Thoroughbreds; height and conformation in Franches-Montagnes[15];

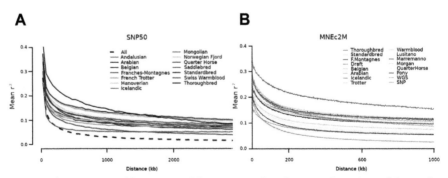

Fig. 1. LD decay measured by average r2 between markers from two iterations of the equine genotyping array: (A) SNP50 BeadChip (McCue et al. [1]) and (B) MNEc2M Axiom array (Schaefer et al. [2]). (*From [A]* McCue ME, Bannasch DL, Petersen JL, et al. A high density SNP array for the domestic horse and extant Perissodactyla: utility for association mapping, genetic diversity, and phylogeny studies. Georges M, ed. *PLoS Genet.* 2012;8(1):e1002451; [*B*] Schaefer RJ, Schubert M, Bailey E, et al. Developing a 670k genotyping array to tag ~2M SNPs across 24 horse breeds. *BMC Genomics.* 2017;18(1):565; with permission.)

semen quality traits[16] and equine recurrent uveitis[17] in German Warmbloods; guttural pouch tympany in both Arabian and German Warmblood Horses[18]; and stallion fertility in Hanoverian Warmblood horses.[19] The SNP50 chip has also been used to concurrently compare multiple breeds, including body size,[20] equine arteritis,[21] and recurrent laryngeal neuropathy.[22]

Similarly, several association studies used the SNP70 array, examining such traits as osteochondrosis in Standardbreds[23]; body weight in Japanese Thoroughbred racehorses[24]; gait[25] and heritable temperament variation in the Tennessee Walking Horse[26]; and height in Shetland Ponies.[27]

Combined SNP50/SNP70

The equine SNP70 array was released shortly after the SNP50 array, leading to several studies using both platforms. This posed some additional complexity owing to different slightly different SNP sets between the arrays, requiring either strict filtering or imputation (see section on Imputation elsewhere in this article). Studies that included both the SNP50 and SNP70 array include those examining: equine herpesvirus type 1–induced myeloencephalopathy susceptibility,[28] susceptibility to immune-mediated myositis in Quarter Horses,[29] and osteochondrosis in multiple horse breeds.[30]

MNEc670k/MNEc2M

The development of the MNEc2M and the commercial release of the MNEc670k array have led to recent studies that have been able to use a much larger SNP set. Similar to the increase in markers seen in the release of the SNP70 array, studies using the MNEc2M and MNEc670k arrays often use genotype imputation to further leverage existing data in previous generation arrays. Using the larger SNP set available in the newest generation SNP chip, studies often are able to use a more complex study design and analyze more complex biological problems, such as expression quantitate trait loci, heritability, and pleiotropy. Recently published studies include: expression quantitate trait loci discovery and their association with severe equine asthma in European Warmblood horses,[31] SNP-based heritability and genetic architecture of tarsal osteochondrosis in North American Standardbred horses,[32] evaluation of an HMGA2 variant for pleiotropic effects on height and metabolic traits in ponies,[33] and heritability of metabolic traits associated with equine metabolic syndrome in Welsh ponies and Morgan horses.[34]

POPULATION GENOMICS

In addition to mapping specific traits of interest, genotyping arrays have also been used to characterize and compare populations of individuals. Depending on the study design, population genomics applications of the array characterized SNPs in a single breed,[35–37] directly compared 2 distinct breeds,[38] or simultaneously compared many different breeds.[39,40]

Population genomics studies leveraging use of equine SNP arrays can be further categorized by the type of analysis that was performed, focusing in on the type of analysis used. Several studies examine runs of homozygosity in and across breeds.[41–43] Furthermore, more sophisticated approaches can be used to compare populations of individuals and can also be used to identify regions or even genes undergoing selection. For example, Avila and colleagues[44] imputed SNPs from the SNP70 array to 2M SNPs in a cohort of 143 elite Quarter Horses representing 6 different subpopulations to identify signatures of selection among the different horse performance types. SNP imputation was crucial in this study for identifying the boundaries of regions and haplotypes of interest from a smaller number of input SNPs, as well as for delineating the candidate genes within each region for downstream pathway and functional analysis.

Domestication and Breed Origins

SNP array-based studies have also been used in examining the historical migration and domestication of the modern-day horse. Jónsson and colleagues[45] examine the gene flow among equids in early speciation and Schubert and colleagues[46] characterize prehistoric genomes, demonstrating the effects and aftermath of domestication. Other studies focus on unraveling the origins and historical foundations of specific breeds including the Persian Arabian horses in Iran,[47] the Debao pony,[48] coastal indigenous horses[49] in China, and the Jeju horse in Korea,[50] as well as breeds of horses across Europe and the Near East.[51]

IMPUTATION

SNP imputation has been a popular strategy to statistically infer genotypes based on haplotypes that are present in a larger reference population. The reference group of haplotypes are inferred based on individuals exhibiting runs of homozygosity (ie, they have 2 copies of the same haplotype) or inferred via expectation maximization algorithms or hidden Markov models.[52] Imputation using a reference population allows for efficient phasing of SNPs from genotyping technologies, such as SNP chips, that are unable to resolve which strand an allele came from. Imputation is also a popular strategy to infer missing genotypes based on haplotype information from the individual (ie, if an SNP is missing, the allele can be inferred from its haplotype).

Although the SNP50 and SNP70 arrays were not explicitly designed for genotype imputation, several studies used imputation, using the legacy arrays in several different scenarios. Corbin and colleagues[53] imputed a very low density panel (1000–3000 markers) to the SNP70 marker set in Thoroughbreds. Frischknecht and colleagues[54] evaluated the possibility of imputing markers from the SNP50 BeadChip to WGS (approximately 13 million SNPs) in Franches-Montagnes horses, a breed with a low effective population size and high genetic relatedness. The study demonstrated the feasibility of imputing from 54,000 to WGS level marker sets with approximately 95% accuracy after correcting for admixture as well as possible annotation errors in EquCab2. McCoy and colleagues[55] used imputation to combine data from individuals genotyped on different arrays, leveraging a high number of shared SNPs between the arrays (approximately 45,000). The study reports an average imputation accuracy of 94.8% on a cohort of 248 horses from 3 breeds (Quarter Horse, Standardbred, and Thoroughbred), noting that breeds with longer LD resulted in more accurate imputation, likely in part owing to fewer number of possible haplotypes.

In contrast with previous arrays, the MNEc670k array was deliberately designed to facilitate genotype imputation to the larger MNEc2M SNP set, as well as to WGS. To decrease the burden of cross-platform imputation and to better leverage existing SNP50 and SNP70 data the MNEc670k SNP chip was designed to be fully backwards compatible with all previous SNP chips. Reference populations generating using the MNEc670 K or MNEc2M can be used to impute datasets generated using the SNP50 or SNP70 arrays. Chassier and colleagues[56] examined this feature on a cohort of 4693 horses representing 5 groupings of horse breeds by imputing legacy SNP data to the MNEc670k SNP set, achieving an overall imputation concordance of greater than 97%.

As presented earlier, SNPs present on the MNEc670 K array were selected to tag haplotypes present in the reference population of 485 horses representing 24 breeds used to design the chip. The strategy in designing the chip for imputation was to identify SNPs that tagged haplotypes using multimarker r^2 statistics. Tagging SNPs were prioritized on the MNEc670k SNP chip based on their ability to tag common haplotypes shared across populations as well as to discern haplotypes common only in a subset of breeds. As described by Schaefer and colleagues,[2] imputation accuracy from the MNEc670 K to the MNEc2M SNP set was evaluated using a cross-validation strategy. Imputation accuracy ranged between 96.6% and 99.4% among the 15 breed groups tested. Although these imputation accuracies may be slightly inflated owing to the lack of an independent dataset (all the data were also used to inform the SNPs selected on the SNP chip), several studies since have performed imputation on independent cohorts showing a high accuracy in imputations. As demonstrated in other species, the prevalence of larger reference populations along with better estimates of allele error rate, average haplotype length, and effective population size will further increase imputation accuracy.[57] These types of data are now being systematically measured in the horse. Recently, Beeson and colleagues[58] used SNPs from a cohort of 485 horses genotyped on the MNEc2M SNP chip to estimate fine scale recombination rates both the entire cohort as well as 12 specific breeds.

FORWARD COMPATIBILITY WITH EquCab3.0

All equine SNP genotyping arrays were developed using EquCab2, a reference genome assembly that was released in 2007.[4] In 2018, an updated reference genome, EquCab3, was publicly released,[59] subsequently resulting in updated SNP orientations and positions across the 2 genome builds. Despite being developed with EquCab2, the MNEc670k SNP chip used an extended reference genome that included an additional 7850 unmapped contigs, designated as ChrUn2, generated from unmapped Twilight genomic DNA reads that were assembled de novo.[2] The inclusion of ChrUn2 was in anticipation that many of the unplaced contigs would be resolved in the next, upcoming reference genome build. Additionally, during development of the MNEc670k array, it was noted that 445,421 SNPs were found to have a 100% alternate allele frequency, even including a large number of reads from Twilight, indicating likely errors in the Sanger sequencing–based EquCab2 genome. These discrepancies would certainly influence the ability to perform imputation. Frischknecht and colleagues[54] note a decreased imputation concordance on ECA12 compared with other chromosomes and discuss the effects of incorrect positions in the reference genome as a possible culprit.

Shortly after EquCab3 was released, Beeson and colleagues[60] released a probe-based remapping of the SNP coordinates of the SNP50, SNP70, MNEc670k, and MNEc2M SNP sets. Although the coordinates and sequence of the reference genome may have changed, the sequence used for the SNP probes of course remained the same. The strategy used by Beeson and colleagues was to identify 100% sequence match coordinates for the SNP the oligonucleotide probe hybridized with. This strategy provided updated SNP coordinates for most probes (>95% in all SNP chips) in addition to providing updated coordinates to many of the markers (37%,204%; 52.8%) from MNEc670k/MNec2M SNP sets that were included from Chrun2. Additionally, a small number of contiguous probes (blocks of 2 or more) were found to be remapped to different chromosomes between assemblies as well as several inversions based on strand flips, both representing errors in EquCab2 that were subsequently fixed in EquCab3. Although most of these SNP positions still need to be validated by remapping WGS, the welcomed updates and corrections in EquCab3 should allow for more precision mapping and imputation given the currently available equine SNP genotyping tools.

ACKNOWLEDGMENTS

The authors would like to thank Jim Mickelson for his thoughtful input and feedback in writing this article.

DISCLOSURE

This work was supported by USDA NIFA project 2012-67015-19432, Minnesota Agricultural Experiment Station Multi-state project MIN-62-090 and the National Animal Genome Project (NRSP8) through the equine genome coordinator: USDA-NRSP8 (2013-2018) horse-technical-committee coordinator funds. The funders had no role in the preparation of this manuscript.

REFERENCES

1. McCue ME, Bannasch DL, Petersen JL, et al. A high density SNP array for the domestic horse and extant Perissodactyla: utility for association mapping, genetic diversity, and phylogeny studies. Georges M, ed. PLoS Genet 2012;8(1): e1002451.
2. Schaefer RJ, Schubert M, Bailey E, et al. Developing a 670k genotyping array to tag ~2M SNPs across 24 horse breeds. BMC Genomics 2017;18(1):565.
3. McCue M, Mickelson J. Genomic tools and resources: development and applications of an equine SNP genotyping array. Equine Genom. John Wiley & Sons 2013;7:113–24. https://doi.org/10.1002/9781118522158.ch7.
4. Wade CM, Giulotto E, Sigurdsson S, et al. Genome sequence, comparative analysis, and population genetics of the domestic horse. Science 2009;326(5954): 865–7.
5. McCue ME, Mickelson JR. Genomic tools and resources: development and applications of an equine SNP genotyping array. In: Chowdhary BP, editor. Equine genomics. 1st edition. John Wiley & Sons, Inc; 2013. p. 113–24.
6. Coleman SJ, Zeng Z, Wang K, et al. Structural annotation of equine protein-coding genes determined by mRNA sequencing. Anim Genet 2010;41:121–30.
7. Lykkjen S, Dolvik NI, McCue ME, et al. Genome-wide association analysis of osteochondrosis of the tibiotarsal joint in Norwegian Standardbred trotters. Anim Genet 2010;41:111–20.
8. Lykkjen S, Dolvik NI, McCue ME, et al. Equine developmental orthopaedic diseases: a genome-wide association study of first phalanx plantar osteochondral fragments in Standardbred trotters. Anim Genet 2013;44(6):766–9.
9. Finno CJ, Stevens C, Young A, et al. SERPINB11 frameshift variant associated with novel hoof specific phenotype in connemara ponies. PLoS Genet 2015; 11(4):1–17.
10. Hauswirth R, Haase B, Blatter M, et al. Mutations in MITF and PAX3 cause "splashed white" and other white spotting phenotypes in horses. Barsh GS, ed. PLoS Genet 2012;8(4):e1002653.
11. Hill EW, Gu J, Eivers SS, et al. A sequence polymorphism in MSTN predicts sprinting ability and racing stamina in thoroughbred horses. PLoS One 2010; 5(1):e8645.

12. Binns MM, Boehler DA, Lambert DH. Identification of the myostatin locus (MSTN) as having a major effect on optimum racing distance in the Thoroughbred horse in the USA. Anim Genet 2010;41:154–8.
13. Corbin LJ, Blott SC, Swinburne JE, et al. A genome-wide association study of osteochondritis dissecans in the Thoroughbred. Mamm Genome 2012;23(3–4): 294–303.
14. Raudsepp T, McCue ME, Das PJ, et al. Genome-wide association study implicates testis-sperm specific FKBP6 as a susceptibility locus for impaired acrosome reaction in stallions. PLoS Genet 2012;8(12). https://doi.org/10.1371/journal.pgen.1003139.
15. Signer-Hasler H, Flury C, Haase B, et al. A genome-wide association study reveals loci influencing height and other conformation traits in horses. Weedon MN. PLoS One 2012;7(5):e37282.
16. Gottschalk M, Metzger J, Martinsson G, et al. Genome-wide association study for semen quality traits in German Warmblood stallions. Anim Reprod Sci 2016; 171:81–6.
17. Kulbrock M, Lehner S, Metzger J, et al. A genome-wide association study identifies risk loci to equine recurrent uveitis in German warmblood horses. Yue GH, ed. PLoS One 2013;8(8):e71619.
18. Metzger J, Ohnesorge B, Distl O. Genome-wide linkage and association analysis identifies major gene loci for guttural pouch tympany in Arabian and German warmblood horses. Veitia RA, ed. PLoS One 2012;7(7):e41640.
19. Schrimpf R, Dierks C, Martinsson G, et al. Genome-wide association study identifies phospholipase C zeta 1 (PLCz1) as a stallion fertility locus in Hanoverian warmblood horses. Wade C, ed. PLoS One 2014;9(10):e109675.
20. Metzger J, Philipp U, Lopes MS, et al. Analysis of copy number variants by three detection algorithms and their association with body size in horses. BMC Genomics 2013;14(1):487.
21. Go YY, Bailey E, Cook DG, et al. Genome-wide association study among four horse breeds identifies a common haplotype associated with in vitro CD3+ T cell susceptibility/resistance to equine arteritis virus infection. J Virol 2011; 85(24):13174–84.
22. Dupuis MC, Zhang Z, Druet T, et al. Results of a haplotype-based GWAS for recurrent laryngeal neuropathy in the horse. Mamm Genome 2011;22(9–10): 613–20.
23. McCoy AM, Beeson SK, Splan RK, et al. Identification and validation of risk loci for osteochondrosis in standardbreds. BMC Genomics 2016;17(1). https://doi.org/10.1186/s12864-016-2385-z.
24. Tozaki T, Kikuchi M, Kakoi H, et al. A genome-wide association study for body weight in Japanese Thoroughbred racehorses clarifies candidate regions on chromosomes 3, 9, 15, and 18. J Equine Sci 2017;28(4):127–34.
25. Staiger EA, Abri MA, Silva CAS, et al. Loci impacting polymorphic gait in the Tennessee Walking Horse1. J Anim Sci 2016;94(4):1377–86.
26. Staiger EA, Albright JD, Brooks SA. Genome-wide association mapping of heritable temperament variation in the Tennessee Walking Horse. Genes Brain Behav 2016;15(5):514–26.
27. Frischknecht M, Jagannathan V, Plattet P, et al. A non-synonymous HMGA2 variant decreases height in Shetland ponies and other small horses. PLoS One 2015;10(10):e0140749.

28. Brosnahan MM, Al Abri MA, Brooks SA, et al. Genome-wide association study of equine herpesvirus type 1-induced myeloencephalopathy identifies a significant single nucleotide polymorphism in a platelet-related gene. Vet J 2019;245:49–54.
29. Finno CJ, Gianino G, Perumbakkam S, et al. A missense mutation in MYH1 is associated with susceptibility to immune-mediated myositis in Quarter Horses. Skelet Muscle 2018;8(1):7.
30. Naccache F, Metzger J, Distl O. Genetic risk factors for osteochondrosis in various horse breeds. Equine Vet J 2018;50(5):556–63.
31. Mason VC, Schaefer RJ, McCue ME, et al. eQTL discovery and their association with severe equine asthma in European Warmblood horses. BMC Genomics 2018;19(1):581.
32. McCoy AM, Norton EM, Kemper AM, et al. SNP-based heritability and genetic architecture of tarsal osteochondrosis in North American Standardbred horses. Anim Genet 2019;50(1):78–81.
33. Norton EM, Avila F, Schultz NE, et al. Evaluation of an HMGA2 variant for pleiotropic effects on height and metabolic traits in ponies. J Vet Intern Med 2019; 33(2):942–52.
34. Norton EM, Schultz NE, Rendahl AK, et al. Heritability of metabolic traits associated with equine metabolic syndrome in Welsh ponies and Morgan horses. Equine Vet J 2019;51(4):475–80.
35. Binns MM, Boehler DA, Bailey E, et al. Inbreeding in the Thoroughbred horse. Anim Genet 2012;43(3):340–2.
36. Kader A, Li Y, Dong K, et al. Population variation reveals independent selection toward small body size in Chinese Debao Pony. Genome Biol Evol 2016;8(1): 42–50.
37. Al Abri MA, König von Borstel U, Strecker V, et al. Application of genomic estimation methods of inbreeding and population structure in an Arabian Horse Herd. J Hered 2017;108(4):361–8.
38. Andersson LS, Swinbune JE, Meadows JRS, et al. The same ELA class II risk factors confer equine insect bite hypersensitivity in two distinct populations. Immunogenetics 2012;64(3):201–8.
39. McCue ME, Bannasch DL, JL P, et al. A high density SNP array for the domestic horse and extant perissodactyla: utility for association mapping, genetic diversity and phylogeny studies. PLoS Genet 2010;8:e1002451.
40. Petersen JL, Mickelson JR, Rendahl AK, et al. Genome-wide analysis reveals selection for important traits in domestic horse breeds. PLoS Genet 2013;9(1). https://doi.org/10.1371/journal.pgen.1003211.
41. Grilz-Seger G, Druml T, Neuditschko M, et al. High-resolution population structure and runs of homozygosity reveal the genetic architecture of complex traits in the Lipizzan horse. BMC Genomics 2019;20(1):174.
42. Grilz-Seger G, Mesarič M, Cotman M, et al. Runs of Homozygosity and population history of three horse breeds with small population size. J Equine Vet Sci 2018;71:27–34.
43. Druml T, Neuditschko M, Grilz-Seger G, et al. Population networks associated with runs of homozygosity reveal new insights into the breeding history of the Haflinger horse. J Hered 2018;109(4):384–92.
44. Avila F, Mickelson JR, Schaefer RJ, et al. Genome-wide signatures of selection reveal genes associated with performance in American quarter horse subpopulations. Front Genet 2018;9:249.

45. Jónsson H, Schubert M, Seguin-Orlando A, et al. Speciation with gene flow in equids despite extensive chromosomal plasticity. Proc Natl Acad Sci U S A 2014;111(52):18655–60.

46. Schubert M, Jónsson H, Chang D, et al. Prehistoric genomes reveal the genetic foundation and cost of horse domestication. Proc Natl Acad Sci U S A 2014; 111(52):201416991.

47. Sadeghi R, Moradi-Shahrbabak M, Miraei Ashtiani SR, et al. Genetic diversity of Persian Arabian horses and their relationship to other native Iranian horse breeds. J Hered 2019;110(2):173–82.

48. Liu X-X, Pan J-F, Zhao Q-J, et al. Detecting selection signatures on the X chromosome of the Chinese Debao pony. J Anim Breed Genet 2018;135(1):84–92.

49. Ma H, Wang S, Zeng G, et al. The origin of a coastal indigenous horse breed in china revealed by genome-wide SNP data. Genes (Basel) 2019;10(3):241.

50. Kim NY, Seong H-S, Kim DC, et al. Genome-wide analyses of the Jeju, Thoroughbred, and Jeju crossbred horse populations using the high density SNP array. Genes Genomics 2018;40(11):1249–58.

51. Grilz-Seger G, Neuditschko M, Ricard A, et al. Genome-wide homozygosity patterns and evidence for selection in a set of European and near eastern horse breeds. Genes (Basel) 2019;10(7):491.

52. Browning S, Browning B. Haplotype phasing: existing methods and new developments. Nat Rev Genet 2011;12(10):703–14.

53. Corbin LJ, Kranis A, Blott SC, et al. The utility of low-density genotyping for imputation in the Thoroughbred horse. Genet Sel Evol 2014;46(1):9.

54. Frischknecht M, Neuditschko M, Jagannathan V, et al. Imputation of sequence level genotypes in the Franches-Montagnes horse breed. Genet Sel Evol 2014; 46(1):63.

55. McCoy AM, McCue ME. Validation of imputation between equine genotyping arrays. Anim Genet 2014;45(1):153.

56. Chassier M, Barrey E, Robert C, et al. Genotype imputation accuracy in multiple equine breeds from medium- to high-density genotypes. J Anim Breed Genet 2018;135(6):420–31.

57. Browning BL, Browning SR. Genotype imputation with millions of reference samples. Am J Hum Genet 2016;98(1):116–26.

58. Beeson SK, Mickelson JR, McCue ME. Exploration of fine-scale recombination rate variation in the domestic horse. Genome Res 2019. https://doi.org/10.1101/gr.243311.118. gr.243311.118.

59. Kalbfleisch TS, Rice ES, DePriest MS, et al. Improved reference genome for the domestic horse increases assembly contiguity and composition. Commun Biol 2018;1(1):197.

60. Beeson SK, Schaefer RJ, Mason VC, et al. Robust remapping of equine SNP array coordinates to EquCab3. Anim Genet 2019;50(1):114–5.

Next-Generation Sequencing in Equine Genomics

Jessica L. Petersen, MS, PhD[a], Stephen J. Coleman, MS, PhD[b],*

KEYWORDS

- Genomics • Equine • RNA sequencing • Transcriptome • Genetic variation

KEY POINTS

- Next-generation sequencing of both DNA and RNA represents a second revolution in equine genetics following publication of the equine genome sequence.
- Technological advancements have resulted in a wide selection of next-generation sequencing platforms capable of completing small targeted experiments or resequencing complete genomes.
- DNA and RNA sequencing have applications in clinical and research environments.
- Standards for the validation and sharing of next-generation sequencing data are critical for the widespread application of the technology and applications discussed herein.
- As researchers and clinicians develop a better understanding of how genetic variation and phenotypic variation are linked, next-generation sequencing could help pave the way to personalized and precision management of horses.

INTRODUCTION

The sequencing and assembly of a reference genome for the horse has been revolutionary for investigation of horse health and performance. Since its publication,[1] the reference genome has enhanced and accelerated genetic research in the horse, led to the development of new ideas regarding management and precision medicine, and has led to the development of powerful tools that increased the scope and resolution of understanding the genetic underpinnings of equine physiology and disease pathology.[2,3] The insights gained into equine health as a result of these new tools and ideas are expertly reviewed in the accompanying articles of this special issue. The advent and application of next-generation sequencing (NGS) methods represent a second revolution for the study of equine genetics, enabling researchers to exploit

[a] Department of Animal Science, University of Nebraska-Lincoln, ANSC A218g, 3940 Fair Street, Lincoln, NE 68583-0908, USA; [b] Department of Animal Sciences, Colorado State University, 1171 Campus Delivery, Fort Collins, CO 80523-1171, USA
* Corresponding author.
E-mail address: stephen.coleman@colostate.edu

Vet Clin Equine 36 (2020) 195–209
https://doi.org/10.1016/j.cveq.2020.03.002
0749-0739/20/© 2020 Elsevier Inc. All rights reserved.

and explore the information encoded in the equine genome through their experiments. NGS has also improved the ability of researchers to translate their discoveries into clinically relevant applications. This article provides an overview of the history and development of NGS, details some of the available sequencing platforms, and describes currently available applications in the context of both discovery and clinical settings (**Fig. 1**).

BUILDING GENOMIC RESOURCES FOR THE HORSE

The use of DNA sequencing to investigate the underlying cause of heritable conditions in the horse dates to the early 1990s. At that time, before the development of an equine reference genome, genetic studies relied on the use of genomic information from other species to inform the investigation for important traits of the horse. Major successes using that approach include the identification of a missense mutation causative of hyperkalemic periodic paralysis in the quarter horse[4] and lethal white overo syndrome in American Paint Horses.[5] In 1995, the scientific communities' focus on generating genomic tools specific to the horse incited the formation of the Horse Genome Project. Through this collaboration, intentional and international partnerships were built across academic and industry institutions resulting in the generation of comparative, linkage, and radiation hybrid maps of the equine genome (reviewed in Chowdhary[6]).

The most notable advancement for equine genomics thus far dates to 2006 when the National Human Genome Research Institute of the National Institutes of Health identified the horse as a species of priority for genome sequence assembly efforts. In 2007, a draft reference equine genome was completed.[1] This reference genome, named EquCab2, was generated with sequencing data from a single thoroughbred mare, Twilight, resulting in an assembly with approximately 6.8-fold coverage. The assembly of these data was complemented by additional sequence information (bacterial artificial chromosome sequencing) of Twilight's half-brother, Bravo. At the time, the

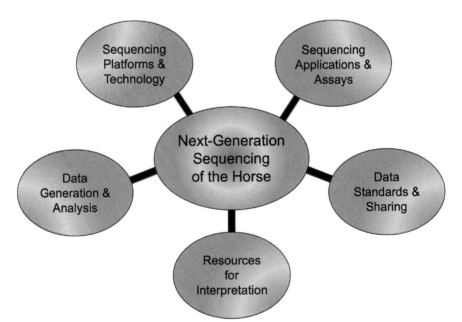

Fig. 1. Visual summary of the key points for NGS application in the horse in both discovery and clinical settings.

accuracy of Sanger sequencing and availability of linkage and physical maps of the genome resulted in EquCab2 being one of the highest-quality reference genomes of any agricultural species. The genome was estimated to be 2.7 billion base pairs (bp), with more than 20,000 protein-coding genes annotated in the initial effort.[1] This resource served as the basis for the development of genomic tools and discovery for the following decade with assays to detect genomic and transcriptomic variation in the horse[2,3,7–9] anchored in EquCab2.

In 2018, a new reference assembly, still based primarily on the sequence of Twilight, was released.[10] This improved reference genome, EquCab3, was the product of new technologies for sequencing of longer reads, helping to characterize repetitive regions of the genome. The EquCab3 assembly also incorporates data generated by methods that use structural proximity of sequences to help build continuity (Chicago[11] and Hi-C[12] libraries). Compared with EquCab2, EquCab3 has 90% fewer gaps, better coverage of GC-rich regions, which often include gene promoters; and more complete coverage of the transcriptome.[10] EquCab3 now serves at the primary reference genome assembly for the horse and should be used for the analysis of future sequence data. It continues to be improved through additional efforts to annotate not only protein-coding regions, but noncoding RNA as well as regulatory features.[13] Both Equ-Cab2 and EquCab3 are available through the National Center for Biotechnology Information (NCBI), Ensembl, and University of California Santa Cruz genome browser utilities.

TECHNOLOGY

The driving force behind many of the developments in equine genetics, including but not limited to the reference genome sequence, has been ever-improving and increasingly accessible DNA sequencing technology. The advancing technologies are generally grouped into distinct generations by the scientific community to recognize the transformational impact they have had on the understanding of genetics. The history and impact of each generation of sequencing technology have been reviewed in detail.[14,15] This article presents a brief overview of each sequencing generation and specifically how it has or can affect studies of the equine genome related to animal health.

The method used to generate the data for assembly of EquCab2, data that were also used for EquCab3, was Sanger sequencing, first published in 1977.[16] Still used for projects concerning a single gene or small portion of DNA, Sanger sequencing produces a high-quality sequence in long fragments. Sanger sequencing relies on the selective incorporation of dideoxy nucleotides during elongation of the nascent DNA strand during in vitro DNA replication. Fragments are then visualized using an electrophoretic system to identify each nucleotide in sequence. This method, which can generate sequence fragments of about 800 bp, may be limited in throughput but remains the gold standard for accuracy (reviewed in Shendure and Ji[17]).

As researchers began to work to develop reference genome assemblies, increasing the throughput of sequencing technologies became a priority. The motivation behind the rapidly evolving technology was to improve access by increasing accuracy and data-generating capacity while at the same time decreasing costs. NGS technologies were designed to increase the rate by which data were generated through platforms that allowed for multiple sequence reads to be collected at 1 time and also by coupling the inclusion of labeled nucleotides with the step of reading their identity. Next-generation, or massively parallel, sequencing, therefore, had an advantage in its ability to generate a significantly greater amount of sequence data at 1 time, although read length was compromised compared with that possible with Sanger sequencing. In the past 10 to 15 years, NGS has become a standard method used in questions regarding the evolution of the species, for discovery of variation associated with phenotypes of interest, for the identification of diversity among individuals and breeds, and for identification of genome function associated with disease.

SEQUENCING PLATFORMS

As sequencing technologies have advanced, sequencing platforms available to generate data have expanded at an astounding rate. Ten years ago, there were only a few types of instruments available; these were expensive and required significant laboratory resources to deploy. At present, there is a wide selection of instruments tailored to generate anywhere from a small amount of targeted sequence data to massive amounts of sequence data capable of characterizing an entire genome in a single experiment. The various platforms use different types of chemistry; those differences have been previously reviewed.[18,19] Now there is an NGS platform for most any job. As this technology continues to become more accessible and manageable, it enhances the opportunities for sequencing and its many applications to find their way into clinical practice.

The available NGS platforms can be classified into 3 main groups: production, benchtop, and portable systems. The choice of which platform to use depends on several variables of interest, the overall throughput needed, the accuracy of base calls, read length, speed of data generation, and budget. Each platform category is described briefly in the following paragraphs and is summarized in **Table 1**.

Table 1
Comparison of production, benchtop, and portable next-generation sequencing platforms

| Descriptors | System Scale | | | | | |
| | Production | | Benchtop | | Portable | |
	Minimum	Maximum	Minimum	Maximum	Minimum	Maximum
Sequence output	7.5 Gbp	6 Tbp	1.2 Gbp	150 Gbp	1.8 Gbp	30 Gbp
Read output	0.5 M	20 B	4 M	400 M	7 M	12 M
Read length	50 bp	1 KB+	50 bp	1 KB+	—	10 Kb+
Platforms	Illumina HiSeq 4000 Illumina HiSeqX Illumina NovaSeq 6000 PacBio Sequel/Sequel II Oxford Nanopore PromethION		Illumina MiSeq Illumina NextSeq Illumina iSeq 100 ThermoFisher Ion S5/ S5 XL Oxford Nanopore GridION		Oxford Nanopore MinION Oxford Nanopore Flongle Oxford Nanopore SmidgION	
Applications	Whole-genome sequencing Exome sequencing Targeted sequencing Epigenetic sequencing DNA-protein interactions Transcriptome sequencing Gene expression profiling Small RNA sequencing		Targeted sequencing Targeted expression profiling Small genome sequencing Small RNA sequencing		Small genome sequencing Targeted sequencing Targeted expression profiling Epigenetic sequencing	

Production systems represent the highest-throughput technology available and are targeted primarily for discovery and research applications. The designation of a production system is derived from the idea that a researcher would need to produce a genome or transcriptome sequence. Systems in this category have sufficient capacity to sequence an entire genome in a single run (realistically many genomes given the coverage needed). They are almost exclusively housed in core or service facilities because of the cost to purchase, deploy, and operate them. The advantage of these platforms is the output. One of the highest-throughput systems currently available, the Illumina NovaSeq 6000, can generate 6 Tb of sequence data or 20 billion reads in less than 2 days (https://www.illumina.com). This amount of data represents enough sequence to characterize the genome of 1 horse more than 300 times. More practically, this amount of data can be used to sequence the genomes of 15 individual horses to coverage sufficient to confidently identify variation unique to an individual in a single run. Other production-level systems, such as those from Pacific Biosystems (https://www.pacb.com/) and Oxford Nanopore (https://nanoporetech.com/) Technologies, produce significantly fewer reads per run than the Illumina systems. Generating long-read output, the reads they produce are generally 10 to 100 times the size, which increases their value for the assembly of complicated genomic or transcriptomic regions. However, long-read sequencing remains expensive for most purposes. At the time of writing, whole-genome sequencing at approximately 15 times coverage using short-read technology can be generated at a core facility for approximately $500 per individual. Overall, these production systems increase sequencing capacity and improve accessibility for researchers by reducing sample costs so that NGS technology can be applied effectively to more research questions.

Benchtop systems represent the category of sequencers, which literally live in a laboratory on the benchtop. In general, they have moderate sequencing capacity (1.2–150 Gbp sequence data and 4–400 million reads per run) but represent an improvement in accessibility for investigators. These instruments serve smaller communities of researchers (or even a single laboratory) compared with the production systems. Therefore, benchtop systems often allow faster data generation because the researchers are not sharing the instrument with as many other users and do not have to wait as long to use the machine. Examples of these include the Illumina MiSeq, iSeq 100, the ThermoFisher Ion Gene Studio S5, and the Oxford Nanopore GridION. Benchtop systems are optimized for investigators who have smaller sample sizes (eg, preliminary studies), who wish to perform transcriptome analyses, which generally require lesser sequence output, or who have targeted sequencing objectives. These systems can also be used by those who want to use sequencing in clinical medicine, although the applications for such sequencing are still developing.

Like much of technology, sequencers are becoming more efficient and are beginning to come in much smaller packages. Portable systems are designed to allow sequencing without the requirement of the support of a full laboratory. Examples of these systems are currently available from Oxford Nanopore and include the MinION and SmidgION (a small-capacity sequencer that can be operated with a smartphone). The amount of data generated is impressive but generally lower than either the benchtop or production systems. Both systems are supported by equally portable sample preparation and analysis tools. Possible applications of these mobile systems include stall-side diagnoses of an infectious pathogen or DNA verification of an individual's identity. Analyses can be conducted in a short amount of time to answer time-sensitive questions (eg, what strain of a virus is present?).

SEQUENCE READS

Just as the number and type of available sequencers have proliferated, so too have the types of data produced. The primary distinction of sequence data is the length of reads generated by the sequencing instrument. There are 2 main categories for NGS data: short and long reads. Short sequence reads (short reads) are usually shorter than 500 bp in length, whereas long sequence reads (long reads) exceed 1000 bp.[20] Sanger sequencing reads are between these 2 classifications.

Short-read sequence is the most common type of NGS data reported in the literature. The main advantage of short-read sequencing is that a single instrument can produce large amounts of data with high-quality base calls in 1 run (see **Table 1**). This ability gives researchers/clinicians options for their sequencing experiments: they can generate high levels of coverage on a few individual samples to support identification of sequence variants in DNA and characterization of gene expression (**Table 2**), or they can pool samples to efficiently and cost-effectively generate data for large sample sets. Short reads can be classified as either single-end or paired-end. This designation refers to whether sequence was generated from both or just 1 end of the captured DNA fragments. Single-end short reads are valuable for rapid and inexpensive characterization of DNA sequence or gene expression. However, their use is limited for the characterization of complex sequence regions such as sequence repeats or alternative splicing. This limitation results from ambiguity in aligning the single-end read back to a reference genome. The advantage of paired-end reads is that sequence from both ends of a DNA fragment of known length is generated. Then, information from both ends of the read can be used in parallel, which enhances the strategies used to address characterization of complex sequences. Paired-end reads, which align to the reference genome at a distance (between the reads) less than or greater to what was expected, can indicate the presence of a sequence variant such as an insertion or deletion, or, in the case of transcriptome data, can reveal

Table 2
Summary of various next-generation sequencing application categories, including the type of variants it is possible to assay and how much sequence data are required

Target	Category	Application/Detection	Coverage/Sequence Required
DNA	Genome sequencing	SNPs, INDELs, CNVs, genotyping	10× to 60× coverage
	Exome sequencing	SNPs	100× coverage
	Targeted sequencing	ChIP, SNPs, chromosome conformation	15–100 million reads
	Methylation	Bisulfite	15–30 million reads
	De novo assembly	SNPs, INDELs, CNVs, genotyping	140× coverage
RNA	Transcriptome sequencing	Differential expression, small RNAs, alternative splicing	10–100 million reads
	Targeted Sequencing	CLIP, transcript panels, tag capture	5–40 million reads
	De novo assembly	Differential expression, small RNAs, alternative splicing	>100 million reads

Abbreviations: ChIP, chromatin immunoprecipitation; CLIP, cross-linking immunoprecipitation; CNVs, copy number variations; INDELs, insertions/deletions; SNPs, single nucleotide polymorphisms.

patterns of alternative splicing. **Fig. 2** shows both single-end and paired-end short reads and the application of those reads to the characterization of DNA and RNA sequences.

Long-read sequence data are increasing in popularity for NGS experiments. The instruments that generate these data generally produce fewer sequence reads per run, but the reads they do provide are significantly longer than those from any short-read NGS platform (see **Table 1**). When first released, reads from these instruments averaged 1100 bp in length. Improvements in chemistry quickly increased the expected read length to 10,000 bp, with some reads spanning 60,000 bp. Genome assembly and the investigation of large-scale structural variation is aided by long-read sequencing because the long reads can sometimes span the length of repetitive regions of the genome, or moderately sized insertions/deletions. The read length achievable has led to the preferential use of this platform for genome assembly and scaffolding, as was the case in the newest assembly of the equine genome, EquCab3.[10] Long-read sequencing has also helped to resolve the structure and sequence of highly repetitive regions such as the equine major histocompatibility complex.[21] Long sequence reads can also be used for annotation of alternative splicing in the

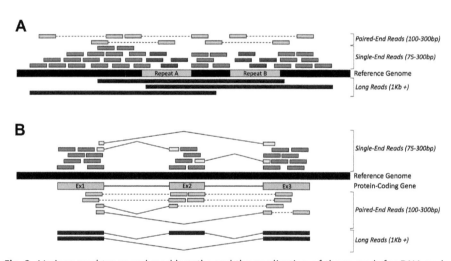

Fig. 2. Various read types and read lengths and the application of those reads for DNA and RNA sequencing. In both cases, the reads are aligned to a reference genome (*black rectangle*) for analysis. (*A*) DNA sequencing: the region of the genome depicted contains 2 copies of a repeated motif (*green rectangles*). Single-end short reads are aligned across the genome at unique locations (*blue rectangles*) or multiple locations (*red rectangles*) if they originated from a repeat sequence. Paired-end short reads (*yellow rectangles joined by dashed lines*) can help to characterize the repeat regions because they align to the repeats and are anchored by alignment to unique sequences. Long reads (*large purple boxes*) align uniquely to the reference genome and can be used to characterize repeat sequence because they span the entire region. (*B*) RNA sequencing: the area of the genome depicted encodes a protein-coding gene (*green boxes connected by solid lines*). Single-end short reads map to sequence representing the exonic regions of the gene and can be mapped with a gapped alignment (*light blue rectangles joined by angled solid lines*) representing the union of 2 exons by splicing. Paired-end short reads also align to the exonic regions of the gene and can be used to define exon order in a transcript by linking multiple exons together. Long reads can help determine full-length transcripts and can be used to separate overlapping transcript structures.

transcriptome because the long reads can span entire transcripts. **Fig. 2** shows how long reads can be used in both DNA and RNA sequencing (RNA-seq) applications. A common strategy is to combine both short-read and long-read data in a single NGS experiment to exploit the advantages offered by each.

APPLICATIONS

With production instruments now capable of producing terabytes of data each run, the sequencing of a horse's entire genome is now arguably the most common use of NGS technologies. This type of sequencing can allow the identification of inherited or de novo variation associated with disease. Whole-genome sequencing in the horse has enabled the discovery of variation that can be assayed to identify the risk of disease or for use in diagnosis. Some findings that resulted from the use of whole-genome sequence include missense variants causative of lavender foal syndrome,[22] immune-mediated myositis,[23] the identification of a locus associated with risk for squamous cell carcinoma in Haflingers,[24] a nonsense mutation associated with hydrocephalus in Friesians,[25] a splice-site mutation in Friesian horses with dwarfism,[26] and a large deletion associated with occipitoatlantoaxial malformation.[27] A practical alternative to whole-genome sequencing can be sequencing of only the exome, the regions of the genome that code for the exons of protein-coding genes. This approach requires that the exonic sequence is captured (either in solution or on an array) to prepare the DNA for sequencing. Because the region to be sequenced is reduced relative to the whole genome, this approach can enable a researcher to generate sequence from a larger number of individuals. The primary limitation in horses is the availability of capture technology. Exome sequencing has been used in the horse to identify variants relative to racing performance in quarter horses.[28] In each of these examples, the sequence generated was aligned to the reference genome and variants differing between affected horses and the reference sequence, or compared with healthy controls, were identified. As part of this process, after variants that either fit the hypothesized mode of inheritance or are found in candidate genes are identified, the possible function of each can be predicted using the genome annotation. In cases where genes may not be annotated, the region can be aligned to orthologous loci of other species. The impact of genomic variants on gene expression can also be assayed through RNA sequencing of the appropriate tissues.

The process of sequencing of the transcriptome (any portion of the DNA actively being transcribed into RNA at the time the tissue is sampled) is similar to that of sequencing DNA. The exception is an initial reverse transcription step, through which the isolated RNA is converted to double-stranded, copy DNA. The library preparation method used for RNA-seq depends on the question at hand. Poly-A$^+$ selected libraries capture most messenger RNA and some long noncoding RNA, as long as a poly-A tail is present on the transcript. Poly-A$^+$ library preparation and paired-end sequencing are the most common means to assess the expression of protein-coding loci. Differential expression can also be assayed using 3′ tag-seq (Quantseq; Lexogen, Greenland, NH), a method in which libraries are created for only the 3′ end of each RNA molecule present in the sample. Tag-seq does not allow the identification of gene isoforms, but, by focusing sequencing efforts on only the terminal end of each transcript, differential expression analyses require significantly lower sequencing depth ($\sim$6 million reads per sample)[29,30] using single-end reads, therefore reducing overall cost. As in whole-genome sequencing, reads from RNA-seq are mapped to the reference genome or, in some cases, the transcriptome. In the horse, RNA-seq data have been used to develop and improve gene annotation.[31–34] The relative abundance of each transcript can then be quantified using the available gene annotation and compared between treatments or disease states.[35–39] The sequencing of mRNA through poly-A$^+$ selection not only allows the quantification of each transcript but can provide insight into splice-site variation. Further, RNA libraries are often stranded, meaning the sequence generated distinguishes the strand of DNA from which the transcript was derived. This technique is a powerful method to identify and distinguish antisense transcripts. The advent of long-read technology can also be applied to studies of the transcriptome. Iso-seq is the use of PacBio sequencing, enabling the profiling of full-length RNA transcripts.[40] This methodology reduces 3′ sequencing bias, which is common in poly-A$^+$ library preparation, and is a powerful means to annotate genomes and identify variation in codon usage. However, as a long-read technology, Iso-seq is thus far too expensive for most clinical investigations. In contrast, Poly-A+ library preparation neglects sequencing of small RNAs such as microRNAs, which can be assayed with a special, small RNA library preparation method. MicroRNAs are small (21–25 nucleotides) RNA fragments encoded by the animal's genome. Although they do not function to create proteins, they can bind to and silence the expression of protein-coding genes; therefore, their activity in posttranscriptional modification can significantly affect genome function.[41] In horses, microRNA profiles have been proposed as useful biomarkers for infection,[42] or other disorders.[43,44]

In addition to the identification of genomic variants and the transcript expression, NGS can be used to understand chemical modifications to the DNA, such as methylation, or to identify regions of the genome interacting with protein. DNA methylation, a chemical modification of cytosine to 5-methylcytosine, is a common epigenetic mechanism involved in silencing gene expression.[45] Although the inheritance of some epigenetic modifications, such as DNA methylation, is not completely understood, like RNA-seq, examining methylation patterns can help to understand differences in gene regulation and expression between diseased and healthy individuals. Similar to chromatin immunoprecipitation (ChIP; discussed later), genome-wide methylation can be assayed by using antibodies to precipitate DNA having 5-methylcytosine modifications; that DNA is then sequenced on a next-generation platform (MeDIP-seq).[46] To the authors' knowledge, this method has not yet been applied in a case of equine disease research; however, this technique has been used to characterize changes in genomic methylation in equine skeletal muscle caused by exercise.[47,48]

ChIP is a method by which regions of the DNA involved in an interaction with protein are isolated.[49] Those regions of DNA can then be sequenced using standard next-generation methodology (ChIP-seq), and the resulting DNA fragments aligned to the reference genome to identify genomic regions involved in the interaction. Similarly, cross-linking immunoprecipitation (CLIP) is a method that enables the isolation of RNA transcripts specifically interacting with a protein.[50] The captured transcripts can be sequenced (CLIP-seq) to identify regulatory aspects of gene expression. Sequence variants in the regions of interaction can alter binding efficiency and thus function. In addition, alteration in protein-DNA or protein-RNA interactions can uncover functional information regarding molecular mechanisms of disease. Therefore, these methods can be used to investigate both the functional significance of genomic variation as well as to identify alterations in genome activity and sequence composition associated with a treatment or disease. Of note, as is the case in transcriptome sequencing, these methods of capturing information on genome function only reveal information about the genome's activity within the tissue or cell population sampled at the time of sampling.

DATA GENERATION AND HANDLING

For most any platform, the process of sequencing is similar. The general workflow of an NGS experiment is presented in **Fig. 3**. The goals for interpretation and application of the data generated can result in alterations of this general approach. The sample necessary depends on the question at hand. For gene expression, RNA must be isolated from a tissue relevant to the phenotype of interest. Because RNA is relatively unstable, care has to be taken to either preserve the sample in an RNA-stabilization solution (eg, RNAlater, Sigma-Aldrich, St Louis, MO; DNA/RNA Shield, Zymo Research, Irvine, CA) or the tissue must be flash-frozen immediate after collection until processing. ChIP data can also be derived from a flash-frozen sample or from samples subjected to a cross-linking protocol, commonly performed with formaldehyde, at the time of collection. If the goal is to identify genomic variation, genomic DNA must first be isolated from a sample of the individual. Blood and tissue are commonly used samples for DNA isolation, although hair follicles can also produce adequate DNA for sequencing of target genes or the whole genome. The isolated DNA is hydrolyzed or sheared to create fragments of similar size and is processed for library preparation. Methods for library preparation are conceptually similar, although there are platform-specific processes to make the input nucleic acid ready for sequencing on a particular instrument. Barcode sequences can be included and allow individual samples to be pooled in a single sequencing run.

The general features of NGS data analysis are similar regardless of the platform used to generate the data (**Fig. 4**). The data received from most sequencing methods are in the form of fastq files. These files encode both the sequence identity of each read as well as an associated quality metric. Data processing then involves an initial step of quality control where any adapter sequences necessary for library preparation are removed, and the sequence is also trimmed to eliminate base calls that do not meet a designated quality threshold. It is standard for the 3' end of each read to be of lesser quality than the 5' end, and thus much of the trimming occurs on this portion of the read. If a paired-end library is sequenced, it is important that the data from the 2 ends of each pair remain associated; if 1 read is completely removed because of poor quality, its paired read must also be removed from the dataset. Once the data are preprocessed for quality control, the reads are aligned with the equine reference genome, or possibly the transcriptome (in the case of RNA-seq efforts). This process is computationally expensive and, depending on available computing resources and amount of data being processed, it could take days to weeks. However, the aligned reads (in bam files) can be visualized in software such as the Integrative Genomics Viewer[51–53] or JBrowse.[54]

Once the sequencing reads are aligned, variants within the newly sequenced individual and between it and the reference genome can be identified. Variant calling identifies single nucleotide polymorphisms (SNPs), insertions/deletions, or structural

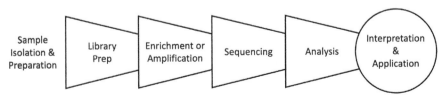

Fig. 3. General workflow of an NGS experiment.

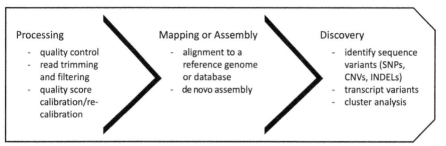

Fig. 4. General features of NGS data analysis. CNV, copy number variation; INDEL, insertion/deletion; SNPs, single nucleotide polymorphisms.

variation that differ between each individual and the reference genome, within an individual (ie, heterozygous sites), or between study individuals. A variety of variant calling software is available and has been reviewed elsewhere.[55,56] The choice of a variant caller depends to some extent on the question asked (eg, rare variant identification vs population frequency). In addition to the selection of variant calling software, the quality of the output also depends on the depth of sequence coverage, sequence quality, and ability to filter false-positive signals. Once variants are identified, the genome annotation provides a means to predict the functional impact (eg, nonsynonymous mutation or splice-site variant) of each. For cases with apparent simple inheritance, several databases exist to help identify candidate genes, or genes previously associated with similar phenotypes. Online Mendelian Inheritance in Man (OMIM; https://www.omim.org/), and Online Mendelian Inheritance in Animals (OMIA; https://omia.org/home/) provide information on thousands of known mendelian traits. Previously annotated variants and quantitative trait loci (loci associated with complex disease) are also often cataloged and can serve as valuable resources when investigating putative functional variation; these are available in databases such as the European Variation Archive (https://www.ebi.ac.uk/eva/). However, not all variants or genes with an essential physiologic function are annotated as such. In contrast, not all loci computationally predicted or modeled to affect gene or protein function necessarily do so. Validation of function of a variant requires significant subsequent work beyond their discovery.

For transcriptomic data, variants can be called in a manner similar to that used for whole-genome sequencing. However, the purpose of RNA-seq is often not to identify variation but altered expression of gene expression between affected versus unaffected tissues. Differential expression analyses are conducted based on the quantification of reads observed per transcript. Data must first be normalized to account for differences in sequencing depth, and, depending on the method used, analyses may also consider transcript length. Reviews of methods for quantification and differential expression analyses of RNA-seq data outline the statistical models used and assumptions underlying each approach.[57,58] Transcriptomic data are often used to investigate the function of putative causative variants or to identify gene pathways associated with disease, such as in the case of stationary night blindness of Appaloosas[35] and Arabian cerebellar abiotrophy.[59]

VALIDATION OF RESULTS

Even though NGS is becoming common, there are currently no standards set forth by the veterinary industry on the interpretation or use of DNA sequencing or RNA-seq data. Therefore, in the use of genetic or genomic information for equine management the onus is on researchers, clinicians, owners, or other end users to evaluate the process by which the data were discovered and validated. In human medicine, various interest groups, such as the Next-Generation Sequencing: Standardization of Clinical testing II informatics workgroup[60] and the American College of Medical Genetics and Genomics,[61] have worked to address the means to ensure that rigorous standards of variant discovery and validation are met. Some of the principles put in place by these entities include outlining a vocabulary useful to classify variant function and assist clinicians in using information regarding genetic tests in practice.[60,61] Another idea shared by both groups emphasizes that variant function and predictive ability need to be validated in individuals unique to those used in the discovery process and the variant frequency within the population (eg, breed in the case of horses) should be described. Toward a similar goal of standardizing how genomics research is implemented, validated, and applied, the international equine genomic research community recently put forth a "Consensus Statement on the Translation and Application of Genomics in the Equine Industry" (Havemeyer Principles 2019: https://horsegenomeworkshop.com/values).[62] In this statement, the researchers acknowledge that genomics and discovery using NGS holds significant promise to improve equine well-being. However, with the complexity of disease and of genome function, the community agreed the most significant benefit of genomics to the horse lies in discovery that encompasses several key elements. These elements include ensuring that genomic research is reproducible and peer reviewed, ethical, and performed and communicated with transparency. As the use of NGS increases, these guidelines will need to become more clearly defined because, although the potential for genomics to improve equine health and well-being is undeniable, its successful application also depends on the rigor of the research behind the discoveries.

FUTURE DIRECTIONS

The degree of advancement of genomic tools for researchers and clinicians in the past 10 years has been tremendous. The accelerated rate of discovery is likely to continue, and, with decreasing costs of NGS, the use of this method in the diagnosis, prevention, and management of disease is likely to become common practice. As researchers build a better understanding of how genetic variation alters an individual's ability to respond to treatment or optimize performance, the idea of personalized or precision management for horses is far reaching. In addition, a greater understanding of genomic relationships among individuals, as well as how genomic variation contributes to complex phenotypes such as disease, lends itself to use in genomic selection, or the incorporation of genomic information with phenotype data to predict an animal's breeding value for a trait or traits of interest. The improved understanding of genome function and disease susceptibility supported by the application of NGS can lead to better horse health and welfare.

DISCLOSURE

The authors have nothing to disclose.

REFERENCES

1. Wade CM, Giulotto E, Sigurdsson S, et al. Genome sequence, comparative analysis, and population genetics of the domestic horse. Science 2009;326:865–7.

2. McCue ME, Bannasch DL, Petersen JL, et al. A high density SNP array for the domestic horse and extant Perissodactyla: utility for association mapping, genetic diversity, and phylogeny studies. PLoS Genet 2012;8:e1002451.

3. Schaefer RJ, Schubert M, Bailey E, et al. Developing a 670k genotyping array to tag ~2M SNPs across 24 horse breeds. BMC Genomics 2017;18:565.

4. Rudolph JA, Spier SJ, Byrns G, et al. Periodic paralysis in quarter horses: a sodium channel mutation disseminated by selective breeding. Nat Genet 1992;2: 144–7.

5. Santschi EM, Purdy AK, Valberg SJ, et al. Endothelin receptor B polymorphism associated with lethal white foal syndrome in horses. Mamm Genome 1998;9: 306–9.

6. Chowdhary BP. Equine genomics. College Station (TX): Wiley-Blackwell; 2013.

7. Ghosh S, Qu Z, Das PJ, et al. Copy number variation in the horse genome. PLoS Genet 2014;10:e1004712.

8. Glaser KE, Sun Q, Wells MT, et al. Development of a novel equine whole transcript oligonucleotide GeneChip microarray and its use in gene expression profiling of normal articular-epiphyseal cartilage. Equine Vet J 2009;41:663–70.

9. Mienaltowski MJ, Huang L, Stromberg AJ, et al. Differential gene expression associated with postnatal equine articular cartilage maturation. BMC Musculoskelet Disord 2008;9:149.

10. Kalbfleisch TS, Rice ES, DePriest MS Jr, et al. Improved reference genome for the domestic horse increases assembly contiguity and composition. Commun Biol 2018;1:197.

11. Putnam NH, O'Connell BL, Stites JC, et al. Chromosome-scale shotgun assembly using an in vitro method for long-range linkage. Genome Res 2016;26:342–50.

12. Belton JM, McCord RP, Gibcus JH, et al. Hi-C: a comprehensive technique to capture the conformation of genomes. Methods 2012;58:268–76.

13. Burns EN, Bordbari MH, Mienaltowski MJ, et al. Generation of an equine biobank to be used for Functional Annotation of Animal Genomes project. Anim Genet 2018;49:564–70.

14. Shendure J, Balasubramanian S, Church GM, et al. DNA sequencing at 40: past, present and future. Nature 2017;550:345–53.

15. Mardis ER. DNA sequencing technologies: 2006-2016. Nat Protoc 2017;12: 213–8.

16. Sanger F, Nicklen S, Coulson AR. DNA sequencing with chain-terminating inhibitors. Proc Natl Acad Sci U S A 1977;74:5463–7.

17. Shendure J, Ji H. Next-generation DNA sequencing. Nat Biotechnol 2008;26: 1135–45.

18. Metzker ML. Sequencing technologies - the next generation. Nat Rev Genet 2010;11:31–46.

19. Goodwin S, McPherson JD, McCombie WR. Coming of age: ten years of next-generation sequencing technologies. Nat Rev Genet 2016;17:333–51.

20. Junemann S, Sedlazeck FJ, Prior K, et al. Updating benchtop sequencing performance comparison. Nat Biotechnol 2013;31:294–6.

21. Viluma A, Mikko S, Hahn D, et al. Genomic structure of the horse major histocompatibility complex class II region resolved using PacBio long-read sequencing technology. Sci Rep 2017;7:45518.

22. Brooks SA, Gabreski N, Miller D, et al. Whole-genome SNP association in the horse: identification of a deletion in myosin Va responsible for Lavender Foal Syndrome. PLoS Genet 2010;6:e1000909.

23. Finno CJ, Gianino G, Perumbakkam S, et al. A missense mutation in MYH1 is associated with susceptibility to immune-mediated myositis in Quarter Horses. Skelet Muscle 2018;8:7.

24. Bellone RR, Liu J, Petersen JL, et al. A missense mutation in damage-specific DNA binding protein 2 is a genetic risk factor for limbal squamous cell carcinoma in horses. Int J Cancer 2017;141:342–53.

25. Ducro BJ, Schurink A, Bastiaansen JW, et al. A nonsense mutation in B3GALNT2 is concordant with hydrocephalus in Friesian horses. BMC Genomics 2015; 16:761.

26. Leegwater PA, Vos-Loohuis M, Ducro BJ, et al. Dwarfism with joint laxity in Friesian horses is associated with a splice site mutation in B4GALT7. BMC Genomics 2016;17:839.

27. Bordbari MH, Penedo MCT, Aleman M, et al. Deletion of 2.7 kb near HOXD3 in an Arabian horse with occipitoatlantoaxial malformation. Anim Genet 2017;48: 287–94.

28. Pereira GL, Malheiros JM, Ospina AMT, et al. Exome sequencing in genomic regions related to racing performance of Quarter Horses. J Appl Genet 2019;60: 79–86.

29. Meyer E, Aglyamova GV, Matz MV. Profiling gene expression responses of coral larvae (Acropora millepora) to elevated temperature and settlement inducers using a novel RNA-Seq procedure. Mol Ecol 2011;20:3599–616.

30. Lohman BK, Weber JN, Bolnick DI. Evaluation of TagSeq, a reliable low-cost alternative for RNAseq. Mol Ecol Resour 2016;16:1315–21.

31. Coleman SJ, Zeng Z, Wang K, et al. Structural annotation of equine protein-coding genes determined by mRNA sequencing. Anim Genet 2010;41(Suppl 2):121–30.

32. Coleman SJ, Zeng Z, Hestand MS, et al. Analysis of unannotated equine transcripts identified by mRNA sequencing. PLoS One 2013;8:e70125.

33. Hestand MS, Kalbfleisch TS, Coleman SJ, et al. Annotation of the Protein Coding Regions of the Equine Genome. PLoS One 2015;10:e0124375.

34. Mansour TA, Scott EY, Finno CJ, et al. Tissue resolved, gene structure refined equine transcriptome. BMC Genomics 2017;18:103.

35. Bellone RR, Holl H, Setaluri V, et al. Evidence for a retroviral insertion in TRPM1 as the cause of congenital stationary night blindness and leopard complex spotting in the horse. PLoS One 2013;8:e78280.

36. Tessier L, Cote O, Clark ME, et al. Impaired response of the bronchial epithelium to inflammation characterizes severe equine asthma. BMC Genomics 2017; 18:708.

37. Pacholewska A, Jagannathan V, Drogemuller M, et al. Impaired Cell Cycle Regulation in a Natural Equine Model of Asthma. PLoS One 2015;10:e0136103.

38. Valberg SJ, Perumbakkam S, McKenzie EC, et al. Proteome and transcriptome profiling of equine myofibrillar myopathy identifies diminished peroxiredoxin 6 and altered cysteine metabolic pathways. Physiol Genomics 2018;50:1036–50.

39. Finno CJ, Bordbari MH, Valberg SJ, et al. Transcriptome profiling of equine vitamin E deficient neuroaxonal dystrophy identifies upregulation of liver X receptor target genes. Free Radic Biol Med 2016;101:261–71.

40. Wang B, Tseng E, Regulski M, et al. Unveiling the complexity of the maize transcriptome by single-molecule long-read sequencing. Nat Commun 2016;7: 11708.

41. He L, Hannon GJ. MicroRNAs: small RNAs with a big role in gene regulation. Nat Rev Genet 2004;5:522–31.

42. Cowled C, Foo CH, Deffrasnes C, et al. Circulating microRNA profiles of Hendra virus infection in horses. Sci Rep 2017;7:7431.
43. Barrey E, Bonnamy B, Barrey EJ, et al. Muscular microRNA expressions in healthy and myopathic horses suffering from polysaccharide storage myopathy or recurrent exertional rhabdomyolysis. Equine Vet J Suppl 2010;(38):303–10.
44. Desjardin C, Vaiman A, Mata X, et al. Next-generation sequencing identifies equine cartilage and subchondral bone miRNAs and suggests their involvement in osteochondrosis physiopathology. BMC Genomics 2014;15:798.
45. Razin A, Riggs AD. DNA methylation and gene function. Science 1980;210: 604–10.
46. Weber M, Davies JJ, Wittig D, et al. Chromosome-wide and promoter-specific analyses identify sites of differential DNA methylation in normal and transformed human cells. Nat Genet 2005;37:853–62.
47. Gim JA, Hong CP, Kim DS, et al. Genome-wide analysis of DNA methylation before-and after exercise in the thoroughbred horse with MeDIP-Seq. Mol Cell 2015;38:210–20.
48. Lee JR, Hong CP, Moon JW, et al. Genome-wide analysis of DNA methylation patterns in horse. BMC Genomics 2014;15:598.
49. Furey TS. ChIP-seq and beyond: new and improved methodologies to detect and characterize protein-DNA interactions. Nat Rev Genet 2012;13:840–52.
50. Licatalosi DD, Mele A, Fak JJ, et al. HITS-CLIP yields genome-wide insights into brain alternative RNA processing. Nature 2008;456:464–9.
51. Robinson JT, Thorvaldsdottir H, Winckler W, et al. Integrative genomics viewer. Nat Biotechnol 2011;29:24–6.
52. Thorvaldsdottir H, Robinson JT, Mesirov JP. Integrative Genomics Viewer (IGV): high-performance genomics data visualization and exploration. Brief Bioinform 2013;14:178–92.
53. Robinson JT, Thorvaldsdottir H, Wenger AM, et al. Variant Review with the Integrative Genomics Viewer. Cancer Res 2017;77:e31–4.
54. Buels R, Yao E, Diesh CM, et al. JBrowse: a dynamic web platform for genome visualization and analysis. Genome Biol 2016;17:66.
55. Bohannan ZS, Mitrofanova A. Calling Variants in the Clinic: Informed Variant Calling Decisions Based on Biological, Clinical, and Laboratory Variables. Comput Struct Biotechnol J 2019;17:561–9.
56. Li Z, Wang Y, Wang F. A study on fast calling variants from next-generation sequencing data using decision tree. BMC Bioinformatics 2018;19:145.
57. Costa-Silva J, Domingues D, Lopes FM. RNA-Seq differential expression analysis: An extended review and a software tool. PLoS One 2017;12:e0190152.
58. Finotello F, Di Camillo B. Measuring differential gene expression with RNA-seq: challenges and strategies for data analysis. Brief Funct Genomics 2015;14: 130–42.
59. Scott EY, Woolard KD, Finno CJ, et al. Variation in MUTYH expression in Arabian horses with Cerebellar Abiotrophy. Brain Res 2018;1678:330–6.
60. Gargis AS, Kalman L, Bick DP, et al. Good laboratory practice for clinical next-generation sequencing informatics pipelines. Nat Biotechnol 2015;33:689–93.
61. Richards S, Aziz N, Bale S, et al. Standards and guidelines for the interpretation of sequence variants: a joint consensus recommendation of the American College of Medical Genetics and Genomics and the Association for Molecular Pathology. Genet Med 2015;17:405–24.
62. Bailey E, Finno C. Translation and application of equine genomics: The Havemeyer principles. Equine Vet J 2019;51:273.

Genetic Testing in the Horse

Rebecca R. Bellone, PhD[a,b,*], Felipe Avila, PhD[b]

KEYWORDS

- Genetics • Horses • Genetic testing • Parentage testing • Coat color testing
- Genetic disease testing • Performance testing

KEY POINTS

- Genetic testing for parentage verification has been used by the horse industry for decades to validate pedigree records and to preserve the genetic integrity of breeds.
- Genetic testing in horses is a powerful tool to inform both breeding and management decisions for genetic diseases and economically important phenotypic traits.
- Screening horses for disease-associated variants can help to confirm clinical diagnosis and assist in clinical management of disease.

INTRODUCTION AND HISTORY OF EQUINE GENETIC TESTING

Genetic testing in horses began with parentage using blood testing (blood group and protein polymorphism tests) in the 1960s. Methods to identify and evaluate genetic variants at the DNA level became available in the late 1990s, and parentage testing subsequently shifted to using DNA markers.[1] Also in the 1990s, advances in molecular techniques led to the discovery of the first genetic disease to be solved in horses (hyperkalemic periodic paralysis [HYPP])[2] and unveiled the first known coat color variant (chestnut).[3] Realizing the need for additional resources and tools to accelerate the pace of discovery of inherited traits in horses, the International Horse Genome Workshop (https://horsegenomeworkshop.com/) was established in 1995, and this collaboration still exists. The goal of this community is to develop tools and resources that empower research to advance knowledge of the biology, evolutionary history, and inherited traits in the horse. This group developed the first horse gene map,[4] the horse reference genome sequence,[5] single nucleotide polymorphism (SNP) arrays to map traits of interest,[6,7] and is currently generating tools that will help to better understand how DNA is regulated in a tissue-specific manner (also referred to as functional annotation).[8]

[a] Department of Population Health and Reproduction Davis, CA 95616, USA; [b] Veterinary Genetics Laboratory, School of Veterinary Medicine, University of California-Davis, One Shields Avenue, Davis, CA 95616, USA
* Corresponding author.
E-mail address: rbellone@ucdavis.edu

Vet Clin Equine 36 (2020) 211–234
https://doi.org/10.1016/j.cveq.2020.03.003
0749-0739/20/© 2020 Elsevier Inc. All rights reserved.

vetequine.theclinics.com

Besides discovering variation in the DNA that contribute to coat color, performance, and health, these tools have enabled the development of genetic tests that assist horse owners, breeders, and breed associations with management and breeding decisions, and that help veterinarians with diagnosis and management of genetic diseases. DNA tests are provided by a growing number of corporate and university service laboratories worldwide. Tests offered by each laboratory vary based on local demand and licensing restrictions (for patented genetic tests). Most genetic tests can be performed with DNA isolated from blood (collected in ethylenediaminetetraacetic acid [EDTA] tubes) or from 20 to 30 hair roots. This article provides an overview of the current application of horse genetic testing for parentage verification and identification, coat color, genetic diseases, and performance traits.

GENETIC TESTING FOR PARENTAGE AND IDENTITY
Basic Principles

Many horse breed registries include parentage verification to validate pedigree records as a requirement for registry. In addition, parentage analysis can be used to solve cases where parents are unknown; for example, in the case of 2 potential sires. Parentage analysis is based on the premise of exclusion. Different genetic factors are evaluated to determine whether there is an exclusion based on 2 genetic principles: (1) every genetic variant (also referred to as an allele) present in the offspring must be present in at least 1 of the parents; and (2) the parent must contribute 1 allele from each of the markers evaluated to their offspring (**Table 1**). When a parent cannot be excluded, it is said to qualify. The number of markers used depends on what is considered sufficient to detect an exclusion. The efficacy of the test also depends on the frequency of the tested alleles in the population; for populations with low genetic diversity, additional markers are needed to reach the same level of efficacy as in populations with greater genetic diversity at the markers being investigated.

DNA Testing Using Short Tandem Repeats

The first DNA markers discovered and validated for parentage testing were microsatellites, also called short tandem repeats (STRs). These short nucleotide sequences (typically 2–4 nucleotides in length) that repeat sequentially are found throughout the genome. For example, AHT5 is an STR located on horse chromosome 8, characterized by a GT dinucleotide that has been observed to range from 14 to 23 repeats in different individuals[9] (**Fig. 1**). Naming of STR markers in the horse is based on where the markers were discovered; AHT5 was discovered at the Animal Health Trust in the United Kingdom, hence the prefix AHT.

Because the alleles differ in size between individuals (based on the number of repeats present), genotyping is performed by determining allele sizes at each locus investigated. The alleles of the offspring are compared with the possible parents and exclusion principles are tested (see **Table 1**; **Table 2**).

Standardization of Parentage DNA Testing

Standardization of both the markers used and nomenclature of alleles was a requirement given the international nature of the horse industry; the movement of horses, semen, and embryos around the world; and the requirement of registries for parentage testing. Standardization for the sharing of genotyping results between laboratories, as well as parentage testing of foals whose parents were tested by another laboratory. In

Table 1
Parentage analysis using International Society of Animal Genetics short tandem repeat panel

Locus	AHT4	AHT5	ASB2	ASB17	ASB23	HMS2	HMS3	HMS6	HMS7	HTG4	HTG10	VGL20
Sire	JO	JK	MN	N	K	KL	MO	M	KM	KM	IO	NO
Offspring	O	KO	MQ	N	KU	KL	MP	MP	LM	KM	OR	MN
Dam	O	NO	OQ	NR	SU	LR	OP	MP	LN	M	OR	MN

Parentage analysis is based on exclusion principles. Genotypes are represented by letters (see description of nomenclature in the text). When available, both the sire and the dam genotypes are evaluated to determine qualification or exclusion. In this example, the sire and the dam qualify as the parents of the offspring, because every allele present in the offspring is present in at least 1 parent and each of the parents can contribute 1 allele from each marker to the offspring. The potential sire contributions are shown in blue and the dam contributions are shown in red.

addition, being able to compare records across laboratories also provides a means to confirm horse identity in cases of transport across countries, or in drug testing for horse racing or other forensic cases.

The standardization of horse STR genotyping is under the auspices of the International Society of Animal Genetics (ISAG; https://www.isag.us/). The first workshop to standardize the marker panel and the naming of alleles occurred in 1996 in Tours, France. A panel of 12 markers, known as the ISAG Panel, was established then and is used across laboratories (**Table 3**).[9–15]

The standardized allele nomenclature designates alleles with alphabetical symbols from smallest to largest. The M allele is represented as the allele whose size is in the middle of the range, whereas the next allele smaller is designated as L, and the next allele larger is designated as N, and so on. Using AHT5 as an example, the M allele corresponds to 19 GT units (see **Fig. 1**, **Table 3**). To ensure allele standardization across laboratories, a biannual comparison test is conducted, in which a duty laboratory provides DNA from approximately 20 animals to all the laboratories participating in the test. In addition, after the test, laboratories are ranked as 1, 2, or 3 based on concordance of their data to reference genotypes. Rank 1 is the highest and is required by the International Studbook Committee to provide parentage testing services to Thoroughbreds.

Although the ISAG panel contains 12 markers, most laboratories routinely test for 17 to 20 markers (or more) that expand on the core panel. Horse breeding practices often involve mating of close relatives, so additional markers are sometimes required to resolve cases. ISAG and the Horse Standing Committee implemented a backup panel for comparison testing, which consists of 14 STRs developed by Tozaki and colleagues[16] (excluding TKY279 reported in that article). Not all laboratories use the backup panel; however, it provides additional resources for parentage exclusion and identity, and enables across-laboratory comparisons and collaborations.

Single Nucleotide Polymorphism Panel Testing

Knowledge of the horse genome has vastly improved since the 1990s, when STR markers were first discovered. Within the last decade, whole-genome data for thousands of horses have unraveled millions of genetic variants.[17] SNPs are the most abundant type of variation that exists, and these are defined as a genomic location where a single nucleotide differs in relation to a reference sequence (eg, adenine or A instead of thymine or T). It is possible to use SNPs instead of, or in addition to, STRs for parentage. However, the number of SNPs needed to achieve the same power of exclusion as STRs is greater, and the exact number depends on the breed and

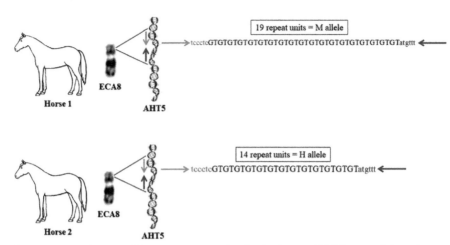

Fig. 1. DNA markers used for parentage testing in the horse. AHT5 is one of the microsatellite markers (STRs) used for parentage testing in horses. This marker is located on horse chromosome 8 (ECA8) and has a GT repeat. The number of GT repeats varies between horses. This repeat is flanked with a unique sequence that is used to amplify this specific region for genotyping. The flanking sequences are denoted in blue and red. The number of repeats determines the size of the allele and hence the genotype at this locus.

allele frequencies for the SNPs investigated. Work by Hirota and colleagues[18] showed that a panel of 53 SNPs could be used for parentage exclusion in a population of Thoroughbred horses, and work by Holl and colleagues[19] showed that 101 SNPs could be used for identity and parentage across several breeds. In 2017, these 154 markers were evaluated in an ISAG comparison test, but SNP genotyping is not yet an official component of ISAG tests for reporting and ranking.

Given the accuracy of STR typing and analysis, and the extensive historical database of STR genotypes that breed organizations have available, most laboratories and the equine industry have not been motivated to switch methodologies to SNP typing. However, as additional genetic variants are identified and the understanding of how this variation is contributing to specific phenotypes increases, the standard use of SNPs for parentage is expected.

GENETIC TESTS FOR COAT COLOR AND ASSOCIATED DISORDERS
Introduction

Since domestication, horses have been selectively bred for a variety of different coat colors and patterns.[20] The Icelandic horse is among those breeds that segregate for many of the known coat color variants. For this breed, DNA testing assists owners with classifying their animals with unique colors that result from a combination of genetic variants. In other breeds, where registration is assigned based on coat color phenotype, DNA testing can assist animal owners in obtaining regular registration papers. For example, in the Appaloosa breed, horses that have the Appaloosa coat pattern (also known as leopard complex spotting) get regular registration papers, whereas those without the coat pattern or other associated characteristics get N/C (noncharacteristic) registration numbers. DNA testing in this case can help to determine coat color when the phenotype is not easily documented by visual inspection. Furthermore, some variants causing pigmentation phenotype have been linked to

Table 2
Horse parentage exclusion example using International Society of Animal Genetics short tandem repeat panel

Locus	AHT4	AHT5	ASB2	ASB17	ASB23	HMS2	HMS3	HMS6	HMS7	HTG4	HTG10	VGL20
Sire A	JO	HI	Q	R	JU	KL	NP	LP	KL	M	O	IN
Sire B	JK	M	MN	O	JS	HK	MP	M	LM	KM	IO	IO
Offspring	KO	M	NR	OP	JS	H	IP	MP	JL	M	IO	IO
Dam	KO	MN	NQ	OP	SU	HR	IO	MP	JN	KM	LO	NO

Horse parentage testing can resolve parentage issues. Sire A is excluded as the sire of offspring in question based on the genotypes at 4 of the 12 markers evaluated (denoted in red: AHT5, ASB2, ASB17, and HMS2). For example, at ASB2, the stallion is homozygous for the Q allele but the offspring is heterozygous NR, thus the allele Q is not present in the foal. Sire B qualifies as the sire of this offspring.

disorders (described later), and thus testing for coat color variants can assist in clinical management decisions.

The first coat color variant to be discovered was the mutation in *melanocortin 1 receptor (MC1R)* which causes the chestnut phenotype, a red body and red points (lower legs, ear rims, mane, and tail).[3] A missense mutation in the coding region of this gene (c.248C>T, p.S83F) was identified using a candidate gene approach. Many of the early discoveries on coat color were made with a similar approach and, as advances in technology and knowledge of the horse genome increased, so did the number of discoveries.

Coat Color Tests Available

Coat color phenotypes can be divided into 3 categories: (1) base coat color, (2) dilutions, and (3) white spotting patterns. Additional pigmentation and hair length variants outside of these categories have also been reported, and their respective tests are described later. For a complete description of horse coat color, please refer to Sponenberg and Bellone.[21] Coat color genes and known causal variants are described in **Tables 4–6**. The coat color variants that have been linked to equine disorders are listed in **Table 7**. Different options for coat color testing range from single tests to panels with multiple tests, as well as larger panels that also include disease markers along with known coat color markers. Panels have the advantage of reducing costs if multiple tests are required but may include tests for colors that are not pertinent to the breed; therefore, relevancy of each test should be considered when choosing tests and interpreting results.

Base Coat Color

The base coat color of a horse can be described as black, bay, or chestnut. Two genes (*agouti signaling protein [ASIP]*, and *melanocortin 1 receptor [MC1R]*) contribute to the base coat color (see **Table 4**). Variants in these genes determine which pigment is produced: eumelanin (black/brown pigment), or pheomelanin (red/yellow pigment) and where it is produced (body or the points).[3,22,23] Chestnut, caused by a recessive mutation in *MC1R*, is epistatic to the *ASIP* locus, meaning if a horse is homozygous recessive at *MC1R (e/e)* it will be chestnut regardless of its *ASIP* genotype. Therefore, if bay or black horses are desired from a particular cross involving a chestnut horse, in order to make informed breeding decisions, genotyping for *ASIP* should also be performed.

Table 3
International Society of Animal Genetics horse short tandem repeat panel for parentage and identification

Locus	Chromosome	Repeat Sequence	Repeat Size of M Allele[a]	References
AHT4	24	$(AC)_nAT(AC)_n$	30	[9]
AHT5	8	$(GT)_n$	19	[9]
ASB2	15	$(GT)_n$	20	[10]
ASB17	2	$(AC)_n$	20	[10]
ASB23	3	$(TG)_n$	21	[11]
HMS2	10	$(CA)_n$	20	[12]
HMS3	9	$(CA)_n$	25	[12]
HMS6	4	$(GT)_n$	15	[12]
HMS7	1	$(CA)_n$	19	[12]
HTG4	9	$(TG)_n$	32	[13]
HTG10	21	$(TG)_n$	21	[14]
VGL20	30	$(TG)_n$	17	[15]

[a] The reported size of the M allele is based on van de Goor and colleagues.[113]

Dilution Variants

Six dilution genes that influence the amount of pigment produced have been identified in the horse (see **Table 5**). Some of these variants only affect either eumelanin or pheomelanin; others reduce the amount of both pigments. Therefore, genotyping becomes important to produce the desired dilution phenotype. For example, the silver phenotype is caused by a missense mutation in the premelanosome protein (*PMEL*, p.R625C). This variant is hypothesized to affect normal deposition of eumelanin in maturing melanosomes, thus diluting the amount of pigment. Black and bay horses with the silver mutation show a dilute phenotype (a lighter mane and tail accompanied by dappling in the coat). However, chestnut-based horses with the silver variant look the same as those without the variant. Therefore, knowing a horse's genotype with respect to silver is important if the owner wants to breed for or away from the silver trait. Further, considering that this allele has been associated with an eye disorder known as multiple congenital ocular anomalies (MCOA),[24] testing chestnut horses for the silver variant in breeds in which this allele is present can help to inform clinical decisions (detailed in Rebecca R. Bellone's article, "Genetics of Equine Ocular Disease," elsewhere in this issue). Aside from silver, other dilution variants include dun, cream, pearl, sunshine, champagne, mushroom, and lavender foal (see **Table 5**).[25–30] Some of these variants are restricted to a particular breed, such as the mushroom variant, which has only been reported in Shetland ponies and miniature horses.[31] Others are found in many breeds; for example, dun, which is considered the wild-type phenotype for equids.[26]

White Patterning Variants

White spotting patterns can occur on any base color and in combination with any dilution genes. More than 40 mutations in 7 different genes have been described that contribute to the white spotting patterns in horses (see **Table 6**). These are frame overo, sabino 1, tobiano, dominant white, splashed white, gray, and leopard complex.[32–43] White spotting phenotypes vary along a continuum, with some animals expressing a minimal phenotype, whereas others with the same variant may express a more pronounced white phenotype. The genetic control of this variability is unknown but is likely the product of an interaction of additional genes that can either enhance or suppress pigment production or pigment cell survival.

Evidence for these additive effects comes from the many mutations already identified. For example, a horse with both splash white 1 (SW1; a mutation in the *MITF* gene) and splash white 2 (SW2; a mutation in *PAX3*) was almost completely white, whereas those with only SW1 or SW2 had less white patterning.[37] Twenty-eight loss-of-functions mutations (W1–W19, W21–W28) in the *KIT* gene that cause a dominant white phenotype have been described; these horses are nearly all white but may retain pigment on the top line and ears.[35–38,44–46] Homozygosity for most of these dominant white mutations is thought to be lethal, and most of these variants have been documented in a single horse or line of horses. W20 is another mutation in *KIT* that has been reported to have a subtler impact on white patterning and is not embryonic lethal.[38] Genetic testing for white spotting patterns can assist breeders in producing horses with desired white patterns, and at the same time avoid health concerns. Studies suggest that most deaf horses have the frame overo pattern and/or the splash white pattern, and therefore horses with these alleles should be evaluated for deafness.[37,47] DNA testing for these mutations in horses with abundant white patterning can assist in mating choices that would avoid producing potentially deaf or embryonic lethal animals and/or those with less desirable phenotypes.

Other Pigmentation and Coat Length–Related Tests

The brindle pattern is a coat color phenotype in which darker vertical stripes appear on any background color. There have been 3 documented causes of brindle: chimerism (the fusion of 2 embryos with different coat color), and genetic variants in 2 X-linked genes.[48,49] Another phenotypic variation in the coat is the curly hair phenotype, a dominant missense variant in the *Keratin 25, type 1* (*KRT25*) gene that has been reported in several breeds, including the American Bashkir, Oldenburger, and Holsteiner.[50,51]

A unique iris color, called tiger eye (in which the iris is bright yellow, amber, or orange) has been reported in the Puerto Rican Paso Fino. Two recessive mutations (denoted at TE1 and TE2) in the *solute carrier family 24 member 5* gene (*SLC24A5*) have been shown to cause this phenotype and DNA testing can help breeders identify

Table 4
Genes, reported alleles, and variant descriptions for horse base coat colors

Base Coat Color/ Gene	Reported Alleles	Mutation Description	Breed	References
Extension/*MC1R*				
Extension or black	*E*	a	—	—
Chestnut	*e*	c.248C>T, p.S83F	Many	3
Chestnut	*e*ᵃ	c.250G>A, p.D84N	Black Forest pony and Knabstrupper	23
Agouti/*ASIP*				
Bay	*A*	a	—	—
Black	*a*	c.191_201del, p.Ala67GlufsTer14	Many	22

ᵃ Denotes wild-type allele.

Table 5
Coat color dilution tests

Gene	Reported Alleles[a]	Phenotype Description	Mutation Description[b]	Breed	References
SLC45A2	Cr	Cream	c.457G>A, p.D153N	Many	27
	Prl	Pearl	c.985G>A, p.A329T	American paint horse, Lusitano, purebred Spanish horse, quarter horse	28
	Sun[c]	Sunshine	c.568G>A, p.G190R	Standardbred × Tennessee walking horse cross	28
TBX3	D	Dun	Wild-type for all equids	—	26
	nd1	Non-dun1	ECA8g.20665796+1067G>T	Many	26
	nd2	Non-dun2	ECA8g.20665796del1617bp	Many	—
SLC36A1	Ch	Champagne	c.188C>G, p.T63R	Spanish Mustang, Tennessee walking horse, quarter horse, Missouri fox trotters, miniature horses, and pony breeds	29
PMEL	Z	Silver	ECA6g.74569773C>T, p.R625C	Miniature horse, Icelandic horse, Rocky Mountain, Kentucky mountain horse, Shetland ponies, Morgan	24,25
MYO5A	LFS	Lavender foal syndrome	c.4309delC p.Arg1396fs	Arabian	30
MFSD12	Mu	Mushroom	c.600dupC, p.Asp201fs	Shetland pony and miniature horse	31

[a] For all genes except *TBX3*, an N allele can also be reported. N is considered the reference/wild-type or the normal allele.
[b] Variants are based on published data or are denoted as EquCab3 coordinates.
[c] Reported in 1 animal.

Table 6
White patterning genetic tests

Phenotype[a]	Gene	Reported Allele[c]	Mutation Description[b]	Breed	References
Frame overo	EDNRB	O	c.353–354TC>AG, p. I118K	American Paint Horse, Miniature Horse, Pinto Horse, Quarter Horse, Thoroughbred, Appaloosa	31
Sabino 1	KIT	SB1	intronic SNP, ECA3g.79544206A>T	Appaloosa, Haflinger, Lipizzaner, Noriker, Quarter Horse	33
Tobiano	KIT (proposed)	To	~43 Mb inversion involving KIT	Many	34
Dominant white	KIT	W4	c.1805C>T, p.A602V	Camarillo White Horse	35
Dominant white	KIT	W5	c.2193delG, p.T732QfsX9	Thoroughbred	36
Dominant white	KIT	W10	c.1126_1129delGAAC, p.E376FfsX3	Quarter Horse	36
Dominant white	KIT	W20	c.2045G>A, p.R682H	American Paint Horse, Appaloosa, German Riding pony, Gipsy, Noriker, Old-Tori, Oldenburg, Quarter horse, Thoroughbred, Warmblood, Welsh Pony	37
Dominant white	KIT	W22	c.1529_1978del, p.E510_G659del	Thoroughbred	38
Splashed white	MITF	SW1	insertion in promoter, ECA16g.21579201Tdelins11	American Miniature Horse, American Paint Horse, Appaloosa, Icelandic, Morgan, Old-Tori, Quarter Horse, Shetland Pony, Trakehner	39
Splashed white	PAX3	SW2	c.209G>A, p.C70Y	Lipizzaner, Noriker, Quarter Horse	39
Splashed white	MITF	SW3	c.519_523delGTGTC, p.C174Sfs*20	Quarter Horse	39
Splashed white	PAX3	SW4	c.95C>G, p.P32R	Appaloosa	37
Splashed white	MITF	SW5	c.555_1260del	American Paint Horse	40
Gray	STX17	G	4.6 kb intronic duplication	Many	41
Leopard Complex Spotting	TRPM1	LP	intronic insertion, ECA1g.g. 109211964_109211965ins1378	American Miniature Horse, Appaloosa, Australian Spotted Pony, British spotted Pony, Knabstrupper, Noriker, Pony of the Americas	42
LP pattern modifier	RFWD3	PATN1	SNP in 3′ UTR, ECA3g.24352525T>G	American Miniature Horse, Appaloosa, Australian Spotted Pony, British Spotted Pony, Knabstrupper, Noriker, pony of the Americas	43

Abbreviation: UTR, untranslated region.
a The most common dominant white alleles are represented.
b Variant information is based on published data or are denoted as EquCab3 coordinates.
c For each locus tested, an N allele (which stands for normal or wild-type/reference allele) may also be reported.

Table 7
Coat color tests important for clinical management decisions

Disorder/Coat Color Phenotype	Genes	Reported Allele	Breed	References
Lethal white foal syndrome /deafness/ frame overo white spotting pattern	EDNRB	O	American paint horse, miniature horse, pinto horse, quarter horse, thoroughbred, Appaloosa	31
Multiple congenital ocular anomalies/ silver dilution[a]	PMEL	Z	American miniature horse, Icelandic Rocky Mountain, Kentucky mountain horse	24,25
Melanoma susceptibility/ gray progressive loss of pigment	STX17	G	Many	41
LFS/lavender foal dilution	MYO5A	LFS	Arabian	30
Congenital stationary night blindness, ERU risk/leopard complex spotting[a]	TRPM1	LP	American miniature horse, Appaloosa, Australian spotted pony, British spotted pony, Knabstrupper, Noriker, pony of the Americas	42
Deafness/splashed white spotting pattern	MITF/PAX3	SW1–SW5	American paint horse, miniature horse, pinto horse, quarter horse, thoroughbred, Appaloosa	37,39,40
Embryonic lethal/ dominant white	KIT	W1–W14, W16–W19, W21–W28	Mutations are breed specific	35–38

Abbreviation: ERU, equine recurrent uveitis; LFS, lavender foal syndrome.
   [a] For more on ocular disorders, see the Rebecca R. Bellone's article, "Genetics of Equine Ocular Disease," elsewhere in this issue.

brown-eyed carriers (individuals with brown eyes but who have 1 copy of 1 of the tiger-eye mutations) for mating.[52]

Testing for Coat Color and Associated Disorders

During embryonic development, melanocytes migrate from the neural crest to the skin, iris, inner ear, and other tissues, such as the heart.[53] Genes important for early melanocyte proliferation and migration are also involved in development of other cells derived from the neural crest. Therefore, mutations in key pigmentation genes can lead to pleiotropic effects (a single gene affects more than 1 phenotype/trait) (see **Table 7**). Genetic testing for these mutations can help confirm clinical diagnosis and identify horses at risk for disease. The first coat color variant to be associated with disease was lethal white overo mutation (LWFS),[31] in 1998. Horses heterozygous for this mutation typically have a white spotting pattern characterized by white patches that occur on the middle of the sides of the body that are framed by pigment; hence, this pattern is called frame overo. In contrast, homozygotes are born completely white and die within a few days after birth. The overo allele is a dinucleotide substitution in the *endothelin receptor B (EDNRB)* gene that affects both melanocyte and neural cell migration, so horses homozygous for this mutation do not develop proper innervation of the intestinal tract. Occasionally, all-white lethal foals result from crossing 2 minimally patterned horses whose owners were unaware they carried the overo allele. Therefore, genetic testing in these cases can detect carrier status, confirm whether lethality is caused by homozygosity for the frame mutation, and inform further breeding decisions.

GENETIC TESTING FOR GENETIC DISEASES
Introduction

Since the discovery of the molecular basis of HYPP in 1992,[2] the number of causal mutations for inherited diseases in horses has been steadily increasing. DNA tests are currently being offered for 21 genetic diseases, which constitutes a significant increase from the 10 tests available just 6 years ago when this topic was last reviewed.[54] Details on disease cause, as well as supporting research findings for the mutations discussed here, are described in detail elsewhere in this issue. A list of specific mutations and breeds in which they occur is provided in **Table 8**.

Testing for genetic diseases is not always a mandatory practice among breed registries. In recent years, more registries are requiring genetic testing for breed-relevant diseases for registration of foals and/or for inspection and licensing of stallions. These include the American Quarter Horse Association (AQHA), American Paint Horse Association (APHA), the Belgian Draft Horse Corporation of America, the Connemara Pony Breeders' Society, The Fell Pony Society, Westfalen Warmblood, Germany Riding Pony, Royal Dutch Warmblood Association of North America, and the New Forest Pony Breeding and Cattle Society. Genetic testing of breeding stock provides essential knowledge for owners, veterinarians, and breed associations to design appropriate breeding strategies that avoid producing affected individuals. Because not all tests are relevant to every breed, this genetic tests available for each breed are described here.

Quarter Horse and Related Breeds

At present, genetic tests are available for 7 inherited diseases found in quarter horses and related breeds: glycogen branching enzyme deficiency (GBED),[55] lethal white foal syndrome (LWFS),[31] hereditary equine regional dermal asthenia (HERDA),[56] HYPP,[2] immune-mediated myositis (IMM),[57] malignant hyperthermia (MH),[58] and polysaccharide storage myopathy type 1 (PSSM1).[59] Allele frequencies in a random sampling of quarter horses submitted for parentage testing at the UC Davis Veterinary Genetics Laboratory (VGL) were reported in 2009 to be 0.055 for PSSM1, 0.054 for GBED, 0.021 for HERDA, and 0.008 for HYPP.[60] The MH mutation is rare in quarter horses; data from more than 24,000 horses genotyped at the University of California (UC), Davis VGL estimates the allelic frequency to be 0.0015. However, it has been shown that horses with both the PSSM1 and MH mutations have a more severe clinical phenotype than those with the PSSM1 mutation alone.[61] The most recent genetic disease test offered for quarter horses detects a missense mutation in *MYH1* associated with IMM, an autoimmune disorder characterized by recurrent and rapid-onset muscle atrophy.[57] Valberg and colleagues[62] showed that this mutation is also associated with nonexertional rhabdomyolysis and determined the allele frequency to be 0.034 in the general quarter horse population and highest among reining, working cow, and halter horses; it was not detected in the barrel racing and racing quarter horse's subpopulations studied.[63]

AQHA regulations mandate that all breeding stallions have a 5-panel genetic disease test on file before registration of foals resulting from breedings after January 1, 2015. This panel includes tests for GBED, HERDA, HYPP, MH, and PSSM1. In addition, after 1/1/2007, foals homozygous for HYPP (H/H) are prohibited from being registered. The APHA also requires breeding stallions to have the 5-panel genetic disease test results on file, plus LWFS, before registration of their foals. The allele frequency of LWFS was estimated to be 0.107 in a random sampling of American paint horses.[60]

Arabian and Related Breeds

Genetic tests are currently being offered for 4 genetic diseases in Arabians and Arabian crosses: cerebellar abiotrophy (CA),[64] lavender foal syndrome (LFS),[30] occipitoatlantoaxial malformation (OAAM),[65] and severe combined immunodeficiency (SCID).[66] Although not mandatory, genetic testing for these conditions is recommended because carriers are phenotypically normal, but 25% of breedings between 2 carrier horses produce an affected foal. With the exception of SCID (a genetic defect of the immune system), all aforementioned diseases cause neurologic dysfunction. Prognosis in all cases is grave, and affected foals usually succumb or need to be euthanized shortly after birth. LFS in Arabians is another pigmentation-related trait with pleiotropic effects.

The CA mutation has been found in low frequency in breeds that have used the Arabian as foundation stock, such as the Danish sport pony, Bashkir curly, Trakehner, and Welsh pony,[64] so genetic testing is recommended in these breeds. Given the use of Arabian blood lines in the German riding pony, recently genetic testing for CA became a requirement for stallions in this breed. In the case of OAAM, a developmental defect that causes vertebral malformation at the craniocervical junction with associated neurologic damage, a genetic test is available for a 2.7-kb intergenic deletion in the homeobox (HOX) gene cluster that was detected in 1 affected individual. This variant was not detected in 2 additional Arabian foals diagnosed with OAAM, thus it is likely that additional variants within the HOX gene cluster and/or other developmental genes may also cause OAAM.[65]

Friesian

Friesian horses are characterized by a high level of inbreeding, and several recessive genetic diseases have been described.[67,68] Testing for known genetic diseases in this breed is essential for proper breeding practices designed to reduce the impact of disease-causing mutations on the overall health of the population. Despite the reported higher incidence of clinical entities in the Friesian horse compared with other breeds,[69] to date genetic tests are available for only 2 genetic disorders: dwarfism and hydrocephalus. The first is a splice site mutation (g.3772591C>T) in the B4GALT7 gene,[70] and the latter is caused by a nonsense mutation (g.76887901C>T) in B3GALNT2.[67] It is estimated that around 12% of the population carry the dwarfism mutation,[69] whereas approximately 17% of Friesians are carriers for the hydrocephalus mutation.[66] These disorders can also affect Friesian crosses. Research is ongoing to elucidate the genetic basis of several other disorders in Frisian horses, including megaesophagus,[71,72] bilateral corneal stroma loss,[73,74] and distichiasis.[75]

Belgian Draft Horse

Genetic testing for junctional epidermolysis bullosa (JEB) became mandatory for Belgian stallions as of November 1, 2002, and for breeding-age mares in 2015. This autosomal recessive disease, caused by a cytosine (C) insertion in exon 10 of the LAMC2 gene, is characterized by extensive and debilitating blistering of the skin and mouth epithelium as well as hoof sloughing. Affected foals eventually

Table 8
Genetic disease tests currently offered for the horse

Disease	Gene	Alleles	Breeds	Mutation Description[a]	References
GBED	GBE1	N, G	Quarter horse and related	ECA26g.8667651C>A	55
HERDA	PPIB	N, HRD	Quarter horse and related	ECA1g.129307092G>A	56
MH	RYR1	N, MH	Quarter horse and related	ECA10g.9678680C>G	58
HYPP	SCN4A	N, H	Quarter horse and related	ECA11g.1547422 8C>G	2
IMM	MYH1	N, My	Quarter horse and related	ECA11g.53345548T>C	57
JEB1	LAMC2	N, J	Belgian and related	ECA5g.17498175_17498176insC	76
JEB2	LAMA3	N, Js	American saddlebred	ECA5g.3724_10749del	89
PSSM1	GYS1	N, P1	Many	ECA10g.19203501G>A	59
NFS	ST14	N, NFS	Akhal-Teke	ECA7g.39711541G>T	87
SA	SHOX, CRLF2	N, Del1, Del2	Shetland Pony and American Miniature Horse	SHOX locus (X/Y PAR)[c]	84
SCID	PRKDC	N, SCID	Arabian and related	ECA9g.36395752_36395759del	66
CA	MUTYH	N, CA	Arabian and related	ECA2g.13122415G>A	64
OAAM	HOXD3	N, OAAM	Arabian and related	ECA18g.54652702_54655412del	65
OSCC	DDB2	N, R	Belgian, Haflinger, Rocky Mountain horse	ECA12g.11726667C>T	80
HWSD	SERPINB11	N, HWSD	Connemara pony	ECA8g.83600643_83600644insC	86
Dwarfism	B4GALT7	N, D	Friesian and related	ECA14g.3772591C>T	70
Hydrocephalus	B3GALT2	N, H	Friesian and related	ECA1g.76887901C>T	67
WFFS	PLOD1	N, WFFS	Warmblood and Thoroughbred	ECA2g.39927817G>A	88
FIS	SLC5A3	N, FIS	Fell and Dales pony	ECA26g.31894278G>T	85
Myotonia	CLCN1	N, Myo[b]	New Forest pony	ECA4g.96518592A>C	78

Abbreviations: CA, cerebellar abiotrophy; FIS, foal immunodeficiency syndrome; GBED, glycogen branching enzyme deficiency; HERDA, hereditary equine regional dermal asthenia; HWSD, hoof wall separation disease; IM, immune-mediated myositis; JEB1, junctional epidermolysis bullosa type 1; JEB2, junctional epidermolysis bullosa type 2; MH, malignant hyperthermia; NFS, naked foal syndrome; OAAM, occipitoatlantoaxial malformation; OSCC, ocular squamous cell carcinoma; PSSM1, polysaccharide storage myopathy type 1; SA, skeletal atavism; SCID, severe combined immunodeficiency; WFFS, warmblood fragile foal syndrome.
a Coordinates are based on EquCab3.
b Proposed.
c Exact genomic coordinates unknown.

succumb to infection or are euthanized before 10 days of age.[76] The same mutation has also been found to be associated with the JEB phenotype in other draft horse breeds, namely the Trait Breton and Trait Comtois,[77,78] Vlaams Paard, Belgische Koudbloed Flander,[78] and the Italian draft horse.[79] Data from the UC Davis VGL suggest that the frequency of JEB carriers in the Belgian horse population has been steadily decreasing since genetic testing for this disorder was established in 2002, from 13% in 2003 to 5% in 2018 (**Table 9**). The use of JEB genetic testing information in breeding decisions may be responsible for the noted reduction in carriers.

In addition, a missense mutation in the *DDB2* gene (c.1013C>T p.Thr338Met) was reported to be strongly associated with ocular squamous cell carcinoma (SCC) status in Haflinger and Belgian horses.[80–82] This risk allele is predicted to impair the ability of DDB2 to recognize and bind to ultraviolet (UV)-damaged DNA, thus leading to cancer, and explained 76% of Belgian cases of ocular SCC.[83] Testing for this risk factor is also recommended in Belgians.

Pony Breeds

Tests are also offered for genetic diseases found in pony breeds. For example, skeletal atavism (SA)[84] is a recessive disorder found in Shetland ponies that is caused by 2 independent, overlapping deletions (160–180 kb and 60–80 kb) that affect the *SHOX* locus in the pseudoautosomal region (PAR) of chromosomes X/Y. Both deletions have been shown to be associated the disease, and it is estimated that 12% of Shetland ponies are carriers. Because these deletions can be inherited independently, individuals that carry 2 copies of either deletion, or 1 copy of each (regardless of sex), are affected. Other genetic diseases found in pony breeds for which tests are available include foal immunodeficiency syndrome (FIS) in the fell and Dales pony,[85] hoof wall separation disease (HWSD) in the Connemara pony,[86] and myotonia in the New Forest pony.[78] Each of these breed organizations have different requirements on genetics testing. For example, genetic testing for FIS is compulsory for colts/stallions in the Fell Pony Society before a stallion license can be issued. Genetic testing is also compulsory for HWSD, and is performed at the time of parentage testing as part of the registration process for the Connemara Pony Breeders' Society. High carrier frequencies have been reported for both FIS and HWSD, and thus genetic testing results should be used to inform breeding decisions to decrease the incidence of these diseases in each pony breed. An anonymous screening of 214 fell ponies and 87 Dales ponies revealed that 38% of the fells and 18% of the Dales were heterozygous for the FIS mutation (no homozygotes were identified)[85]; carrier frequency for HWSD was estimated at 14.8% in Connemara ponies.[87] However, myotonia in the New Forest pony seems to be limited to a single breeding line.[88] Compulsory DNA testing for myotonia ended in 2017 for the New Forest Pony Breeding and Cattle Society, but all approved colts are currently being tested for PSSM1 at the vetting stage.

Other Breeds

Genetic testing is available for a second form of junctional epidermolysis bullosa (termed JEB2), identified in the American Saddlebred. This disorder is associated with a ~6.5-kb deletion spanning exons 24 to 27 of the *LAMA3* gene that was identified exclusively in this breed.[89] The allele frequency of this variant was estimated at 0.026 in the population, with a carrier frequency of 0.051.[89]

Recently, a nonsense mutation (c.388G>T) in the *ST14* gene was found to be associated with naked foal syndrome (NFS) in the Akhal-Teke horse.[87] Besides an almost complete absence of body, mane, and tail hair, individuals affected by NFS show mild ichthyosis and abnormal teeth and digestive system development, and die within days to 2.5 years after birth. The first cases of hairless foals were recorded in 1938, and the number of affected individuals has been steadily increasing. Therefore, genetic testing for this condition helps breeders and owners to identify carriers of this recessive mutation and select mating pairs accordingly.

Warmblood fragile foal syndrome (WFFS) is a fatal recessive disorder characterized by connective tissue fragility found in warmblood horses. Affected foals are born with muscle hypotonia, joint laxity, and extensive skin lesions. A missense mutation in the *PLOD1* gene (ECA2g.39927817G>A) has been associated with this condition.[88] The mutation has been detected in several warmblood breeds and warmblood crosses (https://www.vgl.ucdavis.edu/services/horse/WFFS.php), and work is ongoing to determine breed-specific allelic frequencies. Recently, Bellone and colleagues[90] reported that the *PLOD1* variant is found at a low frequency (1.2%) in the thoroughbred but determined that this variant was not associated with catastrophic breakdown. However, given the presence of the *PLOD1* variant in the breed, testing for WFFS may also be warranted for Thoroughbreds. Several warmblood registries require testing for WFFS; for example, the Royal Dutch Warmblood Association of North America requires testing for all activated approved, licensed, and Foalbook stallions since 2018, and the results of the test are published on the KWPN-NA Web site.

GENETIC TESTING FOR PERFORMANCE TRAITS
Introduction

According to the American Horse Council Foundation, the horse industry had an impact of $122 billion in the US economy in 2017,[91] and approximately 35% of horses owned in the country were used for showing or racing. In 2010, the first mutation associated with a performance trait was reported in the myostatin (*MSTN*)[92] gene in Thoroughbreds and, since then, genetic markers predictive of performance are being recognized as important components of genetic research and testing. Research efforts are currently underway to elucidate the genetic underpinnings of performance in several horse breeds. Such studies are designed to help horse owners, breeders, and trainers to understand the role of genetics, in addition to the environment and training, in contributing to a horse's success in competition. The genetic tests available for performance traits in the horse are discussed here (**Table 10**).

Gaitedness

Gaitedness is a trait present in certain horse breeds that allows them to perform alternative patterns of locomotion, namely ambling and pacing. This ability, present in gaited horses, has been associated with a cytosine (C) to adenine (A) substitution

Table 9
Junctional epidermolysis bullosa carrier frequency in Belgian horses tested in 5 different years at the University of California, Davis Veterinary Genetics Laboratory

Year	N	Carrier Frequency
2003	545	0.13
2004	330	0.13
2009	178	0.11
2017	285	0.07
2018	253	0.05

that causes a premature stop codon in the *DMRT3* gene (DMRT3_Ser301STOP).[93] This so-called 'gait-keeper' mutation has been identified in horses from 68 different breeds, with the frequency of the mutant (A) allele varying from 1.1% to complete fixation (100%) in some gaited breeds, such as the American standardbred.[94]

This variant has also been found to have a strong positive impact on harness racing performance in gaited breeds. Several studies have shown that individuals homozygous for the gait-keeper mutation outperform horses that are heterozygous or homozygous for the wild-type allele.[93,95–97] However, because variation in gait patterns can be observed in breeds fixed or nearly fixed for the gait-keeper mutation (especially in South American breeds),[98,99] it is hypothesized that modifying genes exist that likely influence these gaits, which remain to be discovered. The genetic test for the *DMRT3* gait-keeper mutation is protected by a patent and offered by licensed laboratories worldwide.

Recently, McCoy and colleagues[100] developed an algorithm to predict a standardbred's status as a pacer or trotter based on 7 SNPs identified by a combination of genomics tools. Standardbreds seem to be fixed for the *DMRT3* mutation, but some of them have the ability to pace and others do not. According to the study, the algorithm was greater than 99% accurate in predicting whether an individual was a pacer or a trotter. The biological function of these 7 variants remains to be determined. However, this predictive model will help standardbred owners to make informed breeding and training decisions based on a horse's genotypic profile and will be available commercially in the near future.

Racing Performance

The *myostatin* (*MSTN*) gene encodes a protein that negatively regulates skeletal muscle development, and variants in this gene have been associated with muscle hypertrophy phenotypes in different mammalian species. In 2010, 2 studies identified an SNP (g.66608679C>T) in the first intron of the *MSTN* gene strongly associated with best race distance in thoroughbred racehorses.[92,101] The investigators concluded that C/C horses excel in fast, short-distance races; heterozygous horses (C/T) are more prone to succeeding in middle-distance races; and homozygotes for the mutation (T/T) perform better in longer distance races. Subsequent studies showed that the wild-type (C) allele was associated with a higher proportion of fast-twitch, glycolytic type 2B muscle fibers in gluteal muscle biopsies of Thoroughbreds and racing quarter horses,[102] as well as with increased speed indices in Thoroughbreds.[103] The Speed Gene genetic test for the *MSTN* variant is protected by a patent and offered by PlusVital Inc. Subsequent studies have shown that the causal variant is a 227-bp short interspersed nuclear element (SINE) insertion in the *MSTN* promoter,[102] upstream of the identified SNP and inherited on the same strand of DNA with the C allele.

Recently, a steady stream of studies have identified genes putatively associated with performance traits in different horse breeds.[104–108] It is expected that these promising data will lead to the discovery of additional markers for genetic testing that will help in genomic selection that can be used for breeding and training purposes.

Gene Doping

Gene doping is defined as the use of (1) polymers of nucleic acids or nucleic acid analogues; (2) gene editing to alter genome sequences and/or the transcriptional, post-transcriptional, or epigenetic regulation of gene expression; or (3) normal or genetically modified cells to enhance an individual's performance.[109] The issue of genetic manipulation to improve athletic ability is regarded as a threat in the horse-racing industry, and preventive measures to avoid gene doping are currently being researched in order to ensure fairness. Current technologies are still unable to detect the presence of foreign or edited DNA at the genome level; however, researchers were recently able to successfully detect horse erythropoietin (*EPO*) transgenes extracted from blood (plasma) and urine using droplet digital polymerase chain reaction.[110] This development constitutes an important first step toward the use of molecular tools to monitor gene doping in the equine industry.

STANDARDIZATION FOR DIAGNOSTIC TESTS

Standardization of allele nomenclature and testing parameters, as well as quality control for diagnostic testing (coat color, disease, and performance traits), is not subject to oversight by any organization. As part of the ISAG parentage comparison tests, the duty laboratory may select samples that have variability in coat color and disease traits so that comparisons across laboratories can be made; however, participation is voluntary.

Because no standard nomenclature exists across laboratories to report diagnostic alleles, interpreting results from different laboratories can be difficult. In 2013, Penedo and Raudsepp[54] proposed a standard nomenclature for the 10 tests available at the time by assigning the letter N to the normal allele (wild-type) and a letter symbol associated with each condition for the causative mutation. This article expands this proposed standard to the current tests, based on the allele nomenclature used by the UC Davis VGL (see **Tables 4–10**).

In 2018, the horse genomics research community developed a consensus statement on the application of research for commercial use, which may assist animal owners and clinicians in choosing a laboratory for testing and help in deciding which tests may be most appropriate (https://img1.wsimg.com/blobby/go/3ed25c45-16f5-4198-9333-2dd4d2feeafa/downloads/1cq72554i_382106.pdf?ver=1551977123053). Some key principles identified were that scientific discovery should be reproducible and subject to the peer-review process and that clear differentiation should be made between scientific developments, commercial opportunity, and opinion.

FUTURE DEVELOPMENTS IN EQUINE GENETIC TESTING

Many of the genetic tests available assay simple traits (controlled by 1 or only a few genes). Complex traits are those in which a particular phenotype arises because of an interplay of genetic and environmental factors, and some have a significant negative impact in the horse industry. Only a few tests currently exist for complex traits. For example, ocular SCC involves a genetic risk and environmental exposure to UV light; however, more work is needed to capture the full genetic component of this and other traits. Another important complex trait that affects several breeds is equine metabolic syndrome (EMS). Characterized by obesity and insulin dysregulation, this disorder increases the risk of laminitis in affected individuals. A recent study showed that a

Table 10
Genetic performance tests offered for the horse

Trait	Gene	Alleles	Breeds	Mutation Description[a]	References
Gaitedness	*DMRT3*	C, A	Many (gaited)	ECA23g.22391254C>A	93
Racing distance	*MSTN*	C, T	Thoroughbred	ECA18g.66608679C>T	92

[a] Coordinates are based on EquCab3.

variant in the *HMGA2* gene, previously associated with small stature in pony breeds,[111] also has an effect on EMS traits (and more significantly on baseline insulin levels) in Welsh ponies.[112] The pleiotropic effect of this variant is estimated to contribute ~40% and ~20% of the total heritability for height and baseline insulin, respectively. Ongoing studies will be designed to fully characterize the genetic bases of this disorder, as well as to understand the interaction between genetics and environment on disease onset and severity. Future research on both simple and complex traits will be facilitated by constantly developing technologies, a better understanding of the horse genome, and lower associated costs. One of the promising avenues for equine genetic testing includes precision medicine, which focuses on identifying breed-specific or even individualized health approaches based on the knowledge of the combination of genetic and environmental factors.

DISCLOSURE

R.R. Bellone and F. Avila are affiliated with the VGL, a genetic testing laboratory offering diagnostic tests in horses and other species.

REFERENCES

1. Bowling AT, Eggleston-Stott ML, Byrns G, et al. Validation of microsatellite markers for routine horse parentage testing. Anim Genet 1997;28:247–52.
2. Rudolph JA, Spier SJ, Byrns G, et al. Periodic paralysis in quarter horses: a sodium channel mutation disseminated by selective breeding. Nat Genet 1992;2:144–7.
3. Marklund L, Moller MJ, Sandberg K, et al. A missense mutation in the gene for melanocyte-stimulating hormone receptor (MC1R) is associated with the chestnut coat color in horses. Mamm Genome 1996;7:895–9.
4. Chowdhary BP, Bailey E. Equine genomics: galloping to new frontiers. Cytogenet Genome Res 2003;102:184–8.
5. Wade CM, Giulotto E, Sigurdsson S, et al. Genome sequence, comparative analysis, and population genetics of the domestic horse. Science 2009;326:865–7.
6. Schaefer RJ, Schubert M, Bailey E, et al. Developing a 670k genotyping array to tag ~2M SNPs across 24 horse breeds. BMC Genomics 2017;18:565.
7. McCue ME, Bannasch DL, Petersen JL, et al. A high density SNP array for the domestic horse and extant Perissodactyla: utility for association mapping, genetic diversity, and phylogeny studies. PLoS Genet 2012;8:e1002451.
8. Tuggle CK, Giuffra E, White SN, et al. GO-FAANG meeting: a gathering on functional annotation of animal genomes. Anim Genet 2016;47:528–33.
9. Binns MM, Holmes NG, Holliman A, et al. The identification of polymorphic microsatellite loci in the horse and their use in thoroughbred parentage testing. Br Vet J 1995;151:9–15.
10. Breen M, Lindgren G, Binns MM, et al. Genetical and physical assignments of equine microsatellites–first integration of anchored markers in horse genome mapping. Mamm Genome 1997;8:267–73.
11. Irvin Z, Giffard J, Brandon R, et al. Equine dinucleotide repeat polymorphisms at loci ASB 21, 23, 25 and 37-43. Anim Genet 1998;29:67.
12. Guerin G, Bertaud M, Amigues Y. Characterization of seven new horse microsatellites: HMS1, HMS2, HMS3, HMS5, HMS6, HMS7 and HMS8. Anim Genet 1994;25:62.

13. Ellegren H, Johansson M, Sandberg K, et al. Cloning of highly polymorphic microsatellites in the horse. Anim Genet 1992;23:133–42.

14. Marklund S, Ellegren H, Eriksson S, et al. Parentage testing and linkage analysis in the horse using a set of highly polymorphic microsatellites. Anim Genet 1994; 25:19–23.

15. van Haeringen H, Bowling AT, Stott ML, et al. A highly polymorphic horse microsatellite locus: VHL20. Anim Genet 1994;25:207.

16. Tozaki T, Kakoi H, Mashima S, et al. Population study and validation of paternity testing for Thoroughbred horses by 15 microsatellite loci. J Vet Med Sci 2001; 63:1191–7.

17. Jagannathan V, Gerber V, Rieder S, et al. Comprehensive characterization of horse genome variation by whole-genome sequencing of 88 horses. Anim Genet 2019;50:74–7.

18. Hirota K, Kakoi H, Gawahara H, et al. Construction and validation of parentage testing for thoroughbred horses by 53 single nucleotide polymorphisms. J Vet Med Sci 2010;72:719–26.

19. Holl HM, Vanhnasy J, Everts RE, et al. Single nucleotide polymorphisms for DNA typing in the domestic horse. Anim Genet 2017;48:669–76.

20. Ludwig A, Pruvost M, Reissmann M, et al. Coat color variation at the beginning of horse domestication. Science 2009;324:485.

21. Sponenberg DP, Bellone R. Equine color genetics. 4th edition. Hoboken (NJ): John Wiley & Sons, Inc; 2017.

22. Rieder S, Taourit S, Mariat D, et al. Mutations in the agouti (ASIP), the extension (MC1R), and the brown (TYRP1) loci and their association to coat color phenotypes in horses (Equus caballus). Mamm Genome 2001;12:450–5.

23. Wagner HJ, Reissmann M. New polymorphism detected in the horse MC1R gene. Anim Genet 2000;31:289–90.

24. Andersson LS, Wilbe M, Viluma A, et al. Equine multiple congenital ocular anomalies and silver coat colour result from the pleiotropic effects of mutant PMEL. PLoS One 2013;8:e75639.

25. Andersson LS, Axelsson J, Dubielzig RR, et al. Multiple congenital ocular anomalies in Icelandic horses. BMC Vet Res 2011;7:21.

26. Imsland F, McGowan K, Rubin C-J, et al. Regulatory mutations in TBX3 disrupt asymmetric hair pigmentation that underlies Dun camouflage color in horses. Nat Genet 2016;48:152–8.

27. Mariat D, Taourit S, Guerin G. A mutation in the MATP gene causes the cream coat colour in the horse. Genet Sel Evol 2003;35.

28. Holl HM, Pflug KM, Yates KM, et al. A candidate gene approach identifies variants in SLC45A2 that explain dilute phenotypes, pearl and sunshine, in compound heterozygote horses. Anim Genet 2019;50:271–4.

29. Cook D, Brooks S, Bellone R, et al. Missense mutation in exon 2 of SLC36A1 responsible for champagne dilution in horses. PLoS Genet 2008;4:e1000195.

30. Brooks SA, Gabreski N, Miller D, et al. Whole-genome SNP association in the horse: identification of a deletion in myosin Va responsible for Lavender Foal Syndrome. PLoS Genet 2010;6:e1000909.

31. Tanaka JL, Rushton J, Famula TT, et al. Frameshift Variant in MFSD12 Explains the Mushroom Coat Color Dilution in Shetland Ponies. Genes 2019;10(10):826. https://doi.org/10.3390/genes10100826.

32. Metallinos DL, Bowling AT, Rine J. A missense mutation in the endothelin-B receptor gene is associated with Lethal White Foal Syndrome: an equine version of Hirschsprung disease. Mamm Genome 1998;9:426–31.

33. Brooks SA, Bailey E. Exon skipping in the KIT gene causes a Sabino spotting pattern in horses. Mamm Genome 2005;16:893–902.
34. Brooks SA, Lear TL, Adelson DL, et al. A chromosome inversion near the KIT gene and the Tobiano spotting pattern in horses. Cytogenet Genome Res 2007;119:225–30.
35. Haase B, Brooks SA, Schlumbaum A, et al. Allelic heterogeneity at the equine KIT locus in dominant white (W) horses. PLoS Genet 2007;3:e195.
36. Haase B, Brooks SA, Tozaki T, et al. Seven novel KIT mutations in horses with white coat colour phenotypes. Anim Genet 2009;40:623–9.
37. Hauswirth R, Jude R, Haase B, et al. Novel variants in the KIT and PAX3 genes in horses with white-spotted coat colour phenotypes. Anim Genet 2013;44:763–5.
38. Durig N, Jude R, Holl H, et al. Whole genome sequencing reveals a novel deletion variant in the KIT gene in horses with white spotted coat colour phenotypes. Anim Genet 2017;48:483–5.
39. Hauswirth R, Haase B, Blatter M, et al. Mutations in MITF and PAX3 cause "splashed white" and other white spotting phenotypes in horses. PLoS Genet 2012;8:e1002653.
40. Henkel J, Lafayette C, Brooks SA, et al. Whole-genome sequencing reveals a large deletion in the MITF gene in horses with white spotted coat colour and increased risk of deafness. Anim Genet 2019;50:172–4.
41. Rosengren Pielberg G, Golovko A, Sundström E, et al. A cis-acting regulatory mutation causes premature hair graying and susceptibility to melanoma in the horse. Nat Genet 2008;40.
42. Bellone RR, Holl H, Setaluri V, et al. Evidence for a retroviral insertion in TRPM1 as the cause of congenital stationary night blindness and leopard complex spotting in the horse. PLoS One 2013;8:e78280.
43. Holl HM, Brooks SA, Archer S, et al. Variant in the RFWD3 gene associated with PATN1, a modifier of leopard complex spotting. Anim Genet 2016;47:91–101.
44. Haase B, Signer-Hasler H, Binns MM, et al. Accumulating mutations in series of haplotypes at the KIT and MITF loci are major determinants of white markings in Franches-Montagnes horses. PLoS One 2013;8:e75071.
45. Hoban R, Castle K, Hamilton N, et al. Novel KIT variants for dominant white in the Australian horse population. Anim Genet 2018;49:99–100.
46. Hug P, Jude R, Henkel J, et al. A novel KIT deletion variant in a German Riding Pony with white-spotting coat colour phenotype. Anim Genet 2019;50(6):761–3.
47. Magdesian KG, Williams DC, Aleman M, et al. Evaluation of deafness in American Paint Horses by phenotype, brainstem auditory-evoked responses, and endothelin receptor B genotype. J Am Vet Med Assoc 2009;235:1204–11.
48. Towers RE, Murgiano L, Millar DS, et al. A nonsense mutation in the IKBKG gene in mares with incontinentia pigmenti. PLoS One 2013;8:e81625.
49. Murgiano L, Waluk DP, Towers R, et al. An intronic MBTPS2 variant results in a splicing defect in horses with brindle coat texture. G3 (Bethesda) 2016;6:2963–70.
50. Morgenthaler C, Diribarne M, Capitan A, et al. A missense variant in the coil1A domain of the keratin 25 gene is associated with the dominant curly hair coat trait (Crd) in horse. Genet Sel Evol 2017;49:85.
51. Thomer A, Gottschalk M, Christmann A, et al. An epistatic effect of KRT25 on SP6 is involved in curly coat in horses. Sci Rep 2018;8:6374.
52. Mack M, Kowalski E, Grahn R, et al. Two variants in SLC24A5 are associated with "Tiger-Eye" iris pigmentation in puerto rican paso fino horses. G3 (Bethesda) 2017;7:2799–806.

53. Bardawil T, Khalil S, Bergqvist C, et al. Genetics of inherited cardiocutaneous syndromes: a review. Open Heart 2016;3:e000442.
54. Penedo M, Raudsepp T. Molecular genetic testing and karyotyping in the horse. In: Equine Genomics. 1st edition. Hoboken (NJ): Wiley-Blackwell Publishing Ltd; 2013.
55. Ward TL, Valberg SJ, Adelson DL, et al. Glycogen branching enzyme (GBE1) mutation causing equine glycogen storage disease IV. Mamm Genome 2004; 15:570–7.
56. Tryon RC, White SD, Bannasch DL. Homozygosity mapping approach identifies a missense mutation in equine cyclophilin B (PPIB) associated with HERDA in the American Quarter Horse. Genomics 2007;90:93–102.
57. Finno CJ, Gianino G, Perumbakkam S, et al. A missense mutation in MYH1 is associated with susceptibility to immune-mediated myositis in Quarter Horses. Skelet Muscle 2018;8:7.
58. Aleman M, Riehl J, Aldridge BM, et al. Association of a mutation in the ryanodine receptor 1 gene with equine malignant hyperthermia. Muscle Nerve 2004;30: 356–65.
59. McCue ME, Valberg SJ, Lucio M, et al. Glycogen synthase 1 (GYS1) mutation in diverse breeds with polysaccharide storage myopathy. J Vet Intern Med 2008; 22:1228–33.
60. Tryon RC, Penedo MC, McCue ME, et al. Evaluation of allele frequencies of inherited disease genes in subgroups of American Quarter Horses. J Am Vet Med Assoc 2009;234:120–5.
61. McCue ME, Valberg SJ, Jackson M, et al. Polysaccharide storage myopathy phenotype in quarter horse-related breeds is modified by the presence of an RYR1 mutation. Neuromuscul Disord 2009;19:37–43.
62. Valberg SJ, Henry ML, Perumbakkam S, et al. An E321G MYH1 mutation is strongly associated with nonexertional rhabdomyolysis in Quarter Horses. J Vet Intern Med 2018;32:1718–25.
63. Gianino GM, Valberg SJ, Perumbakkam S, et al. Prevalence of the E321G MYH1 variant for immune-mediated myositis and nonexertional rhabdomyolysis in performance subgroups of American Quarter Horses. J Vet Intern Med 2019;33: 897–901.
64. Brault LS, Cooper CA, Famula TR, et al. Mapping of equine cerebellar abiotrophy to ECA2 and identification of a potential causative mutation affecting expression of MUTYH. Genomics 2011;97:121–9.
65. Bordbari MH, Penedo MCT, Aleman M, et al. Deletion of 2.7 kb near HOXD3 in an Arabian horse with occipitoatlantoaxial malformation. Anim Genet 2017;48: 287–94.
66. Shin EK, Perryman LE, Meek K. A kinase-negative mutation of DNA-PK(CS) in equine SCID results in defective coding and signal joint formation. J Immunol 1997;158:3565–9.
67. Ducro BJ, Schurink A, Bastiaansen JW, et al. A nonsense mutation in B3GALNT2 is concordant with hydrocephalus in Friesian horses. BMC Genomics 2015; 16:761.
68. Ankringa N, Wijnberg ID, Boerma S, et al. Copper-associated hepatic cirrhosis in a Friesian horse. Tijdschr Diergeneeskd 2012;137:310–4.
69. Boerma S, Back W, Sloet van Oldruitenborgh-Ossterbaan MM. The Friesian horse breed: a clinical challenge to the equine veterinarian? Equine Vet Educ 2012;24:66–71.

70. Leegwater PA, Vos-Loohuis M, Ducro BJ, et al. Dwarfism with joint laxity in Friesian horses is associated with a splice site mutation in B4GALT7. BMC Genomics 2016;17:839.

71. Komine M, Langohr IM, Kiupel M. Megaesophagus in Friesian horses associated with muscular hypertrophy of the caudal esophagus. Vet Pathol 2014;51: 979–85.

72. Ploeg M, Grone A, Saey V, et al. Esophageal dysfunction in friesian horses: morphological features. Vet Pathol 2015;52:1142–7.

73. Alberi C, Hisey E, Lassaline M, et al. Ruling out BGN variants as simple X-linked causative mutations for bilateral corneal stromal loss in Friesian horses. Anim Genet 2018;49(6):656–7.

74. Lassaline-Utter M, Gemensky-Metzler AJ, Scherrer NM, et al. Corneal dystrophy in Friesian horses may represent a variant of pellucid marginal degeneration. Vet Ophthalmol 2014;17:186–94.

75. Hermans H, Ensink JM. Treatment and long-term follow-up of distichiasis, with special reference to the Friesian horse: a case series. Equine Vet J 2014;46: 458–62.

76. Spirito F, Charlesworth A, Linder K, et al. Animal models for skin blistering conditions: absence of laminin 5 causes hereditary junctional mechanobullous disease in the Belgian horse. J Invest Dermatol 2002;119:684–91.

77. Milenkovic D, Chaffaux S, Taourit S, et al. A mutation in the LAMC2 gene causes the Herlitz junctional epidermolysis bullosa (H-JEB) in two French draft horse breeds. Genet Sel Evol 2003;35:249–56.

78. Wijnberg ID, Owczarek-Lipska M, Sacchetto R, et al. A missense mutation in the skeletal muscle chloride channel 1 (CLCN1) as candidate causal mutation for congenital myotonia in a New Forest pony. Neuromuscul Disord 2012;22:361–7.

79. Cappelli K, Brachelente C, Passamonti F, et al. First report of junctional epidermolysis bullosa (JEB) in the Italian draft horse. BMC Vet Res 2015;11:55.

80. Bellone RR, Liu J, Petersen JL, et al. A missense mutation in damage-specific DNA binding protein 2 is a genetic risk factor for limbal squamous cell carcinoma in horses. Int J Cancer 2017;141:342–53.

81. Singer-Berk M, Knickelbein KE, Vig S, et al. Genetic risk for squamous cell carcinoma of the nictitating membrane parallels that of the limbus in Haflinger horses. Anim Genet 2018;49:457–60.

82. Singer-Berk MH, Knickelbein KE, Lounsberry ZT, et al. Additional evidence for DDB2 T338M as a genetic risk factor for ocular squamous cell carcinoma in horses. Int J Genomics 2019;2019:3610965.

83. Knickelbein KE, Lassaline ME, Singer-Berk M, et al. A missense mutation in damage-specific DNA binding protein 2 is a genetic risk factor for ocular squamous cell carcinoma in Belgian horses. Equine Vet J 2020;52(1):34–40.

84. Rafati N, Andersson LS, Mikko S, et al. Large deletions at the SHOX locus in the pseudoautosomal region are associated with skeletal atavism in shetland ponies. G3 (Bethesda) 2016;6:2213–23.

85. Fox-Clipsham LY, Carter SD, Goodhead I, et al. Identification of a mutation associated with fatal Foal Immunodeficiency Syndrome in the Fell and Dales pony. PLoS Genet 2011;7:e1002133.

86. Finno CJ, Stevens C, Young A, et al. SERPINB11 frameshift variant associated with novel hoof specific phenotype in Connemara ponies. PLoS Genet 2015; 11:e1005122.

87. Bauer A, Hiemesch T, Jagannathan V, et al. A Nonsense Variant in the ST14 Gene in Akhal-Teke Horses with Naked Foal Syndrome. G3 (Bethesda) 2017; 7:1315–21.

88. Monthoux C, de Brot S, Jackson M, et al. Skin malformations in a neonatal foal tested homozygous positive for Warmblood Fragile Foal Syndrome. BMC Vet Res 2015;11:12.

89. Graves KT, Henney PJ, Ennis RB. Partial deletion of the LAMA3 gene is responsible for hereditary junctional epidermolysis bullosa in the American Saddlebred Horse. Anim Genet 2009;40:35–41.

90. Bellone RR, Ocampo NR, Hughes SS, et al. Warmblood fragile foal syndrome type 1 mutation (PLOD1 c.2032G>A) is not associated with catastrophic breakdown and has a low allele frequency in the Thoroughbred breed. Equine Vet J 2019;52(3):411–4.

91. Foundation AHC. 2017 National Economic Impact Study, 2017. Available at: https://www.horsecouncil.org/press-release/deeper-dive-ahcfs-2017-economic-impact-study/. Accessed September 20, 2019.

92. Hill EW, Gu J, Eivers SS, et al. A sequence polymorphism in MSTN predicts sprinting ability and racing stamina in thoroughbred horses. PLoS One 2010; 5:e8645.

93. Andersson LS, Larhammar M, Memic F, et al. Mutations in DMRT3 affect locomotion in horses and spinal circuit function in mice. Nature 2012;488:642–6.

94. Promerova M, Andersson LS, Juras R, et al. Worldwide frequency distribution of the 'Gait keeper' mutation in the DMRT3 gene. Anim Genet 2014;45:274–82.

95. Jaderkvist K, Andersson LS, Johansson AM, et al. The DMRT3 'Gait keeper' mutation affects performance of Nordic and Standardbred trotters. J Anim Sci 2014;92:4279–86.

96. Kristjansson T, Bjornsdottir S, Sigurdsson A, et al. The effect of the 'Gait keeper' mutation in the DMRT3 gene on gaiting ability in Icelandic horses. J Anim Breed Genet 2014;131:415–25.

97. Jaderkvist Fegraeus K, Johansson L, Maenpaa M, et al. Different DMRT3 genotypes are best adapted for harness racing and riding in finnhorses. J Hered 2015;106:734–40.

98. Patterson L, Staiger EA, Brooks SA. DMRT3 is associated with gait type in Mangalarga Marchador horses, but does not control gait ability. Anim Genet 2015; 46:213–5.

99. Novoa-Bravo M, Jaderkvist Fegraeus K, Rhodin M, et al. Selection on the Colombian paso horse's gaits has produced kinematic differences partly explained by the DMRT3 gene. PLoS One 2018;13:e0202584.

100. McCoy AM, Beeson SK, Rubin CJ, et al. Identification and validation of genetic variants predictive of gait in standardbred horses. PLoS Genet 2019;15: e1008146.

101. Binns MM, Boehler DA, Lambert DH. Identification of the myostatin locus (MSTN) as having a major effect on optimum racing distance in the Thoroughbred horse in the USA. Anim Genet 2010;41(Suppl 2):154–8.

102. Petersen JL, Valberg SJ, Mickelson JR, et al. Haplotype diversity in the equine myostatin gene with focus on variants associated with race distance propensity and muscle fiber type proportions. Anim Genet 2014;45:827–35.

103. Hill EW, Fonseca RG, McGivney BA, et al. MSTN genotype (g.66493737C/T) association with speed indices in Thoroughbred racehorses. J Appl Physiol (1985) 2012;112:86–90.

104. Jaderkvist Fegraeus K, Velie BD, Axelsson J, et al. A potential regulatory region near the EDN3 gene may control both harness racing performance and coat color variation in horses. Physiol Rep 2018;6:e13700.

105. Avila F, Mickelson JR, Schaefer RJ, et al. Genome-wide signatures of selection reveal genes associated with performance in American Quarter Horse Subpopulations. Front Genet 2018;9:249.

106. Velie BD, Fegraeus KJ, Sole M, et al. A genome-wide association study for harness racing success in the Norwegian-Swedish coldblooded trotter reveals genes for learning and energy metabolism. BMC Genet 2018;19:80.

107. Ropka-Molik K, Stefaniuk-Szmukier M, Musial AD, et al. The genetics of racing performance in Arabian horses. Int J Genomics 2019;2019:9013239.

108. Ropka-Molik K, Stefaniuk-Szmukier M, Szmatola T, et al. The use of the SLC16A1 gene as a potential marker to predict race performance in Arabian horses. BMC Genet 2019;20:73.

109. (WADA) WA-DA. Gene and cell doping 2019. Available at: https://www.wada-ama.org/en/content/what-is-prohibited/prohibited-at-all-times/gene-and-cell-doping. Accessed September 20, 2019.

110. Tozaki T, Ohnuma A, Takasu M, et al. Droplet digital PCR detection of the erythropoietin transgene from horse plasma and urine for gene-doping control. Genes (Basel) 2019;10 [pii:E243].

111. Frischknecht M, Jagannathan V, Plattet P, et al. A non-synonymous HMGA2 variant decreases height in shetland ponies and other small horses. PLoS One 2015;10:e0140749.

112. Norton EM, Avila F, Schultz NE, et al. Evaluation of an HMGA2 variant for pleiotropic effects on height and metabolic traits in ponies. J Vet Intern Med 2019;33:942–52.

113. van de Goor LH, Panneman H, van Haeringen WA. A proposal for standardization in forensic equine DNA typing: allele nomenclature for 17 equine-specific STR loci. Anim Genet 2010;41:122–7.

Unraveling the Genetics Behind Equid Cardiac Disease

Samantha L. Fousse[a,b], Joshua A. Stern, DVM, PhD[a,b],*

KEYWORDS

- Ventricular septal defects • Congenital heart disease • Sudden death
- Atrial fibrillation • Aortic rupture • Atrioventricular block • Horse • Donkey

KEY POINTS

- No genetic analyses have been published for aortic rupture in Friesians or atrioventricular block in donkeys despite strong evidence for a genetic cause.
- Arabians have a high predisposition to congenital heart diseases. A significant genome-wide association locus was found on chromosome 25 for ventricular septal defects in Arabians.
- Although a genome-wide association study for sudden death in racehorses was negative, a genetic cause remains a top theory for partially explaining this condition.
- Standardbred horses have a heritability of 29.6% for atrial fibrillation with a complex mode of inheritance, including polygenicity and environmental factors.

INTRODUCTION

The genetics for many cardiac diseases in equids are poorly understood. There are several diseases suspected to have a genetic cause based on increased incidence in a single breed. For example, Friesians are overrepresented for aortic rupture.[1–5] Although a common sire has been implicated for some cases[6] and the Friesian breed has the lowest level of genetic variation among horses due to a severe bottleneck,[7] to date, no genetic studies have been performed to identify the likely genetic cause of aortic rupture in the breed. Similarly, there are several reports for atrioventricular block in donkeys and miniature donkeys.[8,9] It is suspected to be genetic, because of the young age of onset and familial history of similar clinical signs, but not yet proven.[10,11]

[a] Department of Medicine and Epidemiology, School of Veterinary Medicine, University of California Davis, Davis, CA, USA; [b] Stern Comparative Cardiac Genetics Laboratory, UC Davis, 2108 Tupper Hall, One Shields Avenue, Davis, CA 95616, USA
* Corresponding author. Stern Comparative Cardiac Genetics Laboratory, UC Davis, 2108 Tupper Hall, One Shields Avenue, Davis, CA 95616.
E-mail address: jstern@ucdavis.edu

Vet Clin Equine 36 (2020) 235–241
https://doi.org/10.1016/j.cveq.2020.03.004
0749-0739/20/© 2020 Elsevier Inc. All rights reserved.

To date, genetic investigation of equine cardiac disease remains limited to a small number of conditions that are expanded upon in this article.

Ventricular Septal Defects and Other Congenital Heart Defects in Arabians

Ventricular septal defects (VSDs) are the most common congenital heart defects (CHDs) reported in horses.[12–14] VSDs are characterized by an abnormal communication between the left and right ventricles that varies in size, location, and clinical relevance.[15] Even small, high-velocity defects, known as restrictive VSDs, can lead to impaired cardiac function if the cusps of the aortic valve are drawn into the defect, resulting in aortic insufficiency. When severe, these lesions result in volume overload of the left side of the heart and, ultimately, lead to congestive heart failure.

VSDs are suspected based on auscultation of a loud holosystolic murmur with a point of maximal intensity over the right thorax caused by the shunt. In addition, a holosystolic crescendo-decrescendo murmur most audible over the pulmonary valve region may be heard owing to an increased volume of blood leaving the right ventricle.[16] A diagnosis of VSD is confirmed via either echocardiography or necropsy.[15] With cardiac ultrasound, the defect is visualized as a communication between the two ventricles (**Fig. 1**). Velocity and direction of flow through the defect are measured to determine if the defect is restrictive (hemodynamically insignificant) or nonrestrictive. The downstream effects of volume overload, such as dilation of the pulmonary artery, dilation of the left atrium, and eccentric hypertrophy of the left ventricle, may be present.

VSDs had a prevalence of 0.35% in a referral population of horses.[14] Warmbloods, standardbreds, and Arabian horses had a higher predisposition to VSDs, whereas thoroughbreds had a lower predisposition.[14,15] Case reports suggest an association between Arabian horses and CHDs, including VSDs; therefore, a genetic basis in

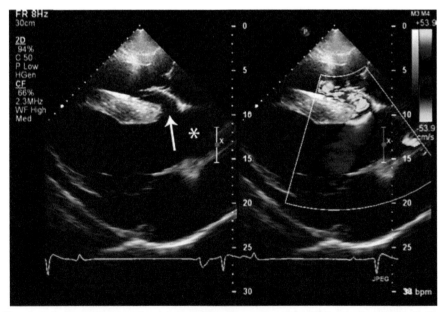

Fig. 1. A 2-dimensional and color Doppler echocardiogram still image is provided of a 2-year-old Arabian gelding diagnosed with a VSD. The image is obtained from the right thorax. The VSD (*arrow*) is visualized with turbulent flow passing into the right ventricle, just below the aortic valve (*asterisk*).

the breed is considered likely.[12,17] A familial form of VSDs has been reported in other veterinary species, including pigs and dogs.[18,19] Familial forms of VSDs occur in humans, with a reported heritability of 0.57.[20] The heritability of VSDs in horses has not been reported. A pilot genome-wide association study in 8 VSD-affected Arabians and 30 unaffected Arabians identified a significant region of association with VSD on chromosome 25; however, a gene has yet to be identified.[21] The results suggest that perimembranous VSDs are genetically distinct from complex VSDs that occur as part of tetralogy of Fallot.[21] In humans, embryologic cardiac genes, such as GATA4, have been associated with VSDs, but further research is required to evaluate if the same genes are involved in horses.[22]

In addition to VSDs, Arabians are predisposed to many other complex CHDs; however, the genetics of other CHDs have not yet been studied. Some of these other defects include isolated or combinations of the following: tricuspid valve dysplasia, mitral valve dysplasia, truncus arteriosus, tetralogy of Fallot, pentalogy of Fallot, patent ductus arteriosus, pulmonic stenosis, tricuspid stenosis, pulmonary atresia, and overriding aorta.[12,23–25] More research is necessary to determine if these defects represent a spectrum of the same genetic mutation or if separate mutations are responsible for each CHD.

Sudden Death in Racehorses

Sudden death is a devastating event that affects the horse-racing industry annually, especially in thoroughbreds.[26–28] Despite a negative result in an early genetic investigation,[28] a genetic cause remains a top theory for explaining this condition. Sudden death represents a rapid and unexpected decline in the condition of an apparently healthy horse.[29] It is the second leading cause of death at racetracks, with the prevalence ranging from 12% to 32% for all postmortem examinations.[28,30,31] Sudden death in horses is suspected to be cardiac related and is often associated with physical activity.[32] One possible cause is a fatal cardiac arrhythmia, because arrhythmias are sometimes associated with exercise in horses.[33–37] Although many horses that die suddenly have negative necropsy findings, common findings include myocardial fibrosis, pulmonary hemorrhage, cardiac lesions, cardiopulmonary failure, and idiopathic blood vessel rupture.[28,32,38,39] Fibrosis could be a contributing factor for promoting an arrhythmogenic substrate and subsequent sudden death in racing horses, but more research is required to confirm this hypothesis.

The cause of many sudden death cases remains unexplained after systematically excluding other causes, such as toxins, infection, and drug administration.[32] This knowledge, combined with the increased incidence in thoroughbred horses, suggests that genetics may play a role. A genome-wide association study performed with 35 horses that died suddenly from presumed cardiac causes and 34 horses that died of other causes did not yield a significant genetic association.[28] If the disease involves multiple genetic and environmental factors, it is likely that this study was dramatically underpowered. Continued case sampling and repeated genome-wide association studies to investigate this condition are warranted. A candidate gene approach may be warranted in racehorse sudden death to investigate some of the human sudden death genetic associations, including genetic variants within ion channels and occult cardiomyopathic genes within the horse.[40]

Atrial Fibrillation in Racehorses

Atrial fibrillation (AF) is the most common arrhythmia in horses.[14] Horses with AF typically present to the clinic with exercise intolerance or poor performance.[41,42] These clinical signs are due to disorganized electrical activity of the atria leading to an "irregularly irregular" heart rhythm. Diagnosis is confirmed with an electrocardiogram indicating the absence of identifiable P waves with irregular R-R intervals.[41] The prevalence of AF is 0.30% to 2.3% in the horse population, with reduced prevalence in studies when the horse is examined at rest.[14,43–45] Certain breeds of horses are more commonly affected than others, including warmbloods and trotters.[14] Specifically, standardbreds have an increased risk of AF, whereas quarterhorses have a reduced risk of AF.[46] There is strong evidence that a particular line of standardbred sires accounts for a high prevalence of AF cases in the breed.[47]

AF is a complex disease with both environmental and genetic causes. This arrhythmia correlates with body weight, with horses weighing more than 550 kg having an increased risk for AF.[14] The genetic component for AF in standardbreds is supported by the high heritably of AF in the breed. In a Canadian standardbred racehorse population, the heritability was 29.6% ± 3.9%.[46] When analyzing the effects of sex and gait in the same population, males had a higher heritability than females, both overall and within the pacer population.[48] Although this work supports a partial genetic role for AF in standardbred horses, it is approximately half of the heritability that is reported for AF in humans[49] and Irish wolfhound dogs.[50] This lower heritability found in horses may be due to differences in study design or may indicate that environmental effects play a larger role in equine AF. The mode of inheritance for AF in standardbred horses is proposed to be complex with multiple genetic variants contributing to the disease.[46,47] Future studies may aim to identify genetic loci associated with equine AF and discover novel pathways for therapeutic intervention.

SUMMARY

There have been some strides made in understanding the genetics behind VSDs in Arabians, sudden death in racehorses, and AF in racehorses. Despite these efforts, no genetic mutation has been identified to date for any equid cardiac disease. With the advancement of genetic tools, including cost-effective whole-genome sequencing, the genetic mechanisms for equid cardiac disorders that appear to have a heritable basis will soon be determined.

DISCLOSURE

Dr JA STERN has nothing to disclose. Dr SL Fousse is funded by the University of California, Davis, National Heart, Lung, and Blood Institute T32HL086350.

REFERENCES

1. Ploeg M, Grone A, van de Lest CHA, et al. Differences in extracellular matrix proteins between Friesian horses with aortic rupture, unaffected Friesians and warmblood horses. Equine Vet J 2017;49(5):609–13.
2. Ploeg M, Saey V, van Loon G, et al. Thoracic aortic rupture in horses. Equine Vet J 2017;49(3):269–74.
3. Ploeg M, Saey V, de Bruijn CM, et al. Aortic rupture and aorto-pulmonary fistulation in the Friesian horse: characterisation of the clinical and gross post mortem findings in 24 cases. Equine Vet J 2013;45(1):101–6.
4. Ploeg M, Saey V, Delesalle C, et al. Thoracic aortic rupture and aortopulmonary fistulation in the Friesian horse: histomorphologic characterization. Vet Pathol 2015;52(1):152–9.
5. Saey V, Vandecasteele T, van Loon G, et al. Friesian horses as a possible model for human acquired aortopulmonary fistulation. BMC Res Notes 2016;9(1):405.

6. van der Linde-Sipman JS, Kroneman J, Meulenaar H, et al. Necrosis and rupture of the aorta and pulmonary trunk in four horses. Vet Pathol 1985;22(1):51–3.

7. Luís C, Juras R, Oom MM, et al. Genetic diversity and relationships of Portuguese and other horse breeds based on protein and microsatellite loci variation. Anim Genet 2007;38(1):20–7.

8. Roberts SL, Dukes-McEwan J. Assessment of cardiovascular disease in the donkey: clinical, echocardiographic and pathological observations. Vet Rec 2016;179(15):1–9.

9. Guccione J, Piantedosi D, Di Loria A, et al. Long-term electrocardiography recording with Holter monitoring in 15 donkeys. J Equine Vet Sci 2014;34(2): 302–6.

10. Pibarot P, Vrins A, Salmon Y, et al. Implantation of a programmable atrioventricular pacemaker in a donkey with complete atrioventricular block and syncope. Equine Vet J 1993;25(3):248–51.

11. Decloedt A. Prevalence of cardiovascular disease in donkeys, vol. 179. England: The Veterinary record; 2016. p. 382–3.

12. Hall TL, Magdesian KG, Kittleson MD. Congenital cardiac defects in neonatal foals: 18 cases (1992-2007). J Vet Intern Med 2010;24(1):206–12.

13. Buergelt CD. Equine cardiovascular pathology: an overview. Anim Health Res Rev 2003;4(2):109–29.

14. Leroux AA, Detilleux J, Sandersen CF, et al. Prevalence and risk factors for cardiac diseases in a hospital-based population of 3,434 horses (1994-2011). J Vet Intern Med 2013;27(6):1563–70.

15. Reef VB. Evaluation of ventricular septal defects in horses using two-dimensional and Doppler echocardiography. Equine Vet J Suppl 1995;19(19):86–95.

16. Hughes KJ. Diagnostic challenge: lethargy and weakness in an Arabian foal with cardiac murmurs. Aust Vet J 2006;84(6):209–12.

17. Crochik SS, Barton MH, Eggleston RB, et al. Cervical vertebral anomaly and ventricular septal defect in an Arabian foal. Equine Vet Educ 2009;21(4):207–11.

18. Ho SY, Thompson RP, Gibbs SR, et al. Ventricular septal defects in a family of Yucatan miniature pigs. Int J Cardiol 1991;33(3):419–25.

19. Patterson DF, Pyle RL, Van Mierop L, et al. Hereditary defects of the conotruncal septum in keeshond dogs: pathologic and genetic studies. Am J Cardiol 1974; 34(2):187–205.

20. Czeizel A, Mészáros M. Two family studies of children with ventricular septal defect. Eur J Pediatr 1981;136(1):81–5.

21. Morgan E, Ontiveros E, Estell K, et al. Identification of genetic markers for ventricular septal defects in Arabian horses. In: Merial-NIH National Veterinary Scholars Symposium. Davis, CA: University of California Davis; 2015.

22. Bellmann K, Perrot A, Rickert-Sperling S. Human genetics of ventricular septal defect. In: Rickert-Sperling S, Kelly RG, Driscoll DJ, editors. Congenital heart diseases: the broken heart: clinical features, human genetics and molecular pathways. Vienna (Austria): Springer Vienna; 2016. p. 307–28.

23. Bayly WM, Reed SM, Leathers CW, et al. Multiple congenital heart anomalies in five Arabian foals. J Am Vet Med Assoc 1982;181(7):684–9.

24. Vitums A, Bayly WM. Pulmonary atresia with dextroposition of the aorta and ventricular septal defect in three Arabian foals. Vet Pathol 1982;19(2):160–8.

25. Krüger MU, Wünschmann A, Ward C, et al. Pulmonary atresia with intact ventricular septum and hypoplastic right ventricle in an Arabian foal. J Vet Cardiol 2016; 18(3):284–9.

26. California Horse Racing Board Postmortem Examination Program 2017-2018 Annual Report. 2019. Available at: http://www.chrb.ca.gov/CHRBDocuments/annual_reports/2018_annual_report.pdf. Accessed November 7, 2019.

27. de Solis CN, Althaus F, Basieux N, et al. Sudden death in sport and riding horses during and immediately after exercise: a case series. Equine Vet J 2018;50(5):644–8.

28. Molesan A, Wang M, Sun Q, et al. Cardiac pathology and genomics of sudden death in racehorses from New York and Maryland racetracks. Vet Pathol 2019;56(4):576–85.

29. Lucke VM. Sudden death. Equine Vet J 1987;19(2):85–91.

30. Physick-Sheard PW, Avison A, Chappell E, et al. Ontario Racehorse Death Registry, 2003–2015: descriptive analysis and rates of mortality. Equine Vet J 2019;51(1):64–76.

31. Boden LA, Charles JA, Slocombe RF, et al. Sudden death in racing thoroughbreds in Victoria, Australia. Equine Vet J 2010;37(3):269–71.

32. Diab SS, Poppenga R, Uzal FA. Sudden death in racehorses: postmortem examination protocol. J Vet Diagn Invest 2017;29(4):442–9.

33. Navas de Solis C. Exercising arrhythmias and sudden cardiac death in horses: review of the literature and comparative aspects. Equine Vet J 2016;48(4):406–13.

34. Gunther-Harrington CT, Arthur R, Estell K, et al. Prospective pre- and post-race evaluation of biochemical, electrophysiologic, and echocardiographic indices in 30 racing thoroughbred horses that received furosemide. BMC Vet Res 2018;14(1):1–10.

35. Ryan N, Marr CM, McGladdery AJ. Survey of cardiac arrhythmias during submaximal and maximal exercise in thoroughbred racehorses. Equine Vet J 2010;37(3):265–8.

36. Buhl R, Petersen EE, Lindholm M, et al. Cardiac arrhythmias in standardbreds during and after racing–possible association between heart size, valvular regurgitations, and arrhythmias. J Equine Vet Sci 2013;33(8):590–6.

37. Physick-Sheard PW, McGurrin MKJ. Ventricular arrhythmias during race recovery in standardbred racehorses and associations with autonomic activity. J Vet Intern Med 2010;24(5):1158–66.

38. Lyle CH, Uzal FA, Mcgorum BC, et al. Sudden death in racing thoroughbred horses: an international multicentre study of post mortem findings. Equine Vet J 2011;43(3):324–31.

39. Nath L, Agbaedeng T, Franklin S, et al. Myocardial fibrosis is present in thoroughbred racehorses with sudden cardiac death. Heart Lung Circ 2019;28:S219.

40. Bezzina CR, Lahrouchi N, Priori SG. Genetics of sudden cardiac death. Circ Res 2015;116(12):1919–36.

41. Bentz BG, Erkert RS, Blaik MA. Evaluation of atrial fibrillation in horses. Compendium Equine: Continuing Education for Veterinarians 2002;24(9):734–40.

42. McGurrin MKJ, Physick-Sheard PW, Kenny DG. Transvenous electrical cardioversion of equine atrial fibrillation: patient factors and clinical results in 72 treatment episodes. J Vet Intern Med 2008;22:609–15.

43. Ohmura H, Hiraga A, Takahashi T, et al. Risk factors for atrial fibrillation during racing in slow-finishing horses. J Am Vet Med Assoc 2003;223(1):84–8.

44. Kriz NG, Hodgson DR, Rose RJ. Prevalence and clinical importance of heart murmurs in racehorses. J Am Vet Med Assoc 2000;216(9):1441–5.

45. Patteson MW, Cripps PJ. A survey of cardiac auscultatory findings in horses. Equine Vet J 1993;25(5):409–15.

46. Physick-Sheard P, Kraus M, Basrur P, et al. Breed predisposition and heritability of atrial fibrillation in the standardbred horse: a retrospective case-control study. J Vet Cardiol 2014;16(3):173–84.
47. Kraus M, Physick-Sheard P, Brito LF, et al. Marginal ancestral contributions to atrial fibrillation in the standardbred racehorse: comparison of cases and controls. PLoS One 2018;13(5):1–17.
48. Kraus M, Physick-Sheard PW, Brito LF, et al. Estimates of heritability of atrial fibrillation in the standardbred racehorse. Equine Vet J 2017;49(6):718–22.
49. Christophersen IE, Ravn LS, Budtz-Joergensen E, et al. Familial aggregation of atrial fibrillation: a study in Danish twins. Circ Arrhythm Electrophysiol 2009; 2(4):378–83.
50. Fousse SL, Tyrrell WD, Dentino ME, et al. Pedigree analysis of atrial fibrillation in Irish wolfhounds supports a high heritability with a dominant mode of inheritance. Canine Genetics and Epidemiology 2019;6(1):11.

Genetics of Equine Respiratory Disease

Vinzenz Gerber, PhD

KEYWORDS

- Genetics • Respiratory disorders • Equine asthma • Guttural pouch tympany
- Recurrent laryngeal neuropathy • Exercise-induced pulmonary hemorrhage • Horses

KEY POINTS

- Respiratory disorders, including guttural pouch tympany, recurrent laryngeal neuropathy, equine asthma, and exercise-induced pulmonary hemorrhage, and some types of airway malformations and infections are influenced by genetic effects.
- The genetic bases of these disorders are likely polygenic, and the clinical expression results from complex interactions between the environment and the genetic make-up of each individual horse.
- Based on the well-documented genetic basis of recurrent laryngeal neuropathy, some breeding associations have successfully adopted selection criteria to remove affected sires from the breeding pool to reduce the risk of producing further affected offspring.
- It is unlikely that single-gene tests will be diagnostically useful for respiratory disorders. Instead, genetic profiling panels that combine genetic factors with an assessment of environmental risk factors may have greater value.

INTRODUCTION

Respiratory tract disorders, such as recurrent laryngeal neuropathy (RLN) and severe equine asthma (sEA), can compromise equine welfare and cause significant economic losses in racehorses and sporthorses.[1] They have long received scientific attention and were among the first equine diseases for which a genetic basis was suspected.[2,3] Further efforts have been made to unravel the genetic basis of these and other respiratory disorders. Estimated heritabilities (often breed-specific) and/or disease-associated chromosomal regions (some of them specific to certain families or dependent on the sex) are now documented for several of these genetically complex and polygenic diseases.[4–7] Furthermore, in some disorders, like sEA, there is an important interaction between the genetic predisposition and environmental risk factors.

Department of Clinical Veterinary Medicine, Vetsuisse Faculty, Swiss Institute of Equine Medicine (ISME), University of Bern, and Agroscope, Laenggassstrasse 124, Berne 3012, Switzerland
E-mail address: vinzenz.gerber@vetsuisse.unibe.ch

Vet Clin Equine 36 (2020) 243–253
https://doi.org/10.1016/j.cveq.2020.03.005
0749-0739/20/© 2020 Elsevier Inc. All rights reserved.

This article aimed to provide an overview of what is presently known on the genetics of respiratory diseases in the horse. Currently, there is evidence that horses may have a genetic predisposition for noninfectious conditions of the upper and lower respiratory tract, including guttural pouch tympany (GPT), RLN, sEA, and exercise-induced pulmonary hemorrhage (EIPH). Genetic factors also may influence specific anatomic airway deformations, such as wry mouth or tracheal collapse, as well as some infectious diseases of the respiratory tract.

TYMPANY OF THE GUTTURAL POUCHES

GPT, an abnormal distension of one or both guttural pouches, affects foals in their first months of life and manifests as a nonpainful, tympanic swelling of the Viborg region that is sometimes accompanied by respiratory obstruction, cough, and dysphagia. The exact nature of the dysfunction at the pharyngeal orifice that leads to air entrapment in the guttural pouch is still unclear.

Breeds that appear predisposed to GPT include thoroughbreds, warmbloods, Arabians, paints, and quarter horses. In four high-risk families, including 276 Arabian individuals, modes of inheritance were polygenic and mixed mono-polygenic and estimated heritabilities were 0.49 ± 0.28 in Arabian foals and 0.81 ± 0.16 in German warmblood foals.[5,8-10]

A genome-wide association study (GWAS) for GPT using microsatellite markers and haplotype analyses in five Arabian and five German warmblood families revealed quantitative trait loci (QTLs) on equine chromosome (ECA) 2 in fillies and on ECA 15 in colts.[5] These sex-specific QTLs agree with the observed higher risk for fillies to develop GPT. An ensuing Illumina (San Diego, CA) equine single-nucleotide polymorphism (SNP) 50 BeadChip-based study narrowed down the QTL on ECA 15 to 64 to 65 Mb in Arabians, and further QTLs were identified on ECA 3 at 16 to 26 Mb and 34 to 55 Mb in warmbloods.[11] The refinement of the breed-specific associated chromosomal regions allowed the identification of potential candidate genes that may influence the formation of cartilage and thereby affect the function at the guttural pouch pharyngeal orifice.

RECURRENT LARYNGEAL NEUROPATHY

Occurring in horses worldwide, RLN is the idiopathic form of laryngeal hemiplegia. It is a bilateral degenerative neuropathy of the recurrent laryngeal nerve, with the left side being more severely affected, and results in lesions of the laryngeal muscles. Consequently, horses suffer from inspiratory stridor and exercise intolerance at higher speeds and workloads. Therefore, RLN is of particular relevance for sporthorses, workhorses, and racehorses, and often leads to surgical intervention, early retirement, or even euthanasia.[12-14]

As early as the sixteenth century [cited in Ref.[3]], investigators have proposed a genetic predisposition for RLN, and evidence for genetic effects has been accumulating in recent years. However, as in other diseases, correct phenotyping has posed challenges in the study of RLN genetics.[15] The gold standard for diagnosing RLN, histologic demonstration of neurogenic atrophy of the abductor and adductor muscles of the larynx, can be effectively performed only *postmortem*. Yet, upper airway endoscopy for the visual assessment of laryngeal function, which is the most common method of phenotyping, may be affected by the observer, the grading system, the sedatives used for the endoscopy, and the time point of examination.[14] Most studies of RLN are cross-sectional, making age another important confounding factor. Sometimes, RLN manifests itself early in foals, but typically, it is first detected in adults and may progress over time.[12,16] Breed, size, and conformation (which are themselves "genetic" factors) also can affect RLN manifestation and diagnosis. Although draft horses are often affected by RLN, an investigation of competing American draft horses reported that prevalence varied considerably between breeds: 42% in Belgians, 31% in Percherons, and 17% in Clydesdales. Interestingly, height at the withers influenced the risk for RLN in Percherons and Belgians, but not in Clydesdales.[17]

Familial aggregation in warmbloods is documented in several studies.[3,12,18] One report describes that 47% of the offspring of an RLN-affected warmblood stallion were affected by RLN, compared with 10% in the control population. In addition to the RLN-status of the parents, age, and height at the withers influenced the incidence and degree of RLN.[18] These studies suggest that RLN has an important genetic basis that is likely due to polygenic inheritance, because no simple recessive or dominant patterns were observed. Subsequent studies have estimated heritabilities between 0.2 (thoroughbred racehorses), 0.4 (Clydesdales), and 0.6 (in German warmblood horses).[19–21]

Early approaches in thoroughbreds, quarter horses, and Swiss warmbloods found no associations of equine lymphocyte antigens (as markers for major histocompatibility complex genotypes) with the RLN phenotypes investigated.[18,22] In contrast, genome-wide linkage and/or association studies have yielded several QTLs related to RLN phenotypes (**Table 1**). A haplotype-based GWAS using the Illumina Equine SNP50 BeadChip in a large cohort (234 RLN-affected cases and 228 unaffected breed-matched controls) identified two genome-wide suggestive loci in warmbloods located on ECA 21 and 31, respectively, displaying a protective effect against RLN. However, only 8% of the observed variation was explained by these loci.[6] Examination of the same genotypes for associations of copy number variants with RLN revealed a suggestive (nonsignificant) effect of a duplication on ECA 10, residing in an 8-Mb inversion shared among three breeds of affected horses.[23]

A subsequent GWAS using the Illumina Equine SNP70 BeadChip in thoroughbred racehorses found a major QTL explaining 6% of the phenotypic variation in RLN, which turned out to be coincident with a known locus for body height on ECA 3, LCORL/NCAPG.[24] The same group showed, in 458 American Belgian draft horses (where the LCORL/NCAPG risk allele is fixed), that RLN risk is related to sexually dimorphic differences in height. The MYPN (ECA 1), a novel locus contributing to height in a sex-specific manner, was identified, but this locus showed little contribution to RLN risk. A further RLN-associated locus on ECA 15 was instead identified in male individuals. Thus, growth traits related to the etiology of RLN appear to display sex-specific gene expression.[7]

In the GWAS of RLN in thoroughbred horses, secondary associations on chromosomes X and ECA 18 revealed further candidate genes, integral membrane protein 2A (ITM2A) and myostatin (MSTN), respectively, which may be involved in muscle tissue physiology and development. Interestingly, the GWAS of RLN in warmblood horses had also identified a QTL in a myosin gene (MYO9B).[6] Together, these current data suggest a complex genetic background of RLN with breed, conformation, and/or sex-dependent effects playing a role. Specifically, the recent progress in genetic research has substantiated previous observations that taller horses are at a greater risk, which may simply reflect the increased length (and thus vulnerability to degenerative changes) of the recurrent laryngeal nerve.[15]

MISCELLANEOUS UPPER AIRWAY DISORDERS

Of the various other functional and structural upper airway disorders described in equids, two have been reported to show breed-specific increased prevalence. Results

Table 1
Summary of reported QTLs in RLN

Method	Population	Results	References
Genome-wide linkage and association analyses using the Illumina Equine SNP50 array (specifically haplotype-based genome-wide association approach)	234 cases (196 warmbloods, 20 trotters, 14 thoroughbreds, and 4 draft horses), 228 breed-matched controls, and 69 parents	Two genome-wide significant loci on ECA 21 and 31, respectively	Dupuis et al,[6] 2011
Genome-wide association study using the Illumina Equine SNP50 array for the detection of copy number variants		Duplication on ECA10	Dupuis et al,[23] 2013
Genome-wide association study using the Illumina Equine SNP70 array	282 thoroughbred cases and 268 unaffected breed-matched controls	A main QTL was found near LCORL/NCAPG on ECA 3, a locus that affects body size; secondary QTLs located on X (candidate gene ITM2A) and ECA18 (candidate gene MSTN)	Boyko et al,[24] 2014
Genome-wide association study using the Illumina Equine SNP70 array	167 RLN-affected and 291 control American Belgian draft horses	Significant locus on ECA 15 contributing to RLN risk in males; growth traits related to the etiology of RLN appear to display sex-specific gene expression	Brooks et al,[7] 2018

Abbreviations: ECA, equine chromosome; QTL, quantitative trait loci; RLN, recurrent laryngeal neuropathy; SNP, single-nucleotide polymorphism.

from a case series of American miniature horses suggests that this breed has an increased risk of tracheal collapse due to primary tracheomalacia.[25] American miniature horses also may suffer more frequently than other breeds from skull malformations including wry nose.[26] Wry nose (campylorrhinus lateralis) is reported to be more prevalent in the Arabian breed,[27] leading to speculations about a genetic basis.

EQUINE ASTHMA

The term EA encompasses mild to moderate manifestations of lower respiratory tract inflammation and hyperreactivity and was previously known as inflammatory airway disease,[28] and the severe phenotype of equine asthma (sEA) was previously referred to as heaves or recurrent airway obstruction.[29-31] Hallmarks of sEA, which mainly affects horses older than 7 years, include marked neutrophilic lower airway inflammation, cholinergic bronchospasm, mucus accumulation with frequent coughing, increased respiratory effort at rest, and exercise intolerance. Another key characteristic of sEA is the reversibility of clinical signs. Changing of the environment, particularly avoidance of hay-dust exposure, as well as corticosteroid and bronchodilator administration, can improve and reverse clinical signs and airway obstruction.

Genetic research in this field has focused on sEA, but the interaction of environment and genetics likely influences the entire spectrum of asthma in the horse. For mild to moderate forms of EA, however, no specific genetic risk factors are reported. Nevertheless, genetic susceptibility to certain bacterial lower airway infections,[32] as discussed later in this article, could potentially be relevant in milder forms of EA, particularly in younger horses. Moreover, persistent respiratory signs such as occasional coughing and nasal discharge associated with hay feeding can be early phenotypic signs for an increased (genetic) risk to later development of sEA,[33] suggesting that the genetics of milder forms of EA may be worth investigating in longitudinal studies.

In contrast, a heritable basis for sEA has been reported in several breeds and subsequently has been the focus of genetic research involving family and epidemiologic studies, whole-genome scans, and investigation of candidate genes. Reports of marked familial aggregation of sEA date back 70 years.[2] Parent, age, and stable environment have significant additive effects that increase the risk for developing sEA, as defined by a history of persistent frequent coughing and/or increased breathing effort.[34,35] This was shown in warmbloods and in Lipizzans, specifically the relative risk (RR, Mantel-Haenszel statistics) of developing sEA was significantly increased in offspring with one parent (RR 3.2) and, even more (RR 4.6), with two affected parents. Interestingly, these findings mirror those of a study on the inheritance of atopy and allergic asthma in children.[36,37] In a study focusing on two families of Swiss warmblood horses with a high prevalence of sEA, offspring of affected sires had a fourfold higher risk of developing sEA compared with offspring of unaffected stallions (maternal half-siblings) and randomly selected warmblood control horses of similar age (**Fig. 1**).[36]

Whole-genome scans in these two high-prevalence families indicated two possible chromosome regions with a genome-wide significant linkage association to sEA.[38] Importantly, the associations differed between the two half-sibling cohorts with the main QTL on ECA 13 in one family and on ECA 15 in another family. Molecular pathway analyses (Ingenuity Pathway Analysis) of genomic and proteomic data showed interactions between interleukin (IL)4R (a candidate gene on ECA 13) and SOCS5 (a candidate gene on ECA 15) upstream of an important inflammatory molecular cascade involving nuclear factor (NF)-κB.[39] Even though no causal genetic variant has been identified in IL-R so far, further association and gene expression studies have

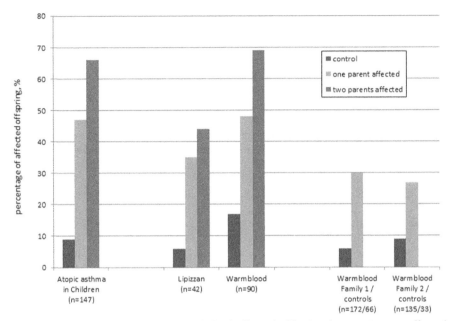

Fig. 1. Comparison of the percentages (%) of affected offspring from 1, 2, or unaffected parents (control) in human children with atopic asthma, and warmbloods and Lipizzans with severe equine asthma based on published data.[35,36,64] (*From* Gerber V, Tessier C, Marti E. Genetics of upper and lower airway diseases in the horse. Equine Vet J 2015;47:390-7; with permission. ©2014 EVJ Ltd.)

strengthened the QTL on ECA 13 (with IL-R and neighboring genes as candidates) in a subset of sEA-affected horses.[40–42] Also, the important role of IL-R in allergic skin diseases and parasite defense in other species has led to the discovery of unexpected relationships of sEA with insect bite hypersensitivity (IBH) and shedding of strongyle eggs. Horses affected with sEA are at an increased risk of developing IBH and urticaria, but conversely, they may have a more efficient defense against intestinal parasites. Depending on infection pressure on the farm and the genetic background (association present in one high-prevalence sEA family, but not the other, and conflicting results in unrelated horses), sEA-affected horses shed fewer strongylid eggs than control animals.[43–45]

An allelic case-control GWAS in more than 600 Swiss warmbloods revealed another QTL on ECA 13. The best-associated marker was located in the protein-coding gene TXNDC11, which may be involved in regulating hydrogen peroxide production in the respiratory tract epithelium, as well as expressing MUC5AC mucin.[4] No genomic copy number variations were found to be associated with sEA,[46] and integrative analyses combining GWAS (including imputed SNP markers), differential expression data, and expression (e)QTLs, did not reveal causative genetic variants that contributed to sEA through gene expression regulation. However, sEA-associated genetic variants appeared to regulate gene expression of DEXI,[47] a gene also implicated in eQTL analyses of human asthma.[48] Furthermore, global gene expression studies of mRNA and microRNA levels in peripheral blood mononuclear cells from these sEA high-prevalence warmblood families and an unrelated cohort that was stimulated in vitro with hay-dust extract have shown sEA-associated impaired cell cycle regulation and CD4+ T-cell differentiation into Th2/Th17 cells, respectively.[49,50]

Many of the findings are based on a limited sample of warmbloods, but even these results suggest that the genetic basis of sEA is robust, but remarkably complex with genetic heterogeneity. This genetic heterogeneity is reflected by differences in the predicted mode of inheritance, sEA-associated chromosomal regions, as well as the dependence of susceptibility and resistance to other allergies and parasites on the (family-) specific genetic background.[38,43,44,51,52] Differences in the genetic background of study cohorts may also explain some conflicting results regarding the immunology of sEA. The polygenic complexity of sEA, potentially with a larger number of genes that each may only contribute small proportions to the total genetic effects, may also make it difficult to discover causative variants.

EXERCISE-INDUCED PULMONARY HEMORRHAGE

Hemorrhage in the lungs caused by pulmonary capillary stress failure during intense exercise mainly affects racehorses. Up to half of racing thoroughbreds develop EIPH, and severe manifestations with frank epistaxis may affect performance, horse health, and welfare.[53]

A study of 1252 cases of EIPH in South African thoroughbred racehorses found an incidence of 2.1% with a calculated heritability of liability of 55.4% in first-degree relatives, 41.3% in second-degree relatives, and 30.4% in third-degree relatives.[54] Another study in Australia, including more than 2000 EIPH cases and more than 115,000 controls based on official data from the Racing Information Services Australia, also showed significant calculated heritabilities (h^2) of 0.27 for lifetime epistaxis risk and 0.50 for individual race epistaxis risk.[55] A candidate gene approach investigating SNPs in CD39/NTPDase-1 and CD39L1/NTPDase-2 found no conclusive associations with EIPH in a very limited number of horses with abnormal hemorrhage or with pathologic changes consistent with EIPH.[56] Clearly, further work is needed to explain these findings and to eventually better understand the genetic basis of EIPH and epistaxis after strenuous exercise.

INFECTIOUS DISEASES OF THE RESPIRATORY TRACT

The immune response of horses to viral pathogens may be influenced by genetic effects, because the humoral response to EHV-1/4 (low vs high anti-EHV-1/4 antibody response) was associated with genetic markers, including an SNP within IL-4R.[57]

Regarding bacterial pathogens, transferrin gene variants appear to be associated with susceptibility to and severity of bacterial disease. Specific alleles of transferrin, an iron-binding protein in the blood with bacteriostatic properties, are associated with protection against *Streptococcus zooepidemicus*[32] or *Rhodococcus equi* infection.[58] Susceptibility to *R equi* pneumonia also may be modulated by further genes including the solute carrier family 11 member 1 (SLC11A1) gene,[59] Casp1 gene (functionally related to IL-1 beta),[60,61] and the IL-7 receptor-encoding gene (IL7R).[61]

Furthermore, as described in the preceding section on sEA genetics, genetic predisposition to this disease and to other hypersensitivities appears to be associated with an increased resistance against intestinal parasites, depending on the genetic background.[43,44]

SUMMARY

Observations (often of breed or familial aggregation of cases) suggesting a heritable basis are reported for a considerable number of respiratory disorders. Studies on the mode of inheritance, heritabilities, candidate genes, and GWAS have been performed to more systematically investigate the genetic basis of GPT, RLN, EA, EIPH, and some infections of the respiratory tract. The current data suggest that most, if not all of these diseases are complex, resulting from the interaction of several genes and environmental factors.

To date, no specific genes and causative mutations have been identified that would allow the development of simple single-gene tests, as has been established for other equine diseases. To avoid "at-risk" matings or for early identification of "at-risk" individuals, genetic profiling panels based on multiple genetic markers combined with an assessment of environmental risk factors (such as hay feeding in sEA) may become available in the future. However, genetic tests are not required for selective breeding with the goal of reducing the prevalence of a disease. When a genetic basis for a disorder is firmly established, affected individuals can be identified phenotypically and removed from the breeding pool to reduce the risk of producing further affected offspring. Such a practice is established for stallions affected with RLN and sometimes even sEA in some European breeding associations.[62] A significant reduction of RLN prevalence was reported in Dutch warmbloods, after the elimination of RLN-affected stallions from breeding programs.[63]

ACKNOWLEDGMENTS

Parts of this article are based on a published review. The author acknowledges coauthors Caroline Tessier and Eliane Marti of that review, and Shannon Axiak Flammer for help with the article. Regarding the work on equine asthma, the author also to acknowledges the contributions of all coinvestigators, graduate students, and horse owners. Major contributions to this work have come from the Institute of Genetics, the Institute of Parasitology of the Vetsuisse Faculty, University of Bern, the Animal Health Trust, the University of Giessen, and Purdue University.

DISCLOSURE

The author has no conflict of interest or relevant financial disclosures.

REFERENCES

1. Smith KC. Lower airway disease, now and in the future. Equine Vet J 2011;43:388–92.

2. Schäper W. Untersuchungen über die Erblichkeit und das Wesen des Lungendampfes beim Pferd. Tierärztliche Rundschau 1939;31:595–9.

3. Schäper W. Über die Erblichkeit des Kehlkopfpfeifens beim Pferd. Dtsch Tierärztl Wochenschr 1939;47:385–8.

4. Schnider D, Rieder S, Leeb T, et al. A genome-wide association study for equine recurrent airway obstruction in European warmblood horses reveals a suggestive new quantitative trait locus on chromosome 13. Anim Genet 2017;48:691–3.

5. Zeitz A, Spotter A, Blazyczek I, et al. Whole-genome scan for guttural pouch tympany in Arabian and German warmblood horses. Anim Genet 2009;40:917–24.

6. Dupuis MC, Zhang Z, Druet T, et al. Results of a haplotype-based GWAS for recurrent laryngeal neuropathy in the horse. Mamm Genome 2011;22:613–20.

7. Brooks SA, Stick J, Braman A, et al. Identification of loci affecting sexually dimorphic patterns for height and recurrent laryngeal neuropathy risk in American Belgian draft horses. Physiol Genomics 2018;50:1051–8.

8. Blazyczek I, Hamann H, Ohnesorge B, et al. Population genetic analysis of the heritability of gutteral pouch tympany in Arabian purebred foals. Dtsch Tierarztl Wochenschr 2003;110:417–9 [in German].

9. Blazyczek I, Hamann H, Ohnesorge B, et al. Gutteral pouch tympany in German warmblood foals: influence of sex, inbreeding and blood proportions of founding breeds as well as estimation of heritability. Berl Munch Tierarztl Wochenschr 2003;116:346–51 [in German].

10. Blazyczek I, Hamann H, Ohnesorge B, et al. Inheritance of guttural pouch tympany in the Arabian horse. J Hered 2004;95:195–9.

11. Metzger J, Ohnesorge B, Distl O. Genome-wide linkage and association analysis identifies major gene loci for guttural pouch tympany in Arabian and German warmblood horses. PLoS One 2012;7:e41640.

12. Ohnesorge B, Deegen E, Miesner K, et al. Laryngeal hemiplegia in warmblood horses–a study of stallions, mares and their offspring. Zentralbl Veterinarmed A 1993;40:134–54 [in German].

13. Rooney J, Delaney F. An hypothesis on the causation of laryngeal hemiplegia in horses. Equine Vet J 1970;2:35–7.

14. Perkins JD, Salz RO, Schumacher J, et al. Variability of resting endoscopic grading for assessment of recurrent laryngeal neuropathy in horses. Equine Vet J 2009;41:342–6.

15. Draper ACE, Piercy RJ. Pathological classification of equine recurrent laryngeal neuropathy. J Vet Intern Med 2018;32:1397–409.

16. Dixon PM, McGorum BC, Railton DI, et al. Clinical and endoscopic evidence of progression in 152 cases of equine recurrent laryngeal neuropathy (RLN). Equine Vet J 2002;34:29–34.

17. Brakenhoff JE, Holcombe SJ, Hauptman JG, et al. The prevalence of laryngeal disease in a large population of competition draft horses. Vet Surg 2006;35:579–83.

18. Poncet PA, Montavon S, Gaillard C, et al. A preliminary report on the possible genetic basis of laryngeal hemiplegia. Equine Vet J 1989;21:137–8.

19. Miesner K. Untersuchung über die abduktorische Funktionsstörung des Kehlkopfes beim Pferd: Genetische und umweltbedingte Einflussfaktoren sowie mögliche züchterische Massnahmen. Bonn, Germany: Agricultural Faculty, Friedrich-Wilhelms University; 1996. Thesis.

20. Barakzsai S. Heritability of recurrent laryngeal neuropathy. Paper presented at: 4th World Equine Airway Symposium (WEAS09). August 5-7, 2009. Berne, Switzerland, 2009.

21. Ibi T, Miyake T, Hobo S, et al. Estimation of heritability of laryngeal hemiplegia in the thoroughbred horse by Gibbs sampling. J Equine Sci 2003;14:81–6.

22. McClure JJ, Koch C, Powell M, et al. Association of arytenoid chondritis with equine lymphocyte antigens but no association with laryngeal hemiplegia, umbilical hernias and cryptorchidism. Anim Genet 1988;19:427–33.

23. Dupuis MC, Zhang Z, Durkin K, et al. Detection of copy number variants in the horse genome and examination of their association with recurrent laryngeal neuropathy. Anim Genet 2013;44(2):206–8.

24. Boyko AR, Brooks SA, Behan-Braman A, et al. Genomic analysis establishes correlation between growth and laryngeal neuropathy in thoroughbreds. BMC Genomics 2014;15:259.

25. Aleman M, Nieto JE, Benak J, et al. Tracheal collapse in American miniature horses: 13 cases (1985-2007). J Am Vet Med Assoc 2008;233:1302–6.

26. Mintz CC. Development of dentition in the small equine breeds and related cases. Paper presented at: IGFP-Kongress March 10-11, 2017, Niederhausern, Germany.

27. Baker GJ. Abnormalities of development and eruption. In: Baker FJ, Easley JR, editors. Equine dentistry. Philadelphia: Saunders; 1999. p. 55.

28. Couetil LL, Hoffman AM, Hodgson J, et al. Inflammatory airway disease of horses. J Vet Intern Med 2007;21:356–61.

29. Lowell FC. Observation on heaves. An asthma like syndrome in the horse. J Allergy 1964;35:322–30.

30. Leclere M, Lavoie-Lamoureux A, Lavoie JP. Heaves, an asthma-like disease of horses. Respirology 2011;16:1027–46.

31. Couetil LL, Cardwell JM, Gerber V, et al. Inflammatory airway disease of horses-revised consensus statement. J Vet Intern Med 2016;30:503–15.

32. Newton JR, Woodt JL, Chanter N. Evidence for transferrin allele as a host-level risk factor in naturally occurring equine respiratory disease: a preliminary study. Equine Vet J 2007;39:164–71.

33. Bosshard S, Gerber V. Evaluation of coughing and nasal discharge as early indicators for an increased risk to develop equine recurrent airway obstruction (RAO). J Vet Intern Med 2014;28:618–23.

34. Gerber H. Sir Frederick Hobday memorial lecture. The genetic basis of some equine diseases. Equine Vet J 1989;21:244–8.

35. Marti E, Gerber H, Essich G, et al. The genetic basis of equine allergic diseases. 1. Chronic hypersensitivity bronchitis. Equine Vet J 1991;23:457–60.

36. Cookson WO, Hopkin JM. Dominant inheritance of atopic immunoglobulin-E responsiveness. Lancet 1988;1:86–8.

37. Cookson WO, Moffatt MF. Genetics of asthma and allergic disease. Hum Mol Genet 2000;9:2359–64.

38. Swinburne JE, Bogle H, Klukowska-Rotzler J, et al. A whole-genome scan for recurrent airway obstruction in Warmblood sport horses indicates two positional candidate regions. Mamm Genome 2009;20:504–15.

39. Racine J, Gerber V, Feutz MM, et al. Comparison of genomic and proteomic data in recurrent airway obstruction affected horses using Ingenuity Pathway Analysis(R). BMC Vet Res 2011;7:48.

40. Lanz S, Gerber V, Marti E, et al. Effect of hay dust extract and cyathostomin antigen stimulation on cytokine expression by PBMC in horses with recurrent airway obstruction. Vet Immunol Immunopathol 2013;155:229–37.

41. Klukowska-Rotzler J, Swinburne JE, Drogemuller C, et al. The interleukin 4 receptor gene and its role in recurrent airway obstruction in Swiss warmblood horses. Anim Genet 2012;43:450–3.

42. Shakhsi-Niaei M, Klukowska-Rotzler J, Drogemuller C, et al. Replication and fine-mapping of a QTL for recurrent airway obstruction in European warmblood horses. Anim Genet 2012;43:627–31.

43. Brundler P, Frey CF, Gottstein B, et al. Lower shedding of strongylid eggs by warmblood horses with recurrent airway obstruction compared to unrelated healthy horses. Vet J 2011;190:e12–5.

44. Neuhaus S, Bruendler P, Frey CF, et al. Increased parasite resistance and recurrent airway obstruction in horses of a high-prevalence family. J Vet Intern Med 2010;24:407–13.

45. Sperl C, Gerber V, Driesslein D, et al. Are respiratory clinical signs in horses associated with Strongyle egg shedding rates on farms with varying egg shedding levels? J Equine Vet Sci 2019;75:104–11.

46. Ghosh S, Das PJ, McQueen CM, et al. Analysis of genomic copy number variation in equine recurrent airway obstruction (heaves). Anim Genet 2016;47:334–44.

47. Mason VC, Schaefer RJ, McCue ME, et al. eQTL discovery and their association with severe equine asthma in European warmblood horses. BMC Genomics 2018;19:581.
48. Li X, Hastie AT, Hawkins GA, et al. eQTL of bronchial epithelial cells and bronchial alveolar lavage deciphers GWAS-identified asthma genes. Allergy 2015;70: 1309–18.
49. Pacholewska A, Jagannathan V, Drogemuller M, et al. Impaired cell cycle regulation in a natural equine model of asthma. PLoS One 2015;10:e0136103.
50. Pacholewska A, Kraft MF, Gerber V, et al. Differential expression of serum microRNAs supports CD4(+) T cell differentiation into Th2/Th17 cells in severe equine asthma. Genes (Basel) 2017;8. https://doi.org/10.3390/genes8120383.
51. Gerber V, Baleri D, Klukowska-Rotzler J, et al. Mixed inheritance of equine recurrent airway obstruction. J Vet Intern Med 2009;23:626–30.
52. Kehrli D, Jandova V, Fey K, et al. Multiple hypersensitivities including recurrent airway obstruction, insect bite hypersensitivity, and urticaria in 2 warmblood horse populations. J Vet Intern Med 2015;29:320–6.
53. Birks EK, Shuler KM, Soma LR, et al. EIPH: postrace endoscopic evaluation of standardbreds and thoroughbreds. Equine Vet J Suppl 2002;375–8.
54. Weideman H, Schoeman SJ, Jordaan GF. The inheritance of liability to epistaxis in the southern African thoroughbred. J S Afr Vet Assoc 2004;75:158–62.
55. Velie BD, Raadsma HW, Wade CM, et al. Heritability of epistaxis in the Australian thoroughbred racehorse population. Vet J 2014;202:274–8.
56. Boudreaux MK, Koehler J, Habecker PL, et al. Evaluation of the genes encoding CD39/NTPDase-1 and CD39L1/NTPDase-2 in horses with and without abnormal hemorrhage and in horses with pathologic evidence of exercise-induced pulmonary hemorrhage. Vet Clin Pathol 2015;44:617–25.
57. Rusek J, Klumplerova M, Molinkova D, et al. Genetics of anti-EHV antibody responses in a horse population. Res Vet Sci 2013;95:137–42.
58. Mousel MR, Harrison L, Donahue JM, et al. *Rhodococcus equi* and genetic susceptibility: assessing transferrin genotypes from paraffin-embedded tissues. J Vet Diagn Invest 2003;15:470–2.
59. Halbert ND, Cohen ND, Slovis NM, et al. Variations in equid SLC11A1 (NRAMP1) genes and associations with *Rhodococcus equi* pneumonia in horses. J Vet Intern Med 2006;20:974–9.
60. Horin P, Osickova J, Necesankova M, et al. Single nucleotide polymorphisms of interleukin-1 beta related genes and their associations with infection in the horse. Dev Biol (Basel) 2008;132:347–51.
61. Horin P, Sabakova K, Futas J, et al. Immunity-related gene single nucleotide polymorphisms associated with *Rhodococcus equi* infection in foals. Int J Immunogenet 2010;37:67–71.
62. Nikolić D. Inherited disorders and their management in some European warmblood sport horse breeds. Uppsala, Sweden: Swedish University of Agricultural Sciences; 2012. Master's Thesis.
63. Sloet van Oldruitenborgh-Oosterbaan M. How do breeding program restrictions influence the incidence of recurrent laryngeal neuropathy. Paper presented at: The 3rd World Equine Airway Symposium July 20-22, 2005, Ithaca, NY.
64. Ramseyer A, Gaillard C, Burger D, et al. Effects of genetic and environmental factors on chronic lower airway disease in horses. J Vet Intern Med 2007;21: 149–56.

Genetics of Equine Neurologic Disease

Lisa Edwards, DVM, Carrie J. Finno, DVM, PhD*

KEYWORDS

- Ataxia • Horse • Inherited • Paresis • Seizure

KEY POINTS

- Neurologic disease in the horse is difficult to diagnose and often carries a poor prognosis for performance.
- To date, there are 5 equine genetic diseases that can be diagnosed with genetic testing: lethal white foal syndrome, lavender foal syndrome, cerebellar abiotrophy, occipitoatlantoaxial malformation, and Friesian hydrocephalus.
- Several additional neurologic diseases likely have an inherited basis, and future genetic tools will enable discovery of putative disease variants.

INTRODUCTION

Neurologic disease in the horse is difficult to diagnose and often carries a poor prognosis for performance. This section focuses on neurologic diseases with known genetic mutations and other neurologic diseases with an underlying genetic cause that are currently being investigated. For each disease, the clinical presentation including typical signalment, age of onset and disease progression, diagnostic tools, treatment options, pathologic findings, and most recent information on the status of the genetic investigation is provided.

NEUROLOGIC DISORDERS WITH KNOWN MUTATIONS

Table 1 provides a summary of equine neurologic disorders with known mutations, including affected breeds and the associated gene.

Ileocolonic Aganglionosis

Ileocolonic aganglionosis, also termed lethal white foal syndrome (LWFS) or overo lethal white syndrome (OLWS), affects American Paint horses, Quarter horses, and has

Department of Veterinary Population Health and Reproduction, School of Veterinary Medicine, University of California Davis, Room 4206 Vet Med 3A One Shields Avenue, Davis, CA 95616, USA
* Corresponding author.
E-mail address: cjfinno@ucdavis.edu

Vet Clin Equine 36 (2020) 255–272
https://doi.org/10.1016/j.cveq.2020.03.006
0749-0739/20/© 2020 Elsevier Inc. All rights reserved.

Table 1
Equine neurologic diseases due to a known genetic mutation

Disease	Breed	Gene	Mode of Inheritance
Cerebellar abiotrophy (CA)	Arabian Carriers identified in Trakehner, Welsh pony, and Bashkir Curly with Arabian ancestry	TOE1/MUTYH	Autosomal recessive
Friesian hydrocephalus	Friesian (1 Belgian)	B3GALNT2	Autosomal recessive
Lavender foal syndrome (LFS) Coat color dilution lethal	Arabian	MYO5A	Autosomal recessive
Lethal white foal syndrome (LWFS)	Paint, Quarter horse, Miniature horse, (rarely) Thoroughbred	EDNRB	Autosomal semi- dominant
Occipitoatlantoaxial malformation (OAAM)	Arabian	HOXD3	Presumed autosomal recessive

been reported in Miniature horses and, rarely, in Thoroughbreds. There is no sex pre-dilection, and clinical signs are usually noted within 24 hours of birth.[1,2] Affected foals are often all white or have nearly an all-white coat and often have blue irides ± hearing deficits (see Sensorineural Deafness in American Paint Horses).[3] Clinical signs include colic, progressive abdominal distension and failure to pass feces despite enema administration. Abdominal ultrasound and radiographs (with or without contrast) can confirm ileus, and a definitive diagnosis is made with genetic testing. There are no treatments available, and the prognosis is invariably grave. Necropsy findings include constrictions of the distal small intestine and complete absence of the intrinsic myen-teric plexus in the distal small intestine, cecum, and colon, with the ileum most severely affected.[1,2,4] The white coat is due to absence of melanocytes from the skin.

Ileocolonic aganglionosis is inherited as an autosomal semidominant trait. The het-erozygous state results in a frame overo phenotype, and the homozygous state is associated with LWFS. The highest incidence of heterozygotes (>94%) are frame overo, highly white calico overo, and frame blend overo. The lowest incidence of het-erozygotes (<21%) are tobiano, sabino, and minimally blend overo and breeding-stock solid.[5] Because inheritance is variably penetrant, heterozygotes may not have the frame overo pattern.[6] The genetic defect responsible for LWFS is a dinucleotide substitution that causes a missense mutation and results in an isoleucine/lysine sub-stitution at codon 118 of the endothelin receptor B gene (EDNRB) located on chromo-some 17.[6,7] An affected foal is homozygous Lys (Lys 118/Lys 118), whereas carriers are heterozygous (Ile 118/Lys 118).[6,7] The mutation causes abnormal development of enteric ganglia and melanocytes within the embryologic neural crest.[1] LWFS is an equine variant of Hirschsprung disease, where children are born with aganglionic megacolon.[4]

A genetic test for LWFS is available. This test is useful in confirming suspect LWFS cases and determining carrier status, especially in horses that cannot be recognized by the overt phenotype (ie, tobiano Paint horses, Thoroughbreds, and Quarter horses). According to the 2017 American Paint Horse Association Rule Book, "...all breeding stallions are required to have a Genetic Health Panel test on file with APHA prior to the registration of their foals that result from breedings occurring after January 1, 2018." The Genetic Health Panel test includes OLWS (LWFS).

Lavender Foal Syndrome

Lavender foal syndrome (LFS), also referred to as lethal LFS or coat color dilution lethal, affects Egyptian lineage Arabian neonates. Foals have a silver, pewter, lavender, or pale chestnut (pink) coat color and demonstrate tetanic episodes with opisthotonus, paddling, and extensor rigidity from birth. Foals cannot become sternal or stand and suckling may be strong, weak, or absent.[8,9] Direct and indirect pupillary light responses are generally present, although ventral strabismus and nystagmus may be observed.[10,11] Reflexes may be present but result in an exaggerated response characterized by increased paddling and rigidity. It is unclear if paddling episodes are due to seizure activity[11] or attempts of the foal to stand[9] because electroencephalograms (EEG) have not been performed. There are no specific clinicopathologic abnormalities, unless other conditions are present. Radiographs of skull and cervical spine are normal. A definitive diagnosis requires genetic testing. Treatment consists mainly of supportive care. Diazepam and phenobarbital may provide temporary relief; however, whether this is due to sedative or anticonvulsant effects of these drugs is unknown.[11] The clinical condition deteriorates despite treatment, necessitating euthanasia. At necropsy, histopathological examination may reveal no central nervous system (CNS) lesions[9,11]; however, an anomalous choroid plexus[10] and vacuolization of CNS neurons[12] have been described. Skin biopsies may reveal no notable pathology[11] or abnormal clumping of melanin.[9] The lack of consistent pathologic lesions in the CNS suggests a potential biochemical lesion.

LFS is inherited as an autosomal recessive trait and was the first equine disease to have the molecular genetic mutation mapped using a single nucleotide polymorphism (SNP)-based genome-wide association study approach with the EquineSNP50 Beadchip (Illumina, San Diego, CA).[13] Six LFS-affected and 30 healthy relatives were genotyped and 14 highly significant SNPs were identified on chromosome 1, spanning a region of 10.5 Mb. Homozygosity mapping further narrowed the region to a 1.6 Mb block that was homozygous in all 6 affected horses and heterozygous in obligate carriers. Ten genes fell into this region, including 1 of the 2 candidate genes for the disease, myosin Va (MYO5A). Sequencing of the 39 exons of MYO5A revealed a single base pair deletion in exon 30, causing the reading frame to shift and creating a premature stop codon in the translation of exon 30.[13,14] Based on the known function of the gene in other species and high conservation across the mutated region, it is hypothesized that the mutation impairs binding of myosin Va to organelles with appropriate receptors, which leads to the loss of vesicle traffic (melanosomes and dendritic cargo) and interferes with the function of melanocytes and neurons.[13]

Preliminary carrier frequencies were estimated to be 10.3% in Egyptian Arabian (58 horses tested) and 1.8% in non-Arabians (56 tested).[13] Carrier frequency of LFS in a population of Arabians in South Africa was slightly higher at 11.7%.[15] A possible relationship between LFS and juvenile idiopathic epilepsy (JIE) has been postulated, as both conditions occur in Arabian foals of Egyptian breeding, and overlap between mares producing both LFS- and JIE-affected foals has been reported.[9] In a study investigating known genetic mutations of Arabians, the MYO5A mutation was not found in 10 Egyptian Arabian foals with confirmed JIE via EEG.[16] However, a low number of foals were genotyped. LFS seems to be an equine variant of Griscelli syndrome, although the mutations of MYO5A that have been associated with Griscelli syndrome in humans are often due to changes in a single amino acid rather than loss of a large portion of the transcript.[17] The clinical signs observed in foals with LFS are more severe than those observed in humans with mutations in the MYO5A gene.

A genetic test for LFS is available. This test can be used to definitively diagnose LFS and determine carrier status, especially of Egyptian lineage Arabian horses. The Arabian Horse Association Code of Ethics requires members to disclose LFS status, if known, for any horse capable of reproducing that is being offered for breeding, sale, or lease. In addition, an owner of a mare that produces affected offspring should immediately notify the stallion owner.

Cerebellar Abiotrophy

Cerebellar abiotrophy (CA) primarily affects Arabian horses[18–20] but has also been reported in the Oldenburg,[21] Gottland pony,[22] and Eriskay pony.[23] There is no sex predilection and clinical signs typically appear between 6 weeks and 6 months of age. Affected foals show intention tremors, ataxia, spasticity, dysmetria, and an absent or inconsistent menace response. The dysmetria is typically more pronounced in the thoracic limbs than in the pelvic limbs. Conscious proprioceptive deficits are observed as a base-wide or base-narrow stance. Until the development of a genetic test, definitive diagnosis required histopathological examination of the cerebellum.[19] Genetic testing can now be performed to definitively diagnose CA. There is no treatment of CA, although affected horses may stabilize with time due to a learned accommodation.[24] At necropsy, gross postmortem examination typically reveals a cerebellum of roughly normal size, although a study analyzing morphometric MRI data found that CA-affected horses had a relatively smaller cerebellum compared with total brain mass than control horses.[25] Histologic evaluation reveals degenerative Purkinje cells, which have undergone apoptosis,[18] along with variable gliosis and thinning of the granular and molecular layers. Mineralized cell bodies have been reported in the thalamus of affected cases.[20]

CA is inherited as an autosomal recessive trait.[26] In 2010, CA in Arabians was mapped to a region on equine chromosome 2 and a putative mutation was identified.[27] The mutation is an SNP (EquCab3.0 chr2:13,122,415 G > A) located in exon 4 of *TOE1* (*Target of EGR1*) and approximately 1200 bp upstream from *MUTYH (MutY Homolog)*. *TOE1* is expressed in the CNS, although not at high levels in the cerebellum, and is involved in cell-cycle regulation.[28,29] As the missense mutation does not seem to cause a deleterious amino acid change (arginine to histidine), its role in the development of the CA phenotype is the subject of ongoing research. *MUTYH*, which is located on the opposite strand, is highly expressed in the cerebellum and encodes for a DNA glycosylase involved in postreplicative repair in the nuclei of rapidly proliferating Purkinje cells as well as DNA repair due to oxidative damage of mitochondrial genomes.[30,31]

Previously, it was proposed that total *MUTYH* expression was downregulated[27] or unchanged[32] in CA-affected horses. Total RNA sequencing to investigate the underlying molecular mechanism of CA revealed that *TOE1* and *MUTYH* were not differentially expressed in CA-affected horses. However, genes involved in calcium homeostasis and specifically expressed in Purkinje cells were downregulated in CA-affected cerebella, whereas markers for microglial phagocytosis were found to upregulated. These findings correlate to the characteristic histopathologic abnormalities of CA.[32] It has now been determined that specific *MUTYH* isoforms are differentially expressed in the equine cerebellum. Expression of isoforms 1 and 2 were significantly increased in CA-affected cerebella compared with healthy controls. Healthy horses seem to express isoforms 3 and 4 but further work is needed regarding expression of these isoforms. In addition, it was found that the CA-associated SNP results in loss of methylation in the *MUTYH* promoter, which causes binding of a unique transcription factor, myelin transcription factor-1-like protein (*MYT1L*). The effects of

MYT1L on *MUTYH* and its role in CA have not yet been elucidated. *MUTYH* gene expression corresponds to differential localization in the Purkinje (mitochondrial) and granular neurons (nuclear) of the cerebellum as well as the spectrum of onset and severity of disease.[32,33]

A genetic test for CA is available. Initial CA testing in Arabians was based on the conserved haplotype (50 kb) identified in affected Arabians as compared with controls. This haplotype block contains 22 mutations, with only the SNP described earlier (g.13122415G > A) identified in the Arabian breed and breeds with Arabian ancestry. In 2011, the CA mutation was documented in a Danish Sport Horse as well as Bashkir Curly horses (carrier frequency 5.6%), Trakehners (carrier frequency 1.4%), and Welsh Ponies (carrier frequency 0.7%) with confirmed Arabian ancestry.[34] Initially, the carrier frequency in Arabians was reported to be 19.7%; however, this finding was likely biased, as samples were submitted specifically for CA testing. The carrier frequency of CA reported in a South African population of Arabians was 5.1% and no co-mutations between CA, LFS, or severe combined immunodeficiency were identified.[15] In another study investigating known genetic mutations of Arabians, the CA mutation (carrier) was found in one Egyptian Arabian foal with confirmed JIE.[16] The CA-affected genotype was identified, to date, in 9 apparently unaffected Arabian horses, which researchers attribute to variable expression of the disease due to varying amounts of DNA damage in the Purkinje cells of the cerebellum or the existence of a potential suppressor mutation.[27] Additional work to define the roles of *TOE1*, *MUTYH*, and *MYT1L* in the molecular mechanism of the disease is ongoing.

The Arabian Horse Association Code of Ethics requires members to disclose CA status, if known, for any horse capable of reproducing that is being offered for breeding, sale, or lease. In addition, an owner of a mare that produces affected offspring should immediately notify the stallion owner.

Familial Occipitoatlantoaxial Malformation of Arabians

Congenital malformations of the occiput, atlas, and axis (occipitoatlantoaxial malformations [OAAM]) were initially classified into 3 disease groups by Mayhew and colleagues.[35] Subsequently, 3 additional disease entities have been recognized; thus dividing these malformations into a total of 6 classes.

1. Familial occipitalization of the atlas with atlantalization of the axis in Arabian horses (**Fig. 1**)
   • Pedigree analysis in cases described by Mayhew and colleagues[35] and Watson and colleagues[36] revealed common ancestry among affected foals
2. Congenital asymmetrical OAAM
   • Non-Arabian breeds (Standardbred, Morgan, Miniature Horse[37])
3. Asymmetric atlantooccipital fusion
   • Single reported case, unknown breed[35]
4. Duplication of the axis and/or atlas
   • Half-Arabian foal[38] and Arabian horse[39]
5. Symmetric OAAM in non-Arabian horses
   • Appaloosa, Quarter horse, Friesian, Miniature horse[40,41]
6. Subluxation of the atlantooccipital joint, fusion of the atlas and axis with lateral deviation of the atlantoaxial joint, and 20° rotation of the atlas
   • Half-Arabian colt[42]

There is no sex predilection for OAAM, and affected foals may be stillborn or demonstrate neurologic abnormalities at birth. Clinical signs include symmetric upper motor neuron signs and general proprioceptive deficits. An extended neck

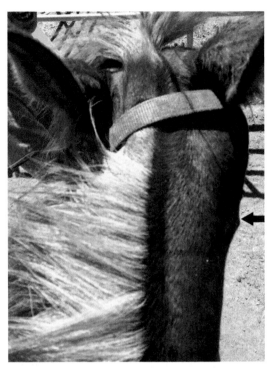

Fig. 1. An Arabian foal affected with occipitoatlantoaxial malformation (OAAM). The arrow indicates the asymmetric atlas.

posture may be observed, with an audible "click" heard during neck movement due to movement of the dens. A diagnosis can be made using cervical radiography. For one variant of OAAM, a genetic test is available. Although surgical stabilization by fusion of the axis to the atlas was attempted in select cases, the overall prognosis for OAAM is poor. At necropsy, occipitalization of the atlas and atlantalization of the axis with bilaterally symmetric compression of the cervical spinal cord may be identified.

OAAM is suspected to be inherited as an autosomal recessive trait in the Arabian breed. The familial OAAM seen in Arabian horses is very similar to that described in Hoxd-3$^{-/-}$ mice, which are homozygous for a targeted disruption of the homeobox containing gene, Hoxd3.[43] Mice homozygous for this mutation demonstrate occipitilization of the atlas and atlantization of the axis, an aspect of the phenotype that is fully penetrant. The homeobox (HOX) gene cluster is involved in the development of the axial and appendicular skeleton. In 2017, whole-genome sequencing was performed in an OAAM-affected Arabian horse, and a 2.7-kb deletion was identified 4.4 kb downstream of the end of HOXD4 and 8.2 kb upstream of the start of HOXD3. Both parents of the OAAM-affected horse were heterozygous for the deletion, whereas the affected foal was homozygous. The deletion was not found in 371 horses of other breeds. Although the variant was found in the carrier state in 2 other unaffected Arabians, 2 additional Arabian OAAM-affected foals did not have the 2.7-kb deletion. In-depth examination of the foals' phenotypes revealed notable variation, including cardiac deformities, and it is postulated that genetic heterogeneity may exist across the HOXD locus in Arabian foals with OAAM.[44]

A genetic test for the OAAM1 mutation in Arabians is available. Further work is necessary to characterize the genetic basis for other forms of OAAM as well as possible inheritance in non-Arabian breeds.

Friesian Hydrocephalus

Friesian hydrocephalus affects Friesian fetuses and foals, with no sex predilection.[45] Isolated reports of hydrocephalus exist in other breeds, including Miniature horses,[46] Quarter horses,[47] Standardbreds,[48] Warmbloods,[49] and a Belgian Draft.[50] However, these may be genetically distinct from the genetic variant described here. Affected Friesian foals are aborted, stillborn, or born with severe neurologic debilitation and cranial distention. The phenotype is clinically apparent, and radiographs can support a diagnosis. Definitive diagnosis can be achieved through genetic testing. There are no treatment options available. However, there is a report of attempted treatment of a 3-day old Quarter horse foal with hydrocephalus using a ventriculoperitoneal shunt. The foal euthanized due to shunt complications.[51] At necropsy, a communicative hydrocephalus, leading to decreased cerebrospinal fluid (CSF) absorption secondary to a distorted jugular foramen, is identified. Tetraventricular and venous dilatations and malformation of the petrosal bone have been noted.[45]

Hydrocephalus, an accumulation of CSF within the CNS, is rarely encountered in the horse. It is associated with known genetic mutations in mice, cattle, and humans. Friesian hydrocephalus is inherited as an autosomal recessive trait. In 2015, a GWA study of hydrocephalus in 13 affected Friesians and 69 control Friesians found that a nonsense mutation (c.1423C > T, p.Gln475*) in exon 12 of the β-1,3-N-acetylgalacto-saminyltransferase 2 (*B3GALNT2*) gene on chromosome 1 was associated with Friesian hydrocephalus. The mutation is identical to a *B3GALNT2* mutation identified in a human case of muscular dystrophy-dystroglycanopathy with hydrocephalus. *B3GALNT2* is involved in glycosylation of dystroglycans, which are present in skeletal muscle but also in many tissues as the brain where it affects morphogenesis and early development. Immunohistochemical examination of muscle biopsies from Friesians with hydrocephalus would need to be performed to determine if muscular dystrophy is also present in these horses. From this study, the estimated allele frequency in Friesian was determined to be 8.5%.[52] The frequency of the mutant allele in a population of Friesian stallions in Mexico was found to be 9.6%, with a carrier prevalence of 19.2%.[53]

Genetic testing for hydrocephalus in Friesians is available. Recently, the *B3GALNT2* mutation was identified in an aborted Belgian draft horse fetus.[50] Further work is necessary to evaluate the inheritance of hydrocephalus across other breeds.

Neurologic disorders with ongoing mapping efforts

In-depth discussion of all equine neurologic diseases suspected to be inherited is beyond the scope of this text. Selected diseases with recent genetic studies are presented later. **Table 2** provides a list of additional neurologic diseases with ongoing genetic studies and associated references.

Equine Neuroaxonal Dystrophy/Equine Degenerative Myeloencephalopathy

Equine neuroaxonal dystrophy (eNAD) is a neurodegenerative disease associated with vitamin E deficiency in the early life of genetically predisposed horses. In horses, eNAD is considered the underlying basis of equine degenerative myeloencephalopathy (EDM), which is more severe pathologic variant.[54] Multiple breeds are affected,[54–65] and an inherited basis is supported by pedigree analysis in Quarter horses[54] and prospective breeding trials in Morgans[64] and Appaloosa horses.[65] There is no sex

Table 2
Equine neurologic diseases with suspected inheritance that wasnot included in the text

Disease	Breed	Reference
Cervical vertebral compressive myelopathy (CVCM)	Multiple including TB, WB, QH	95–98
Equine motor neuron disease (EMND)	Multiple, QH at higher risk	99–101
Holoprosencephaly	Morgan (1 report)	102
Equine-inherited myoclonus	Peruvian Paso Fino	103
Leukoencephalomyelopathy, spongiform	QH	104
Narcolepsy	Miniature Horses, Lipizzaner, Shetland pony, Suffolk pony	105–110
Neuronal ceroid lipofuscinosis	Icelandic x Peruvian Paso crossbred (3 distantly related cases)	111
Photic head shaking	Multiple, most commonly QH, Warmblood, TB	112
Shivers	Multiple, draft breeds (overrepresented), WB, TB, QH, light breeds (rarely)	113–116

Abbreviations: QH, American Quarter Horse; TB, thoroughbred; WB, warmblood.

predilection. Clinical signs of symmetric ataxia, often more severe in the pelvic limbs, and varying degrees of pelvic limb paresis typically develop within the first year of life.[57,62,64] Hyporeflexia of the cervicofacial and cutaneous trunci as well as an absent laryngeal adductor reflex have been reported.[55,56] Stance may be abnormal at rest (**Fig. 2**). An inconsistent menace and varying degrees of obtundation have been reported in Quarter horses.[54] Neurologic abnormalities typically stabilize by 2 to 3 years of age and remain static. Equine NAD and EDM are not clinically distinguishable. There is no definitive antemortem diagnostic at this time. Antemortem suspicion based on clinical signs, elimination of other causes of neurologic disease, and possible association with a low-serum vitamin E concentration. Currently, there is no treatment of eNAD/EDM. Vitamin E supplementation, in the form of RRR-alpha-tocopherol, may stabilize clinical cases in addition to preventing severe signs in genetically predisposed individuals.[54,55,61] Supplementation with a water-dispersible formulation of RRR-alpha-tocopherol is highly recommended for late gestation mares and genetically susceptible foals throughout the first year of life.[66] At necropsy, the distinction between eNAD and EDM is based on location of lesions. Histologic features include dystrophic neurons and axons, vacuolization, and spheroid formation.[67] With eNAD, lesions are confined strictly and bilaterally to the lateral (accessory) cuneate, medial cuneate, and gracilis nuclei of the caudal myeloencephalon and the nucleus thoracicus (Clarke nucleus) of the spinal cord from the first thoracic vertebrae to the third lumbar vertebrae.[67,68] With EDM, lesions are similar to eNAD, and in addition, bilateral axonal degeneration of the dorsal spinocerebellar and ventromedial tracts is identified.

There is an association of vitamin E deficiency in cases of eNAD/EDM, although low vitamin E levels are not consistently present in all cases. It seems that vitamin E is a factor in the development of eNAD/EDM in the first year of life in genetically predisposed foals.[65] Tocopherol transfer protein alpha (*TTPA*) was excluded as a candidate gene for eNAD in the Quarter horse.[69] There is strong evidence that eNAD/EDM is inherited as either an autosomal dominant or polygenic trait, and environmental

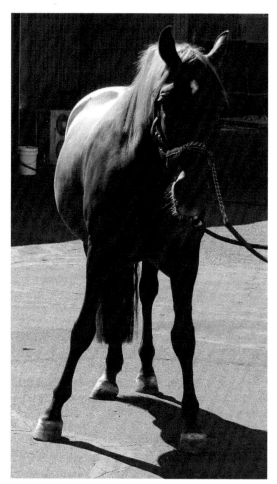

Fig. 2. An Andalusian gelding affected with equine neuroaxonal dystrophy/degenerative myeloencephalopathy (eNAD/EDM) demonstrating an abnormal base-wide stance.

effects, specifically the amount of alpha-tocopherol received during early life, play a role in determining the overall phenotype.[54,64,70]

NAD has been associated with neurologic disease in many mammalian species including humans, sheep, cattle, cats, and dogs; however, the clinical and specific histopathological findings vary. In most of the NAD cases in various species, dystrophic neurons and axons are most commonly found in specific nuclear areas of the gray matter in brain and spinal cord.[71] In canine and feline NAD, there is involvement of the cerebellum, which is not observed in horses.[72–74] Specific genetic mutations for NAD have been identified in the Papillon[75] and Rottweiler[76] dog breeds. In humans, an underlying genetic basis for the disease has been identified in 2 of the 5 NAD disorders: infantile NAD (mutations in *PLA2G6*) and juvenile/adult Hallervorden-Spatz disease (mutations in *PANK2* gene).[77–79] Equine NAD/EDM varies considerably from human NAD in both clinical signs and affected neuroanatomical pathways and therefore a candidate gene approach is unlikely to identify a putative mutation for the disease in horses.

Genotyping of 133 horses was performed using the EquineSNP50 Beadchip (Illumina, San Diego, CA) in a genome-wide association study. Variants uncovered in this investigation (*PIK3C3*, *RIT2*, and *STY4*) were not causative for eNAD/EDM.[80] In 2018, a missense mutation (EquCab3.0 chr3:73,781,733 C > T) within adhesion G-protein-coupled receptor L3 (*ADGRL3*) was associated with risk for EDM in the Caspian breed.[81] However, this study was refuted in 2019, where there was no significant association found between the *ADGRL3* mutation, along with 3 other associated SNPs, in 31 confirmed cases of eNAD/EDM across various breeds.[82] RNA-sequencing performed to investigate the underlying molecular mechanism of eNAD/EDM identified downregulated glutamate receptor and synaptic vesicle trafficking pathways in affected horses.In addition, upregulation of specific genes targeted by a nuclear transcription factor, the liver X receptor (LXR), was identified.[83] The natural ligands for LXR activation are oxysterols. Preliminary evaluation of eNAD/EDM affected horses identified a trend toward increased spinal cord oxysterols that result from autooxidation of cholesterol and oxidation of 7-dehydrocholesterol by cytochrome P450 7A1 (CYP7A1; 7-alpha-hydroxylase). Concentrations of spinal cord 7-ketocholesterol, 7-hydroxycholesterol, and 7-keto-27-hydrocholesterol, the markers of cholesterol oxidation, were found to be higher in eNAD/EDM-affected horse compared with healthy controls. No significant difference was found between the concentration of oxysterols in the CSF and serum of eNAD/EDM and healthy horses.[84] These findings suggest a potential dysregulation of cholesterol homeostasis in the CNS of eNAD/EDM-affected horses leading to neurodegeneration. The protective role of α-tocopherol may be due to prevention of oxysterol accumulation within specific somatosensory neurons.[83]

A genome-wide association study was recently successful at mapping eNAD in Quarter horses to a 2.5 Mb region on chr7. This region included a strong candidate gene, caytaxin (*ATCAY*), which has been associated with Cayman ataxia in humans. *ATCAY* was excluded as a candidate gene through whole-genome sequencing and experiments using the *Atcay*[ji-hes] mouse model.[85] The associated region on chr7 therefore requires further investigation.

Juvenile Idiopathic Epilepsy

Juvenile idiopathic epilepsy (JIE) affects Arabian foals of Egyptian lineage, with no sex predilection. Median age at onset is 2 months of age, with a range from 2 days to 6 months.[86] Clinical signs consist of multiple generalized or partial seizures lasting less than 1 minute. In the preictal phase, there may be no clinical signs or mild behavior changes. During the ictal phase, tonic seizures are followed by clonic motor activity in severe cases or focal head twitches and nystagmus in milder cases. During the postictal phase, blindness, lethargy, and obtundation are observed. A decreased to absent menace response may be present. At this time, a definitive diagnosis requires an EEG, with spikes, sharp waves, spike and wave discharges, or multiple spike complexes supporting a diagnosis of JIE.[86] Seizures are responsive to treatment with benzodiazepines (diazepam, midazolam),[86,87] and phenobarbital is often used for long-term control of seizures.[86] Potassium bromide may be added in some cases. Additional therapies include supportive care for seizure-induced trauma and antimicrobials for aspiration pneumonia.[86] Seizures are self-limiting and resolve by 1 to 2 years of age.[86,87]

JIE displays an autosomal dominant mode of inheritance in Arabian foals from Egyptian lineage. In humans, many of the rare Mendelian idiopathic generalized epilepsies are ion voltage- and receptor-mediated channelopathies.[88] There are 3 types of neonatal and infancy epilepsy syndromes in humans that are characterized by afebrile focal motor seizures that remit after weeks or months with administration of standard antiepileptic drugs. All 3 syndromes have an autosomal dominant mode of inheritance with high penetrance.[89]

1. Benign familial neonatal convulsions
   - Mutations in *KCNQ2* or *KCNQ3*, both voltage-gated potassium channels that regulate neuronal excitability
2. Benign familial neonatal-infantile seizures
   - Mutations in *SCN2A*, a subunit of the neuronal voltage-gated sodium channel
3. Benign familial infantile seizures
   - No causative genes identified

Recently, whole-genome comparisons between 9 JIE-affected foals and 27 non-Arabian controls in Israel identified variants unique to the JIE-affected group. Further investigation revealed a single 19 bp deletion coupled with a triple-C insertion (Δ19InsCCC) within *TRIM39-RPP21*. The allele was present in all JIE-affected foals but absent from 3 unaffected Arabian controls in the study.[90] Subsequent work has refuted its significance across EEG-confirmed cases of JIE in Egyptian Arabians,[91] and studies are ongoing to identify a mutation.

Sensory Deafness in American Paint Horses

Sensory deafness in American Paint horses has no apparent sex predilection. Affected horses have extensive white facial markings and one or more blue irides. Palpebral skin may be partially pigmented and white markings are often found on the legs. Associated coat colors affected with sensory deafness include the splashed white overo and frame-splashed white overo blends. Clinical signs of sensory deafness include a decreased or absent response to auditory stimuli; however, definitive diagnosis requires brainstem auditory-evoked response (BAER) testing.[3,92] There is currently no treatment of the condition and owners should be counseled regarding management and handling of deaf horses.

There is a small population of melanocytes within the inner ear that are essential for the development of the stria vascularis, which is a blood-vessel–rich zone of the cochlea that plays a role in modulating the chemical composition of endolymph and the resultant production of an endocochlear potential. In mice that have been genetically engineered to have no melanocytes in the stria (viable dominant spotting mice), the endocochlear potential is close to zero (wild type +100 mV) at all stages of development, and the mice are profoundly hearing impaired.[93] In many species, congenital deafness is associated with abnormal migration of these melanocytes from the neural crest and poor survival within the inner ears of some animals with coat and iris pigmentation alterations.[93,94]

A case-control series evaluating 14 confirmed deaf, 20 suspected deaf, and 13 non-deaf American Paint horses was performed to further evaluate deafness by phenotype, clinical findings, BAERs, and endothelin B receptor (*EDNBR*) genotype.[3] Horses were confirmed to be bilaterally deaf through BAER testing. Phenotypes of the confirmed and suspected deaf groups were as described earlier. Otoscopic examination, routine clinicopathological analysis of whole blood and serum, skull radiographs, and neurologic examinations revealed no abnormalities in the confirmed deaf horses. When evaluating the confirmed deaf horses for the *EDNRB* mutation that is causative for LWFS (I118K), 7/8 confirmed deaf horses were carriers for the mutation and 1/8 was not.[3] Therefore, a relationship between the mutation and deafness was established; however, this could represent 2 independent mutations that are prevalent in certain overo horses.

In humans, there are several conditions that cause hypopigmentation and deafness. Type II Waardenburg syndrome is limited to hypopigmentation and deafness without any craniofacial deficits and is caused by a mutation in the *Mitf* gene, which is a central mediator of melanocyte development.[94] Type IV Waardenburg syndrome includes deafness and hypopigmentation in conjunction with Hirschsprung's disease and is associated with a mutation of the *SOX10, EDN3,* or *EDNRB* genes.[94] Based on likely candidate genes, additional investigation into the genetics of deafness in horses is currently being pursued.

SUMMARY

A variety of neurologic disorders in horses have demonstrated to be heritable. With the sequencing of the equine genome and molecular tools currently available to perform whole genome interrogation, the identification of quantitative trait loci for multifactorial traits in addition to mapping of simple Mendelian genetic traits is possible. Equine genetic research will continue to advance, and the molecular discoveries will provide insight into disease pathophysiology and allow veterinarians the ability to definitively diagnose particular conditions while advising breeders in order to decrease the overall prevalence of certain inherited diseases in the equine population.

ACKNOWLEDGMENTS

Support for C.J.F. was provided by NIH L40 TR001136.

DISCLOSURE

The authors have nothing to disclose.

REFERENCES

1. Hultgren BD. Ileocolonic aganglionosis in white progeny of overo spotted horses. J Am Vet Med Assoc 1982;180(3):289–92.
2. Vonderfecht SL, Bowling AT, Cohen M. Congenital intestinal aganglionosis in white foals. Vet Pathol 1983;20(1):65–70.
3. Magdesian KG, Williams DC, Aleman M, et al. Evaluation of deafness in American Paint Horses by phenotype, brainstem auditory-evoked responses, and endothelin receptor B genotype. J Am Vet Med Assoc 2009;235(10):1204–11.
4. McCabe L, Griffin LD, Kinzer A, et al. Ovetrolethal white foal syndrome: equine model of aganglionic megacolon (Hirschsprung Disease). Am J Med Genet 1990;36:336–40.
5. Santschi EM, Vrotsos PD, Purdy AK, et al. Incidence of the endothelin receptor B mutation that causes lethal white foal syndrome in white-patterned horses. Am J Vet Res 2001;62(1):97–103.
6. Metallinos DL, Bowling AT, Rine J. A missense mutation in the endothelin-B receptor gene is associated with Lethal White Foal Syndrome: an equine version of Hirschsprung disease. Mamm Genome 1998;9(6):426–31.
7. Santschi EM, Purdy AK, Valberg SJ, et al. Endothelin receptor B polymorphism associated with lethal white foal syndrome in horses. Mamm Genome 1998;9(4):306–9.
8. Pascoe RR, Knottenbelt DC. Congenital/Developmental diseases. In: Pascoe RR, Knottenbelt DC, editors. Manual of equine dermatology. London: W.B. Saunders; 1999. p. 148–9.

9. Fanelli HH. Coat colour dilution lethal ('lavender foal syndrome'): a tetany syndrome of Arabian foals. Equine Vet Education 2005;17(5):260–3.

10. Bowling AT. Medical genetics. In: Bowling AT, editor. Horse Genetics. Wallingford (England): CAB International; 1996. p. 105–6.

11. Page P, Parker R, Harper C, et al. Clinical, clinicopathologic, postmortem examination findings and familial history of 3 Arabians with lavender foal syndrome. J Vet Intern Med 2006;20(6):1491–4.

12. Madigan J. Congenital anomalies and genetic disorders. In: Madigan J, editor. Manual of equine neonatal medicine. Woodland (CA): Saunders Co; 1997. p. 148–9.

13. Brooks SA, Gabreski N, Miller D, et al. Whole-genome SNP association in the horse: identification of a deletion in myosin Va responsible for Lavender Foal Syndrome. PLoS Genet 2010;6(4):e1000909.

14. Bierman A, Guthrie AJ, Harper CK. Lavender foal syndrome in Arabian horses is caused by a single-base deletion in the MYO5A gene. Anim Genet 2010;41: 199–201.

15. Tarr CJ, Thompson PN, Guthrie AJ, et al. The carrier prevalence of severe combined immunodeficiency, lavender foal syndrome and cerebellar abiotrophy in Arabian horses in South Africa. Equine Vet J 2014;46(4):512–4.

16. Aleman M, Finno CJ, Weich K, et al. Investigation of known genetic mutations of Arabian Horses in Egyptian Arabian Foals with Juvenile Idiopathic Epilepsy. J Vet Intern Med 2018;32(1):465–8.

17. Sanal O, Ersoy F, Tezcan I, et al. Griscelli disease: genotype-phenotype correlation in an array of clinical heterogeneity. J Clin Immunol 2002;22(4):237–43.

18. Blanco A, Moyano R, Vivo J, et al. Purkinje cell apoptosis in arabian horses with cerebellar abiotrophy. J Vet Med A Physiol Pathol Clin Med 2006;53(6):286–7.

19. Palmer AC, Blakemore WF, Cook WR, et al. Cerebellar hypoplasia and degeneration in the young Arab horse: clinical and neuropathological features. Vet Rec 1973;93(3):62–6.

20. Turner Beatty M, Leipold HW, Cash W, et al. Cerebellar disease in Arabian Horses. In 31st Annual Proceedings of the American association of equine Practitioners. Toronto, Canada, 1985;241-55.

21. Koch P, Fischer H. Die Oldenburger Fohlen Taxie als Erbkrankeit. Tierarztl Umschau 1950;5:317–20.

22. Bjorck G, Everz KE, Hansen HJ, et al. Congenital cerebellar ataxia in the gotland pony breed. Zentralbl Veterinarmed A 1973;20(4):341–54.

23. Hahn CN, Mayhew IG, MacKay RJ. Nervous system. In: Calahan PT, Merritt AM, Moore JN, et al, editors. Equine medicine and surgery. St Louis (MO): Mosby; 1999. p. 904–96.

24. DeBowes RM, Leipold HW, Turner-Beatty M. Cerebellar abiotrophy. Vet Clin North Am Equine Pract 1987;3(2):345–52.

25. Cavalleri JM, Metzger J, Hellige M, et al. Morphometric magnetic resonance imaging and genetic testing in cerebellar abiotrophy in Arabian horses. BMC Vet Res 2013;9:105.

26. Brault LS, Famula TR, Penedo MCT. Inheritance of equine cerellar abiotrophy in Arabian horses. Am J Vet Res 2011;72(7):940-4.

27. Brault LS, Cooper CA, Famula TR, et al. Mapping of equine cerebellar abiotrophy to ECA2 and identification of a potential causative mutation affecting expression of MUTYH. Genomics 2011;97(2):121–9.

28. De Belle I, Wu JX, Sperandio S, et al. In vivo cloning and characterization of a new growth suppressor protein TOE1 as a direct target gene of Egr1. J Biol Chem 2003;278(16):14306–12.

29. Sperandio S, Tardito S, Surzycki A, et al. TOE1 interacts with p53 to modulate its transactivation potential. FEBS Lett 2009;583(13):2165–70.

30. Lee HM, Wang C, Hu Z, et al. Hypoxia induces mitochondrial DNA damage and stimulates expression of a DNA repair enzyme, the Escherichia coli MutY DNA glycosylase homolog (MYH), in vivo, in the rat brain. J Neurochem 2002;80(5): 928–37.

31. Gu Y, Parker A, Wilson TM, et al. Human MutY homolog, a DNA glycosylase involved in base excision repair, physically and functionally interacts with mismatch repair proteins human MutS homolog 2/human MutS homolog 6. J Biol Chem 2002;277(13):11135–42.

32. Scott EY, Penedo MCT, Murray JD, et al. Defining trends in global gene expression in Arabian Horses with cerebellar abiotrophy. Cerebellum 2017;16(2): 462–72.

33. Scott EY, Woolard KD, Finno CJ, et al. Variation in MUTYH expression in Arabian horses with cerebellar abiotrophy. Brain Res 2018;1678:330–6.

34. Brault LS, Penedo MC. The frequency of the equine cerebellar abiotrophy mutation in non-Arabian horse breeds. Equine Vet J 2011;43(6):727–31.

35. Mayhew IG, Watson AG, Heissan JA. Congenital occipitoatlantoaxial malformations in the horse. Equine Vet J 1978;10(2):103–13.

36. Watson AG, Mayhew IG. Familial congenital occipitoatlantoaxial malformation (OAAM) in the Arabian horse. Spine (Phila Pa 1976) 1986;11(4):334–9.

37. Rosenstein DS, Schott HC 2nd, Stickle RL. Imaging diagnosis–occipitoatlantoaxial malformation in a miniature horse foal. Vet Radiol Ultrasound 2000; 41(3):218–9.

38. de Lahunta A, Hatfield C, Dietz A. Occipitoatlantoaxial malformation with duplication of the atlas and axis in a half Arabian foal. Cornell Vet 1989;79(2):185–93.

39. Watson AG, Quick CB, DeLahunta A. Congenital occipitoatlantoaxial malformation (OAAM) with two atlases in a young Arabian horse. Anat Histol Embryol 1978;7:354.

40. Wilson WD, Hughes SJ, Ghoshal NG, et al. Occipitoatlantoaxial malformation in two non-Arabian horses. J Am Vet Med Assoc 1985;187(1):36–40.

41. Bell S, Detweiler D, Benak J, et al. What is your diagnosis? Occipitoatlantoaxial malformation. J Am Vet Med Assoc 2007;231(7):1033–4.

42. Blikslager AT, Wilson DA, Constantinescu GM, et al. Atlantoaxial malformation in a half-Arabian colt. Cornell Vet 1991;81(1):67–75.

43. Condie BG, Capecchi MR. Mice homozygous for a targeted disruption of Hoxd-3 (Hox-4.1) exhibit anterior transformations of the first and second cervical vertebrae, the atlas and the axis. Development 1993;119(3):579–95.

44. Bordbari MH, Penedo MCT, Aleman M, et al. Deletion of 2.7 kb near HOXD3 in an Arabian horse with occipitoatlantoaxial malformation. Anim Genet 2017; 48(3):287–94.

45. Sipma KD, Cornillie P, Saulez MN, et al. Phenotypic characteristics of hydrocephalus in stillborn Friesian foals. Vet Pathol 2013;50(6):1037–42.

46. Ferris RA, Sonnis J, Webb B, et al. Hydrocephalus in an American Miniature Horse Foal: a case report and review. J Equine Vet Sci 2011;31(11):611–4.

47. Foreman JH, Reed SM, Rantanen NW, et al. Congenital internal hydrocephalus in a quarter horse foal. J Equine Vet Sci 1983;3(5):154–64.

48. Ojala M, Ala-Huikku J. Inheritance of hydrocephalus in horses. Equine Vet J 1992;24(2):140–3.
49. Oey L, Muller JM, von Klopmann T, et al. Diagnosis of internal and external hydrocephalus in a warmblood foal using magnetic resonance imaging. Tierarztl Prax Ausg G Grosstiere Nutztiere 2011;39(1):41–5.
50. Kolb DS, Klein C. Congenital hydrocephalus in a Belgian draft horse associated with a nonsense mutation in B3GALNT2. Can Vet J 2019;60(2):197–8.
51. Bentz BG, Moll HD. Treatment of congenital hydrocephalus in a foal using a ventriculoperitoneal shunt. J Vet Emerg Crit Care 2008;18(2):170–6.
52. Ducro BJ, Schurink A, Bastiaansen JW, et al. A nonsense mutation in B3GALNT2 is concordant with hydrocephalus in Friesian horses. BMC Genomics 2015; 16:761.
53. Ayala-Valdovinos MA, Galindo-Garcia J, Sanchez-Chipres D, et al. Genotyping of friesian horses to detect a hydrocephalus-associated c.1423C>T mutation in B3GALNT2 using PCR-RFLP and PCR-PIRA methods: frequency in stallion horses in Mexico. Mol Cell Probes 2017;32:69–71.
54. Aleman M, Finno CJ, Higgins RJ, et al. Evaluation of epidemiological, clinical, and pathological features of neuroaxonal dystrophy in Quarter Horses. J Am Vet Med Assoc 2011;239(6):823–33.
55. Mayhew IG, Brown CM, Stowe HD, et al. Equine degenerative myeloencephalopathy: a vitamin E deficiency that may be familial. J Vet Intern Med 1987;1(1): 45–50.
56. Gandini G, Fatzer R, Mariscoli M, et al. Equine degenerative myeloencephalopathy in five Quarter Horses: clinical and neuropathological findings. Equine Vet J 2004;36(1):83–5.
57. Mayhew IG, deLahunta A, Whitlock RH, et al. Spinal cord disease in the horse. Cornell Vet 1978;68(Suppl 6):1–207.
58. Liu SK, Dolensek EP, Adams CR, et al. Myelopathy and vitamin E deficiency in six Mongolian wild horses. J Am Vet Med Assoc 1983;183(11):1266–8.
59. Siso S, Ferrer I, Pumarola M. Abnormal synaptic protein expression in two Arabian horses with equine degenerative myeloencephalopathy. Vet J 2003; 166(3):238–43.
60. Cummings JF, de Lahunta A, Mohammed HO, et al. Endothelial lipopigment as an indicator of alpha-tocopherol deficiency in two equine neurodegenerative diseases. Acta Neuropathol 1995;90(3):266–72.
61. Dill SG, Correa MT, Erb HN, et al. Factors associated with the development of equine degenerative myeloencephalopathy. Am J Vet Res 1990;51(8):1300–5.
62. Adams AP, Collatos C, Fuentealba C, et al. Neuroaxonal dystrophy in a two-year-old quarter horse filly. Can Vet J 1996;37(1):43–4.
63. Baumgartner W, Frese K, Elmadfa I. Neuroaxonal dystrophy associated with vitamin E deficiency in two Haflinger horses. J Comp Pathol 1990;103(1):114–9.
64. Beech J, Haskins M. Genetic studies of neuraxonal dystrophy in the Morgan. Am J Vet Res 1987;48(1):109–13.
65. Blythe LL, Hultgren BD, Craig AM, et al. Clinical, viral, and genetic evaluation of equine degenerative myeloencephalopathy in a family of Appaloosas. J Am Vet Med Assoc 1991;198(6):1005–13.
66. Finno CJ, Estell KE, Katzman S, et al. Blood and cerebrospinal fluid alpha-tocopherol and selenium concentrations in neonatal foals with neuroaxonal dystrophy. J Vet Intern Med 2015;29(6):1667–75.
67. Beech J. Neuroaxonal dystrophy of the accessory cuneate nucleus in horses. Vet Pathol 1984;21(4):384–93.

68. Miller MM, Collatos C. Equine degenerative myeloencephalopathy. Vet Clin North Am Equine Pract 1997;13(1):43–52.

69. Finno CJ, Famula T, Aleman M, et al. Pedigree analysis and exclusion of alpha-tocopherol transfer protein (TTPA) as a candidate gene for neuroaxonal dystrophy in the American Quarter Horse. J Vet Intern Med 2013;27(1):177–85.

70. Blythe LL, Craig AM, Lassen ED, et al. Serially determined plasma alpha-tocopherol concentrations and results of the oral vitamin E absorption test in clinically normal horses and in horses with degenerative myeloencephalopathy. Am J Vet Res 1991;52(6):908–11.

71. Siso S, Hanzlicek D, Fluehmann G, et al. Neurodegenerative diseases in domestic animals: a comparative review. Vet J 2006;171(1):20–38.

72. Carmichael KP, Howerth EW, Oliver JE Jr, et al. Neuroaxonal dystrophy in a group of related cats. J Vet Diagn Invest 1993;5(4):585–90.

73. Cork LC, Troncoso JC, Price DL, et al. Canine neuroaxonal dystrophy. J Neuropathol Exp Neurol 1983;42(3):286–96.

74. Chrisman CL, Cork LC, Gamble DA. Neuroaxonal dystrophy of Rottweiler dogs. J Am Vet Med Assoc 1984;184(4):464–7.

75. Tsuboi M, Watanabe M, Nibe K, et al. Identification of the PLA2G6 c.1579G>A missense mutation in papillon dog neuroaxonal dystrophy using whole exome sequencing analysis. PLoS One 2017;12(1):e0169002.

76. Lucot KL, Dickinson PJ, Finno CJ, et al. A missense mutation in the vacuolar protein sorting 11 (VPS11) gene is associated with neuroaxonal dystrophy in rottweiler dogs. G3 (Bethesda) 2018;8(8):2773–80.

77. Khateeb S, Dickinson PJ, Finno CJ, et al. PLA2G6 mutation underlies infantile neuroaxonal dystrophy. Am J Hum Genet 2006;79(5):942–8.

78. Morgan NV, Westaway SK, Morton JE, et al. PLA2G6, encoding a phospholipase A2, is mutated in neurodegenerative disorders with high brain iron. Nat Genet 2006;38(7):752–4.

79. Zhou B, Westaway SK, Levinson B, et al. A novel pantothenate kinase gene (PANK2) is defective in Hallervorden-Spatz syndrome. Nat Genet 2001;28(4):345–9.

80. Finno CJ, Aleman M, Higgins RJ, et al. Risk of false positive genetic associations in complex traits with underlying population structure: a case study. Vet J 2014;202(3):543–9.

81. Posbergh CJ, Pollott GE, Southard TL, et al. A nonsynonymous change in adhesion G protein-coupled receptor L3 associated with risk for equine degenerative myeloencephalopathy in the Caspian Horse. J Equine Vet Sci 2018;70:96–100.

82. Marquardt SA, Wilcox CV, Burns EN, et al. Previously identified genetic variants in ADGRL3 are not associated with risk for equine degenerative myeloencephalopathy across breeds. Genes (Basel) 2019;10(9).

83. Finno CJ, Bordbari MH, Valberg SJ, et al. Transcriptome profiling of equine vitamin E deficient neuroaxonal dystrophy identifies upregulation of liver X receptor target genes. Free Radic Biol Med 2016;101:261–71.

84. Finno CJ, Estell KE, Winfield L, et al. Lipid peroxidation biomarkers for evaluating oxidative stress in equine neuroaxonal dystrophy. J Vet Intern Med 2018;32(5):1740–7.

85. Hales EN, Esparza C, Peng S, et al. Genome-wide association study and subsequent exclusion of ATCAY as a candidate gene involved in equine neuroaxonal dystrophy using two animal models. Genes (Basel) 2020;11(1).

86. Aleman M, Gray LC, Williams DC, et al. Juvenile idiopathic epilepsy in Egyptian Arabian foals: 22 cases (1985-2005). J Vet Intern Med 2006;20(6):1443–9.

87. Mittel L. Seizures in the horse. Vet Clin North Am Equine Pract 1987;3(2):323–32.
88. Panayiotopoulos CP. Idiopathic generalized epilepsies: a review and modern approach. Epilepsia 2005;46(Suppl 9):1–6.
89. Baulac S, Baulac M. Advances on the genetics of mendelian idiopathic epilepsies. Neurol Clin 2009;27(4):1041–61.
90. Polani S, Dean M, Lichter-Peled A, et al. Sequence variant in the TRIM 39-RPP21 gene readthrough is shared across a cohort of arabian foals diagnosed with juvenile idiopathic epilepsy. J Genet Mutat Disord 2018;1(1).
91. Rivas VN, Aleman M, Peterson JA, et al. TRIM39-RPP21 variants (19InsCCC) are not associated with juvenile idiopathic epilepsy in Egyptian Arabian Horses. Genes (Basel) 2019;10(10).
92. Harland MM, Stewart AJ, Marshall AE, et al. Diagnosis of deafness in a horse by brainstem auditory evoked potential. Can Vet J 2006;47(2):151–4.
93. Steel KP, Barkway C. Another role for melanocytes: their importance for normal stria vascularis development in the mammalian inner ear. Development 1989;107(3):453–63.
94. Price ER, Fisher DE. Sensorineural deafness and pigmentation genes: melanocytes and the Mitf transcriptional network. Neuron 2001;30(1):15–8.
95. Dimock WW. "Wobbles" an hereditary disease in horses. J Hered 1950;41(12):319–23.
96. Falco MJ, Whitwell K, Palmer AC. An investigation into the genetics of 'wobbler disease' in thoroughbred horses in Britain. Equine Vet J 1976;8(4):165–9.
97. Wagner PC, Grant BD, Watrous BJ, et al. A study of the heritability of cervical vertebral malformation in horses. In: 31st Annual Convetion of the American association of equine Practitioners. Toronto, Canada, 1985;43-50.
98. Stewart RH, Reed SM, Weisbrode SE. Frequency and severity of osteochondrosis in horses with cervical stenotic myelopathy. Am J Vet Res 1991;52(6):873–9.
99. Delaruadomenech R, Mohammed HO, Atwill ER, et al. Epidemiologic evidence for clustering of equine motor-neuron disease in the United-States. Am J Vet Res 1995;56(11):1433–9.
100. de la Rua-Domenech R, Mohammed HO, Cummings JF, et al. Incidence and risk-factors of equine motor-neuron disease - an ambidirectional study. Neuroepidemiology 1995;14(2):54–64.
101. de la Rua-Domenech R, Wiedmann M, Mohammed HO, et al. Equine motor neuron disease is not linked to Cu/Zn superoxide dismutase mutations: sequence analysis of the equine Cu/Zn superoxide dismutase cDNA. Gene 1996;178(1–2):83–8.
102. Koch TG, Loretti AP, de Lahunta A, et al. Semilobar holoprosencephaly in a Morgan horse. J Vet Intern Med 2005;19(3):367–72.
103. Gundlach AL, Kortz G, Burazin TC, et al. Deficit of inhibitory glycine receptors in spinal cord from Peruvian Pasos: evidence for an equine form of inherited myoclonus. Brain Res 1993;628(1–2):263–70.
104. Seahorn TL, Fuentealba IC, Illanes OG, et al. Congenital encephalomyelopathy in a quarter horse. Equine Vet J 1991;23(5):394–6.
105. Lunn DP, Cuddon PA, Shaftoe S, et al. Familial occurrence of narcolepsy in miniature horses. Equine Vet J 1993;25(6):483–7.
106. Ludvikova E, Nishino S, Sakai N, et al. Familial narcolepsy in the Lipizzaner horse: a report of three fillies born to the same sire. Vet Q 2012;32(2):99–102.
107. Sheather AL. Fainting in foals. J Comp Pathol Ther 1924;37:106–13.
108. Dreifuss FE, Flynn DV. Narcolepsy in a horse. J Am Vet Med Assoc 1984;184(2):131–2.

109. Sweeney CR, Hendricks JC, Beech J, et al. Narcolepsy in a horse. J Am Vet Med Assoc 1983;183(1):126–8.
110. Bathen-Nothen A, Heider C, Fernandez AJ, et al. Hypocretin measurement in an Icelandic foal with narcolepsy. J Vet Intern Med 2009;23(6):1299–302.
111. Url A, Bauder B, Thalhammer J, et al. Equine neuronal ceroid lipofuscinosis. Acta Neuropathol 2001;101(4):410–4.
112. Chowdhary BP. Equine Genomics 2013.
113. Draper AC, Bender JB, Firshman AM, et al. Epidemiology of shivering (shivers) in horses. Equine Vet J 2015;47(2):182–7.
114. Valberg SJ, Lewis SS, Shivers JL, et al. The equine movement disorder "shivers" is associated with selective cerebellar purkinje cell axonal degeneration. Vet Pathol 2015;52(6):1087–98.
115. Draper ACE, Trumble TN, Firshman AM, et al. Posture and movement characteristics of forward and backward walking in horses with shivering and acquired bilateral stringhalt. Equine Vet J 2015;47(2):175–81.
116. Baird JD, Firshman AM, Valberg SJ. Shivers (Shivering) in the horse: a review. In: Proceedings of the Annual Convention of the American Asssociation of equine Practitioners. San Antonia, TX, 2006;359-64.

Genetics of Immune Disease in the Horse

Rebecca L. Tallmadge, PhD[a], Douglas F. Antczak, VMD, PhD[b],*,
Maria Julia Bevilaqua Felippe, MV, MS, PhD[c]

KEYWORDS

- Horse • Equine • Genetics • Immunity • Disease

KEY POINTS

- Mutations in essential immune system genes that lead to catastrophic consequences, such as inability to fight off infections, are rare. Evolution operates to eliminate profound immunodeficiencies through natural selection.
- Genetic variants that have a large influence on the outcome of specific infectious diseases caused by one or a few similar microorganisms are rare, likely because of the redundancy in immune defense mechanisms.
- Examples of autoimmune and allergic diseases with a genetic basis are relatively common. Such conditions are often not life threatening, and they can arise through production of an inappropriate immune response to a self-antigen or environmental antigen, rather than the lack of specific responses that characterize immunodeficiency diseases.

INTRODUCTION AND SCOPE

Through the processes of evolution, vertebrates have made a major investment in the mechanisms that afford protection against infection. The estimated 7% of coding genes of mammals that are related to immunity and infection total between 1500 and 2000 genes,[1] which provides hundreds of opportunities for mutations to arise in structural genes or associated regulatory regions that can result in disease states or in increased predisposition to disease. Such mutations have been recognized as genetically determined immunodeficiencies, allergies, and autoimmune conditions, and increased susceptibility to infections, with hundreds of genetic loci implicated in humans and laboratory rodents.[2] A similar range of disease conditions has been described in the horse, but the number of specific genes identified is lower. Genetic

[a] Animal Health Diagnostic Center, College of Veterinary Medicine, Cornell University, 240 Farrier Road, Ithaca, NY 14853, USA; [b] Baker Institute for Animal Health, College of Veterinary Medicine, Cornell University, 235 Hungerford Hill Road, Ithaca, NY 14853, USA; [c] Department of Clinical Sciences, College of Veterinary Medicine, Cornell University, 930 Campus Road, Ithaca, NY 14853, USA
* Corresponding author.
E-mail address: dfa1@cornell.edu

Vet Clin Equine 36 (2020) 273–288
https://doi.org/10.1016/j.cveq.2020.03.007
0749-0739/20/© 2020 Elsevier Inc. All rights reserved.

vetequine.theclinics.com

diseases that involve the equine immune system occur in several organ systems, including the respiratory system, the skin, the muscles, and the eye. The reader is referred to separate articles in this issue on those systems for additional information. Here, the authors focus on immunodeficiencies, infectious diseases, and a few other conditions that share an association with the major histocompatibility complex (MHC).

Immunodeficiencies of the Horse with Known Genetic Cause

Reported primary immunodeficiencies with known genetic cause in the horse include foal immunodeficiency syndrome (FIS) and severe combined immunodeficiency (SCID) syndrome. In addition, common variable immunodeficiency (CVID) has been shown to at least involve epigenetic mechanisms of gene silencing. Other humoral and cellular immunodeficiencies clinically described in the horse have not yet been associated with genetic defects to date.[3–5]

Foal immunodeficiency syndrome

FIS is an autosomal-recessive hereditary fatal condition characterized by profound anemia and septicemia in young male and female foals of the Fell pony and Dales breeds.[6–9] Affected foals are born apparently healthy but dullness, weight loss, and signs of infection (necrotizing enterocolitis and/or bronchopneumonia, septicemia) involving bacteria, virus, and opportunistic organisms develop rapidly within the first weeks of age.[10]

Profound nonregenerative anemia owing to paucity of hematopoietic precursors in the bone marrow, B-cell lymphopenia, and plasma cell depletion rapidly develop after birth has been reported.[11–14] The medullary cavities of bones are filled with pale or tan fatty tissue; the thymus is hypoplastic, and secondary lymphoid tissues are poorly developed and lack germinal centers. Serum immunoglobulin M (IgM) concentration is markedly low or undetectable, and serum IgG concentration reflects solely colostrum-derived antibodies. In addition, peripheral ganglionopathy, characterized by neuronal chromatolysis involving trigeminal, cranial mesenteric and dorsal root ganglia, has been reported.[10,11]

The Fell pony breed experienced loss of genetic diversity owing to the small numbers of animals and overuse of prominent stallions. Pedigree analysis of the Fell pony breed suggests that FIS has an autosomal-recessive inheritance, in which affected foals are homozygous for the defective gene, and heterozygous carriers are asymptomatic.[15] Linkage and homozygosity mapping, followed by haplotype analysis of samples from FIS-affected, FIS-carrier, and unknown carrier status Fell pony horses, mapped a mutation to chromosome 26 (ECA26). A genome-wide association study (GWAS) identified 2 statistically significant single nucleotide polymorphisms (SNPs), BIEC2-692674 and BIEC2-69138. Sequencing of the denoted chromosome region revealed an amino acid substitution mutation in the sodium/myoinositol cotransporter gene SLC5A3. Although this mutation has been associated with FIS, the mechanistic or biologic effect of this mutation on the bone marrow function has not been fully resolved.

A DNA-based test was developed by the Animal Health Trust (Newmarket, UK), which allows reproductive management planning in order to avoid the mating of heterozygous carriers for the genetic defect, which would result in a 25% chance of producing an affected homozygous offspring. Using the genetic test, the frequency of carriers with the mutation was calculated as 39% in the Fell pony, 18% in Dales, and 1% in colored pony horses; other common breeds (Welsh, part-bred Welsh, Highland, Exmoor, and Clydesdale) of the United Kingdom were tested but did not reveal positive carriers.[16] Two years after the genetic test became available, a publication indicated a reduction in the number of FIS-affected Fell foals, and none diagnosed in the Dales population, supporting the use of the genetic test for appropriate breeding planning.[17] The exclusive use of carrier-negative horses in breeding is challenged by the limited number of horses and genetic pool of Fell and Dales populations, and the high frequency of heterozygotes. Consequently, the use of carriers in breeding has been adopted by some breeders, which may be a necessary delay in the removal of this genetic mutation from these rare breeds.

Severe combined immunodeficiency

SCID is an autosomal-recessive hereditary condition that affects the development of B and T cells in male and female foals of the Arabian breed,[18] and potentially other breed lines that carry Arabian ancestors in their pedigree, as described in an Appaloosa foal.[19] Affected foals are apparently normal at birth, but infections of the respiratory and gastrointestinal tracts involving bacteria, virus, and opportunistic organisms manifest within 2 months of age.[19–21] In affected foals, the thymus has a paucity of lymphocytes and is infiltrated by adipose tissue instead.[22] The lymph nodes and spleen are hypocellular and lack germinal centers and periarteriolar lymphocytic sheaths, respectively.[23,24] These foals present with severe and persistent peripheral blood lymphopenia (<1000 cells/uL); serum IgM is undetectable, and serum IgG concentration reflects solely colostrum-derived antibodies.[25]

Treatment of infections in SCID-affected foals is challenging, and the condition is always fatal.[18] Nevertheless, a functional immune system was achieved in an SCID-affected foal after a successful experimental transplantation of bone marrow and thymic cells from a healthy histocompatible full sibling.[26]

The absence of B and T cells in SCID-affected foals is caused by failure of V(D)J gene recombination during B and T development. A 5-base-pair deletion (TCTCA) in the gene encoding DNA-dependent protein kinase catalytic subunit (DNA-PKc) on chromosome 9 results in a frame-shift mutation and premature stop codon, which prevents translation of the 967 C-terminal amino acids of the protein.[27,28] The inactive DNA-PKc protein prevents B- and T-receptor variable region development, and the formation of coding joints and signal joints. The gene must be disrupted in both chromosome alleles in the affected foal (homozygous). Carrier horses are heterozygous for the defective gene and are immunocompetent. However, there may be some immunologic deficit in SCID heterozygotes, because it has been reported that there is a higher incidence of sarcoid tumors in Arabian horses carrying 1 copy of the mutant SCID gene.[29]

The definitive diagnosis of affected foals and carriers is made by DNA testing using whole blood, cheek swab, or pulled hair samples.[30] Several commercial laboratories offer this test. The test should be performed in all Arabian and Arabian-crossbred horses used for breeding. The mating of heterozygous carriers will produce an affected foal in 25% of the offspring. Therefore, in order to decrease the prevalence of the defective gene in the horse population, only horses without the genetic defect should be used in breeding.

Indeed, the prevalence of carriers in the Arabian breed seems to be decreasing: using the genetic test in random samples from a population of Arabian horses, the calculated prevalence of SCID-carriers was 8.4% (21 out of 250) in the United States[31] and 2.8% (3 out of 106) in the United Kingdom decades ago.[32] More recently, the single-allele SCID mutation was diagnosed in 3 out of 808 (q = 0.00185) Arabian horses in Poland[33]; no carriers were diagnosed in a random population of Arabian horses in Egypt.[34] Different causal SCID-associated mutations have been described in other species and could potentially be involved in unexplained SCID of other horse breeds.[33,35]

Common variable immunodeficiency

CVID in the horse is caused by a rare late-onset B-cell lymphopenia and consequent inadequate antibody production.[36,37] Clinical signs of fevers and recurrent infections and septicemia with encapsulated bacteria manifest often in adulthood (average age 10 years, range 2–23 years).[36] Affected animals are unrelated adult horses of both sexes, different breeds (including thoroughbred, quarter horse, Arabian, warm-blood, paint, pony), living in distinct geographic areas. Short-term medical management of CVID-affected horses is possible, but euthanasia is often elected because of high costs of care, unavailable immunoglobulin replacement, and poor quality of life.

Peripheral blood lymphocyte immunophenotyping reveals persistent severe B-cell lymphopenia (distribution <2% of total lymphocytes).[36] Secondary lymphoid tissues are hypoplastic and lack germinal centers; peripheral absolute lymphopenia can be intermittent or persistent. Serum IgG concentration is often less than protective levels (<800 mg/dL), and serum IgM concentration is often less than normal reference interval (<25 mg/dL).

B-cell depletion is caused by impaired B-cell differentiation, which is coordinated by a network of transcription factors with epigenetic regulation at promoter or regulatory gene expression sites.[38] Using transcriptome analysis and real-time quantitative reverse transcription polymerase chain reaction (PCR) of bone marrow samples, the expression of key early B-cell commitment genes, including *E2A* and *PAX5*, was found to be significantly decreased in CVID-affected horses when compared with healthy horses. In addition, *PAX5* downstream target genes are also significantly reduced in CVID-affected horses, including *CD19*, *IGHM*, and *IGHD*.[39] Hypermethylation of the enhancer region of the *PAX5* gene has been shown in CVID-affected bone marrow samples using genome-wide reduced representation bisulfate sequencing and bisulfate PCR sequencing.[40] Developmental failure in the transition between pre-pro-B cells and pro-B cells in the bone marrow seems progressive, which leads to total B-cell depletion in secondary lymphoid tissues and blood. No genetic mutations have been identified to date, and events that affect upstream gene expression are under investigation.

Infectious Diseases with a Genetic Immune Component

The prior section dealt with 2 genetic diseases, Fell pony immunodeficiency syndrome and SCID disease of Arabians, and a third condition, common variable immunodeficiency disease, that result in profound reductions in the ability of affected horses to fight off many types of pathogens, and which also render the horses susceptible to opportunistic infections. In this section, the authors consider the role of genetics in infection by specific pathogens.

Variants of the CXCL16 chemokine gene associated with equine arteritis virus susceptibility

Infection with equine arteritis virus (EAV) usually causes a mild or unapparent disease in adult horses, but it can lead to abortion in pregnant mares, fatal infections in foals, and a state of persistent infection in stallions with continual shedding of virus in semen.[41–43] A disparity in EAV infection rates has been observed between breeds; EAV is considered to be endemic in standardbreds, whereas only 5% of thoroughbreds are seropositive for EAV (reviewed in Refs.[42,44]).

Based on this extreme breed bias in EAV prevalence, a GWAS was undertaken to identify possible genetic factors that might influence EAV infections. With the use of an in vitro assay for EAV cellular infection, a small cohort of horses was sorted into susceptible or resistant groups and then genotyped with the Equine SNP50 BeadChip array.[45] One SNP on chromosome ECA11, BIEC2-157867, was significantly different between the groups.[45] The genetic association was confirmed using an independent assay, with additional horses tested that represented American saddlebreds, quarter horses, standardbreds, and thoroughbreds. The investigators observed that, among the 60 standardbred horses studied, almost all carried the susceptibility haplotype,[45] consistent with the observation of the high prevalence of EAV infection in the breed.[42,44,45]

Sequencing of the region surrounding the BIEC2-157867 SNP in DNA from 1 resistant and 2 susceptible horses revealed a characteristic set of linked differences (haplotypes) that distinguished the resistant and susceptible horses.[46] These informative SNPs were located in exon 1 of the gene encoding the *CXCL16* chemokine. The EqCXCL16S (S for susceptibility) haplotype was 100% associated with EAV infection phenotypes.[46] Stallions with known EAV carrier status were then genotyped, and 86% of those with long-term EAV carrier status carried at least 1 copy of the EqCXCL16S genotype, whereas 73% of EAV noncarriers were homozygous for the EqCXCL16R genotype.[46] In all genotype versus phenotype comparisons, it became apparent that the susceptibility allele (EqCXCL16S genotype) was dominant over the resistant EqCXCL16R genotype.[46] The EqCXCL16 chemokine exists as a cell membrane–bound form and as a secreted form. Elegant transfection experiments demonstrated that the EqCXCL16S transmembrane protein acts as a receptor for EAV.[47] These landmark studies have advanced the understanding of the pathogenesis of equine viral arteritis and also its peculiar breed distribution.

Immune gene variation link to West Nile virus susceptibility

West Nile virus (WNV) is a flavivirus that is transmitted to horses by mosquitoes that have fed on infected birds.[48] WNV has been detected on every continent except Antarctica, and many horse breeds are susceptible to disease.[48,49] Although most horses endure subclinical disease accompanied by seroconversion, nearly 10% of horses develop encephalomyelitis with ataxia, and fatality rates greater than 20% have been reported.[48,50–52] Fortunately, several effective licensed vaccines are available.[48,50]

Studies in humans[53] and mice[54] have linked variations in the *OAS1* gene, which encodes 2′-5′ oligoadenylate synthase 1, to susceptibility to flavivirus infections. As part of the innate immune system, OAS proteins are induced by interferons and activated by double-stranded RNA and trigger the breakdown of viral and cellular RNA by ribonuclease L (RNASEL).[55,56] Rios and colleagues[57] described the equine *OAS1* and *RNASEL* genes, including several polymorphic sites. Subsequently, genotyping for SNPs in equine *OAS1* and *RNASEL* was performed in horses that were exposed to WNV and either developed subclinical (control population) or clinical encephalitis (case population).[58] A single common haplotype comprising 6 SNPs was significantly ($P = 4.953E-06$) associated with WNV susceptibility.[58] Functional assays to measure the effect of these SNPs on the ability of the *OAS1* promoter to respond to interferon induction suggested that promoter activity might be decreased when the susceptible SNP haplotype is present.[58]

Two other studies sought genetic associations between WNV pathogenesis and selected candidate immune system genes. The first study assessed horses in the Camargue region of France, where WNV is endemic.[59,60] Horses were phenotyped into 3 categories (seronegative; seropositive with subclinical disease; or seropositive with clinical disease) and further grouped by breed (Camargue or other breeds).[60] No significant associations were identified with single-genetic markers but, when markers were combined into compound 2-gene genotypes, several associations were detected. The second study focused on Romanian semiferal horses in the Danube Delta Biosphere Reserve.[61] In this study, horses were phenotyped for IgG antibodies specific for the WNV envelope protein and classified as seropositive or seronegative. As in the previous study, no markers were significantly associated with WNV individually; however, analysis of compound genotypes identified some significant associations.

Genotypes comprising MHC and LY49 alleles were associated with WNV in both studies, although the particular markers differed among the comparisons.[60,61] MHC and LY49 represent large and complicated loci, and so further refinement is needed to appreciate the biological role of the association detected. The markers associated with only 1 population require additional research to confirm their validity.

Genetic predisposition to Rhodococcus equi pneumonia

Pneumonia in young foals is commonly caused by R equi, a gram-positive facultative intracellular bacterium.[62] Clinical manifestations vary, ranging from subclinical disease detected only by the use of ultrasonography to clinical disease manifesting in pyogranulomatous pneumonia, with some lethal infections.[62,63] A confounding aspect of R equi epidemiology is that, although virulent R equi is easily found in the soil of many horse-breeding farms, the incidence of R equi pneumonia in foals is variable.[62,64] The variability of disease given the pathogen prevalence combined with anecdotal evidence of familial susceptibility or resistance to developing R equi pneumonia has led to the suggestion of a polygenic genetic basis contributing to disease manifestation.[65]

A GWAS using the EquineSNP70 array was performed on foals with clinical pneumonia caused by R equi, foals with subclinical pneumonia, and unaffected foals.[66] A region on equine chromosome 26 was associated with R equi infection ($P \leq 6.78E-05$) that included SNP UKUL3936.[66] This genomic region encompasses the TRPM2 gene, which encodes the transient receptor potential cation channel subfamily M member 2 protein. TRPM2 participates in forming neutrophil extracellular traps and contributes to antimicrobial control of pneumonic bacterial infection.[67] Although loss of TRPM2 function could be consistent with increased susceptibility to R equi infection, the UKUL3936 SNP is a synonymous variant that does not change the amino acid sequence and so is likely to be a disease marker rather than a causal variant.[68] Although a small RNA-seq study focused on TRPM2 was performed, the functional role of the UKUL3936 SNP has not yet been defined.[68]

The equine solute carrier family 11 member 1 (SLC11A1) gene (also known as Nramp1) is a robust candidate for a genetic marker of resistance to R equi infection because (1) SLC11A1 gene variants are associated with disease and reduced control of bacterial growth in other species; (2) SLC11A1 is expressed in macrophages, the cell type used for R equi replication; and (3) SLC11A1 has a role in regulating intracellular iron concentrations, which are essential for R equi survival.[69–71] SNPs in the equine SLC11A1 gene were identified, and then these SNP allele genotypes were determined for foals with and without R equi pneumonia on 3 unrelated farms. One SLC11A1 variant, SNP-57, the -57C allele was found more frequently in control foals on 2 of the farms.[72] The functional consequence of this SNP is not known.

Transferrin is responsible for iron transport and the homeostasis of iron levels in plasma.[73] It has been shown that iron sequestration mediated by transferrin can restrict the growth of gram-negative and gram-positive bacteria, as well as fungi.[74]

At least 15 transferrin polymorphisms can be identified in horses with biochemical and SNP typing.[75–77] Transferrin allele frequencies were measured in a cohort of foals that died as a consequence of *R equi* infection.[76] When compared with healthy control populations, the group of *R equi*–affected foals harbored an overrepresentation of the transferrin *F* allele, whereas the *D* allele was underrepresented (*P*<.05).[76] A separate study compared transferrin types with the incidence and severity of clinical respiratory disease in foals.[77] The transferrin *F2* allele was associated with foals that exhibited more severe disease (*P*<.0001), and the *D* allele was associated with foals that exhibited less severe disease (*P*<.0001).[77] These independent studies suggest that the transferrin *D* allele may impart a protective effect on foals with bacterial respiratory infections, whereas those carrying the *F* or *F2* alleles are more likely to incur severe clinical disease. The mechanism underlying the association between equine transferrin alleles and disease susceptibility may be due to differences in the capacity of iron sequestration between transferrin variants leading to differences in microbial growth restriction.

An effort to identify associations between polymorphisms near immune genes and susceptibility to *R equi* infection was made using microsatellite typing on a cohort of thoroughbred foals on a single farm. No significant associations were found when infected foal genotypes were compared with those of controls. However, a subsequent analysis stratified foals into "extreme phenotypes" based on the sum of clinical signs, when *R equi* was detected and the number of *R equi* colonies was detected in transtracheal aspirate. By this phenotyping method, the 6 most-susceptible and 25 least-susceptible foals were compared, and a significant difference in HMS01 microsatellite genotypes was detected.[78] A subsequent study of the same extreme phenotypes foal cohort identified an association between *R equi* infection and interleukin-7 receptor variant IL7R168T/C.[79]

Lawsonia intracellularis susceptibility linked to variation near immune genes
Associations between polymorphic genetic markers and *L intracellularis* infection were identified in a group of thoroughbred foals.[78] Individually, polymorphic microsatellites HTG06, HTG10, and HMS03 were significantly linked to *L intracellularis* infection (*P*≤.03), and the combination of HTG10 allele 101 with HMS03 allele 160 demonstrated a higher level of significance (*P* = .005). Several immune genes are located near these microsatellite markers, including β-defensins, granzyme A (CTLA3), complement component C9, cytokine IL-1B, and cytokine receptors IL-1RN and IL-7R. The authors posit that these immune genes are responsible for the differences in fecal shedding of *L intracellularis*.[78]

Genetic predisposition bacterial, viral, and fungal infections
An investigation into the potential for genetic variation in the collagenous lectin gene family to predispose horses to increased susceptibility to bacterial, viral, and fungal pathogens was performed using targeted resequencing on 89 horses, 37 of which had infectious or autoinflammatory disease and the remaining 52 were healthy.[80] Analysis of coding regions, introns, and flanking regions of 12 genes from 89 horses yielded 4174 SNPs and 385 small insertions or deletions. Of these, 113 variants exhibited significant differences in allele frequency between healthy horses and those with disease. Although more work is needed to establish significant associations between individual variants and specific pathogens or clinical presentations, this report provides an abundant starting point.

The family of collagenous lectin genes encompasses secreted pattern recognition proteins of the innate immune system, such as mannose binding lectins 1 and 2

(MBL1 and MBL2, respectively), ficolins, collectins, surfactant proteins A and D (SFTPA1 and SFTPD, respectively), as well as proteins responsible for activating the proteolytic cascade such as MBL-associated serine proteases (MASP-1, 2, 3).[81] Thus, mutations in collagenous lectin genes could impair pathogen detection and/or lysis of pathogens or infected host cells. Collagenous lectin gene mutations have been associated with susceptibility to sepsis, atypical pneumonia, and bacteremia in humans as well as mastitis in cattle.[82–86] Other than the report of a significant reduction in MBL serum levels in sick horses, little is known about collagenous lectins in the horse.[87]

The Major Histocompatibility Complex and Equine Disease

The MHC is one of the most important genetic regions governing immune responses in vertebrates. The MHC region contains clusters of closely related genes (the MHC class I and class II genes) that encode proteins that function in antigen presentation to thymus-derived lymphocytes (T cells).[2] The genes of the MHC display an enormous amount of variability within species, a property that is thought to contribute to species survival and immune capacity against infectious disease through heterozygote advantage.[88]

Since the first description of an association between human MHC genes and disease 50 years ago, thousands of studies have probed the relationship between the MHC region and susceptibility or resistance to a large number of conditions.[89] The human MHC region is called HLA, for human leukocyte antigen. Most of the investigations involved case-control studies in which individuals were phenotyped for a disease and genotyped for specific HLA alleles. A typical outcome of such research demonstrates that a particular HLA allele is found more frequently in cases versus controls. The interpretation is that the associated HLA allele appears to lead to increased predisposition for the condition under study. Despite tremendous efforts, few mechanisms of MHC disease associations have been elucidated.

It was natural for equine researchers to seek similar linkages between the equine MHC region and diseases of the horse. MHC region associations have been reported and confirmed in 3 conditions: sarcoid tumors, insect bite hypersensitivity (IBH; also known as sweet itch), and uveitis.

The equine major histocompatibility complex and sarcoid tumors

The earliest linkage between the equine MHC and sarcoid tumors was reported more than 30 years ago, when Lazary and colleagues[90] described associations between 3 serologically detected equine leukocyte antigen (ELA) alleles in riding horses of Irish, Swiss, and French breeding. Subsequent research identified an association with one of those ELA alleles and sarcoid in thoroughbreds,[91] and in Swedish half-breds.[92] Very strong evidence of transmission of sarcoid susceptibility with particular ELA alleles was later shown in a family study of paternal half-siblings.[93]

A GWAS using an equine SNP array in a large cohort of several breeds, including American quarter horses and thoroughbreds from the United Kingdom, confirmed the earlier MHC region association that had been detected using serologic techniques.[94] However, a separate GWAS study identified a region on ECA20, but not within the MHC.[95] The reason for this discrepancy is not clear. At the level of breed predisposition, in a retrospective study of more than 19,000 equine cases, it was observed that sarcoid was rarely diagnosed in standardbred horses.[96] This finding supports the MHC association with sarcoid susceptibility because the ELA-A3 haplotype that was often linked to sarcoid is very rare in standardbreds.[97]

The sarcoid-MHC association is of interest for several reasons. It is now widely considered that sarcoid tumors are caused by infection with bovine papillomavirus or a closely related equine virus.[98] Thus, sarcoid is an example of a virus-induced cancer with a strong host genetic component. Sarcoid is also the most common neoplasm of the horse. Its course can be highly variable, and sarcoids are challenging to treat.[99] Associations between HLA region alleles and human papillomavirus–induced cervical carcinoma have been shown in many populations.[100–102] Furthermore, linkage between rabbit MHC class II genes and progression of tumors caused by cottontail rabbit papillomavirus has also been shown.[103] It seems likely that a common mechanism may underlie these MHC-tumor associations in 3 distinct species.

The major histocompatibility complex and insect bite hypersensitivity

Similar to the situation with sarcoid, veterinary geneticists have explored associations between equine MHC alleles and susceptibility to IBH, a severe allergic immune reaction induced by bites of midges of the genus *Culicoides*. This condition is particularly important in Icelandic horses that have been exported as adults to Europe, but it also occurs in their offspring, although at lower incidence.[104] The initial reports of linkage between ELA alleles and IBH in Icelandic horses determined using serologic techniques[93,105] were later confirmed and extended to another breed (Exmoor ponies) using intra-MHC microsatellites.[106] IBH was also linked to the MHC using the SNP670 array in Friesian horses.[107] Other studies using SNP arrays in Icelandic horses,[108] Exmoor ponies,[109] and Dutch Shetland ponies[110] failed to identify associations within the MHC region. Thus, the validity of the MHC association with IBH remains unresolved.

The major histocompatibility complex and spontaneous recurrent uveitis: a moving target

The first evidence for a genetic predisposition to spontaneous recurrent uveitis in the horse was reported 1988, in a large retrospective study of more than 16,000 equine cases from the Cornell Large Animal Hospital and more than 3000 samples from the New York State Veterinary Diagnostic Laboratory obtained during the same period.[96] In that study, the Appaloosa was overrepresented among uveitis cases compared with other breeds, suggesting a genetic basis for susceptibility. Deeg and colleagues[111] reported an association between the ELA-A9 MHC haplotype and the occurrence of uveitis in a population of German warmblood horses. A decade later, Fritz and colleagues[112] reported an association between intra-MHC microsatellite markers and the presence of uveitis in 2 populations of Appaloosa horses. More recent studies using SNP arrays identified genomic regions associated with recurrent uveitis in German warmbloods[113] and Appaloosas,[114] but neither study confirmed the previously reported MHC association. Thus, as for IBH, the evidence for a genetic predisposition and immune system involvement in pathogenesis is clear, but the specific genetic mechanisms are unknown.

SUMMARY

Genetic studies in the horse are always challenging because of the small number of animals usually available for testing, the long generation time of horses, and the rarity of large full-sibling families for segregation studies. The well-known redundancy of immune defense mechanisms adds to those challenges in investigations of genetic factors in equine diseases involving the immune system. Despite these difficulties, the characterization of SCID disease in Arabian horses stands out as a tremendous accomplishment for equine science. Hence, too, the MHC-disease associations pioneered by the equine immunology group at the University of Bern in Switzerland have largely stood the test of time. The new genome-level assays and tools now available to equine geneticists and clinicians hold promise for more discoveries in the years to come.

ACKNOWLEDGMENTS

The authors thank the horse owners who kindly provided samples for some of the studies described here. This research was supported in part by the Harry M. Zweig Memorial Fund for Equine Research and by NIH grants AI079796 and NIH OD007216 to M.J.B. Felippe. D.F. Antczak is an investigator of the Dorothy Russell Havemeyer Foundation, Inc.

DISCLOSURE

The authors have nothing to disclose.

REFERENCES

1. Kelley J, de Bono B, Trowsdale J. IRIS: a database surveying known human immune system genes. Genomics 2005;85:503–11.
2. Murphy K, Weaver C. Janeway's immunobiology. New York: Garland Science; 2017.
3. Banks KL, McGuire TC, Jerrells TR. Absence of B lymphocytes in a horse with primary agammaglobulinemia. Clin Immunol Immunopathol 1976;5:282–90.
4. Perryman LE, McGuire TC, Hilbert BJ. Selective immunoglobulin M deficiency in foals. J Am Vet Med Assoc 1977;170:212–5.
5. Flaminio MJ, Rush BR, Cox JH, et al. CD4+ and CD8+ T-lymphocytopenia in a filly with Pneumocystis carinii pneumonia. Aust Vet J 1998;76:399–402.
6. Scholes SF, Holliman A, May PD, et al. A syndrome of anaemia, immunodeficiency and peripheral ganglionopathy in Fell pony foals. Vet Rec 1998;142:128–34.
7. Richards AJ, Kelly DF, Knottenbelt DC, et al. Anaemia, diarrhoea and opportunistic infections in Fell ponies. Equine Vet J 2000;32:386–91.
8. Dixon JB, Savage M, Wattret A, et al. Discriminant and multiple regression analysis of anemia and opportunistic infection in Fell pony foals. Vet Clin Pathol 2000;29:84–6.
9. Fox-Clipsham L, Swinburne JE, Papoula-Pereira RI, et al. Immunodeficiency/anaemia syndrome in a Dales pony. Vet Rec 2009;165:289–90.
10. Thomas GW, Bell SC, Phythian C, et al. Aid to the antemortem diagnosis of Fell pony foal syndrome by the analysis of B lymphocytes. Vet Rec 2003;152:618–21.
11. Gardner RB, Hart KA, Stokol T, et al. Fell Pony syndrome in a pony in North America. J Vet Intern Med 2006;20:198–203.
12. Tallmadge RL, Stokol T, Gould-Earley MJ, et al. Fell Pony syndrome: characterization of developmental hematopoiesis failure and associated gene expression profiles. Clin Vaccin Immunol 2012;19:1054–64.
13. Bell SC, Savidge C, Taylor P, et al. An immunodeficiency in Fell ponies: a preliminary study into cellular responses. Equine Vet J 2001;33:687–92.
14. Thomas GW, Bell SC, Carter SD. Immunoglobulin and peripheral B-lymphocyte concentrations in Fell pony foal syndrome. Equine Vet J 2005;37:48–52.

15. Fox-Clipsham LY, Carter SD, Goodhead I, et al. Identification of a mutation associated with fatal foal immunodeficiency syndrome in the Fell and Dales pony. PLoS Genet 2011;7:e1002133.

16. Fox-Clipsham LY, Brown EE, Carter SD, et al. Population screening of endangered horse breeds for the foal immunodeficiency syndrome mutation. Vet Rec 2011;169:655.

17. Carter SD, Fox-Clipsham LY, Christley R, et al. Foal immunodeficiency syndrome: carrier testing has markedly reduced disease incidence. Vet Rec 2013;172:398.

18. McGuire TC, Poppie MJ, Banks KL. Combined (B- and T-lymphocyte) immunodeficiency: a fatal genetic disease in Arabian foals. J Am Vet Med Assoc 1974; 164:70–6.

19. Perryman LE, Boreson CR, Conaway MW, et al. Combined immunodeficiency in an Appaloosa foal. Vet Pathol 1984;21:547–8.

20. Mair TS, Taylor FG, Harbour DA, et al. Concurrent cryptosporidium and coronavirus infections in an Arabian foal with combined immunodeficiency syndrome. Vet Rec 1990;126:127–30.

21. Thompson DB, Spradborw PB, Studdert M. Isolation of an adenovirus from an Arab foal with a combined immunodeficiency disease. Aust Vet J 1976;52: 435–7.

22. McGuire TC, Banks KL, Davis WC. Alterations of the thymus and other lymphoid tissue in young horses with combined immunodeficiency. Am J Pathol 1976;84: 39–54.

23. Wyatt CR, Magnuson NS, Perryman LE. Defective thymocyte maturation in horses with severe combined immunodeficiency. J Immunol 1987;139:4072–6.

24. McGuire TC, Banks KL, Poppie MJ. Combined immunodeficiency in horses: characterization of the lymphocyte defect. Clin Immunol Immunopathol 1975; 3:555–66.

25. Lew AM, Hosking CS, Studdert MJ. Immunologic aspects of combined immunodeficiency disease in Arabian foals. Am J Vet Res 1980;41:1161–6.

26. Bue CM, Davis WC, Magnuson NS, et al. Correction of equine severe combined immunodeficiency by bone marrow transplantation. Transplantation 1986; 42:14–9.

27. Wiler R, Leber R, Moore BB, et al. Equine severe combined immunodeficiency: a defect in V(D)J recombination and DNA-dependent protein kinase activity. Proc Natl Acad Sci U S A 1995;92:11485–9.

28. Shin EK, Perryman LE, Meek K. A kinase-negative mutation of DNA-PK(CS) in equine SCID results in defective coding and signal joint formation. J Immunol 1997;158:3565–9.

29. Ding Q, Bramble L, Yuzbasiyan-Gurkan V, et al. DNA-PKcs mutations in dogs and horses: allele frequency and association with neoplasia. Gene 2002;283: 263–9.

30. Shin EK, Perryman LE, Meek K. Evaluation of a test for identification of Arabian horses heterozygous for the severe combined immunodeficiency trait. J Am Vet Med Assoc 1997;211:1268–70.

31. Bernoco D, Bailey E. Frequency of the SCID gene among Arabian horses in the USA. Anim Genet 1998;29:41–2.

32. Swinburne J, Lockhart L, Scott M, et al. Estimation of the prevalence of severe combined immunodeficiency disease in UK Arab horses as determined by a DNA-based test. Vet Rec 1999;145:22–3.

33. Bugno-Poniewierska M, Stefaniuk-Szmukier M, Kajtoch AP, et al. Genetic screening for cerebellar abiotrophy, severe combined immunodeficiency and lavender foal syndrome in Arabian horses in Poland. Vet J 2019;248:71–3.

34. AbouEl Ela NA, El-Nesr KA, Ahmed HA, et al. Molecular detection of severe combined immunodeficiency disorder in Arabian horses in Egypt. J Equine Vet Sci 2018;68:55–8.

35. Larson J, Buechner-Maxwell V, Crisman MV, et al. Severe combined immunodeficiency in a Caspian filly. J Vet Intern Med 2011;25:954–8.

36. Flaminio MJ, LaCombe V, Kohn CW, et al. Common variable immunodeficiency in a horse. J Am Vet Med Assoc 2002;221:1296–302, 1267.

37. Flaminio MJ, Tallmadge RL, Salles-Gomes CO, et al. Common variable immunodeficiency in horses is characterized by B cell depletion in primary and secondary lymphoid tissues. J Clin Immunol 2009;29:107–16.

38. Hagman J, Lukin K. Transcription factors drive B cell development. Curr Opin Immunol 2006;18:127–34.

39. Tallmadge RL, Such KA, Miller KC, et al. Expression of essential B cell development genes in horses with common variable immunodeficiency. Mol Immunol 2012;51:169–76.

40. Tallmadge RL, Shen L, Tseng CT, et al. Bone marrow transcriptome and epigenome profiles of equine common variable immunodeficiency patients unveil block of B lymphocyte differentiation. Clin Immunol 2015;160:261–76.

41. Balasuriya UBR, MacLachlan NJ. The immune response to equine arteritis virus: potential lessons for other arteriviruses. Vet Immunol Immunopathol 2004;102:107–29.

42. Timoney PJ, McCollum WH. Equine viral arteritis. Vet Clin North Am Equine Pract 1993;9:295–309.

43. Timoney PJ, McCollum WH, Roberts AW, et al. Demonstration of the carrier state in naturally acquired equine arteritis virus infection in the stallion. Res Vet Sci 1986;41:279–80.

44. Balasuriya UBR, MacLachlan NJ. Chapter 14–Equine viral arteritis. In: Sellon DC, Long MT, editors. Equine infectious diseases. Saint Louis (MO): W.B. Saunders; 2007. p. 153–64.

45. Go YY, Bailey E, Cook DG, et al. Genome-wide association study among four horse breeds identifies a common haplotype associated with in vitro CD3+ T cell susceptibility/resistance to equine arteritis virus infection. J Virol 2011; 85:13174–84.

46. Sarkar S, Bailey E, Go YY, et al. Allelic variation in CXCL16 determines CD3+ T lymphocyte susceptibility to equine arteritis virus infection and establishment of long-term carrier state in the stallion. PLoS Genet 2016;12:e1006467.

47. Sarkar S, Chelvarajan L, Go YY, et al. Equine arteritis virus uses equine CXCL16 as an entry receptor. J Virol 2016;90:3366–84.

48. Angenvoort J, Brault AC, Bowen RA, et al. West Nile viral infection of equids. Vet Microbiol 2013;167:168–80.

49. Chancey C, Grinev A, Volkova E, et al. The global ecology and epidemiology of West Nile virus. Biomed Res Int 2015;2015:376230.

50. Gardner IA, Wong SJ, Ferraro GL, et al. Incidence and effects of West Nile virus infection in vaccinated and unvaccinated horses in California. Vet Res 2007;38:109–16.

51. Ostlund EN, Crom RL, Pedersen DD, et al. Equine West Nile encephalitis, United States. Emerg Infect Dis 2001;7:665–9.

52. Schuler LA, Khaitsa ML, Dyer NW, et al. Evaluation of an outbreak of West Nile virus infection in horses: 569 cases (2002). J Am Vet Med Assoc 2004;225: 1084–9.

53. Lim JK, Lisco A, McDermott DH, et al. Genetic variation in OAS1 is a risk factor for initial infection with West Nile virus in man. PLoS Pathog 2009;5:e1000321.

54. Mashimo T, Lucas M, Simon-Chazottes D, et al. A nonsense mutation in the gene encoding 2'-5'-oligoadenylate synthetase/L1 isoform is associated with West Nile virus susceptibility in laboratory mice. Proc Natl Acad Sci U S A 2002;99: 11311–6.

55. Hovanessian AG, Brown RE, Kerr IM. Synthesis of low molecular weight inhibitor of protein synthesis with enzyme from interferon-treated cells. Nature 1977;268: 537–40.

56. Kerr IM, Brown RE, Hovanessian AG. Nature of inhibitor of cell-free protein synthesis formed in response to interferon and double-stranded RNA. Nature 1977; 268:540–2.

57. Rios JJ, Perelygin AA, Long MT, et al. Characterization of the equine 2'-5' oligoadenylate synthetase 1 (OAS1) and ribonuclease L (RNASEL) innate immunity genes. BMC Genomics 2007;8:313.

58. Rios JJ, Fleming JGW, Bryant UK, et al. OAS1 polymorphisms are associated with susceptibility to West Nile encephalitis in horses. PLoS One 2010;5:e10537.

59. Bahuon C, Marcillaud-Pitel C, Bournez L, et al. West Nile virus epizootics in the Camargue (France) in 2015 and reinforcement of surveillance and control networks. Rev Sci Tech 2016;35:811–24.

60. Stejskalova K, Cvanova M, Oppelt J, et al. Genetic susceptibility to West Nile virus infection in Camargue horses. Res Vet Sci 2019;124:284–92.

61. Stejskalova K, Janova E, Horecky C, et al. Associations between the presence of specific antibodies to the West Nile virus infection and candidate genes in Romanian horses from the Danube Delta. Mol Biol Rep 2019;46:4453–61.

62. Giguère S, Cohen ND, Chaffin MK, et al. Diagnosis, treatment, control, and prevention of infections caused by Rhodococcus equi in foals. J Vet Intern Med 2011;25:1209–20.

63. Giguère S. Treatment of infections caused by Rhodococcus equi. Vet Clin North Am Equine Pract 2017;33:67–85.

64. Cohen ND, Carter CN, Scott HM, et al. Association of soil concentrations of Rhodococcus equi and incidence of pneumonia attributable to Rhodococcus equi in foals on farms in central Kentucky. Am J Vet Res 2008;69:385–95.

65. McQueen CM, Dindot SV, Foster MJ, et al. Genetic susceptibility to Rhodococcus equi. J Vet Intern Med 2015;29:1648–59.

66. McQueen CM, Doan R, Dindot SV, et al. Identification of genomic loci associated with Rhodococcus equi susceptibility in foals. PLoS One 2014;9:e98710.

67. Tripathi JK, Sharma A, Sukumaran P, et al. Oxidant sensor cation channel TRPM2 regulates neutrophil extracellular trap formation and protects against pneumoseptic bacterial infection. FASEB J 2018;32:6848–59.

68. McQueen CM, Whitfield-Cargile CM, Konganti K, et al. TRPM2 SNP genotype previously associated with susceptibility to Rhodococcus equi pneumonia in quarter horse foals displays differential gene expression identified using RNA-Seq. BMC Genomics 2016;17:993.

69. Govoni G, Canonne-Hergaux F, Pfeifer CG, et al. Functional expression of Nramp1 in vitro in the murine macrophage line RAW264.7. Infect Immun 1999;67:2225–32.

70. Jordan MC, Harrington JR, Cohen ND, et al. Effects of iron modulation on growth and viability of Rhodococcus equi and expression of virulence-associated protein A. Am J Vet Res 2003;64:1337–46.

71. Hondalus MK, Mosser DM. Survival and replication of Rhodococcus equi in macrophages. Infect Immun 1994;62:4167–75.

72. Halbert ND, Cohen ND, Slovis NM, et al. Variations in equid SLC11A1 (NRAMP1) genes and associations with Rhodococcus equi pneumonia in horses. J Vet Intern Med 2006;20:974–9.

73. Gkouvatsos K, Papanikolaou G, Pantopoulos K. Regulation of iron transport and the role of transferrin. Biochim Biophys Acta 2012;1820:188–202.

74. Bruhn KW, Spellberg B. Transferrin-mediated iron sequestration as a novel therapy for bacterial and fungal infections. Curr Opin Microbiol 2015;27:57–61.

75. Brandon RB, Giffard JM, Bell K. Single nucleotide polymorphisms in the equine transferrin gene. Anim Genet 1999;30:439–43.

76. Mousel MR, Harrison L, Donahue JM, et al. Rhodococcus equi and genetic susceptibility: assessing transferrin genotypes from paraffin-embedded tissues. J Vet Diagn Invest 2003;15:470–2.

77. Newton JR, Woodt JLN, Chanter N. Evidence for transferrin allele as a host-level risk factor in naturally occurring equine respiratory disease: a preliminary study. Equine Vet J 2007;39:164–71.

78. Horin P, Smola J, Matiasovic J, et al. Polymorphisms in equine immune response genes and their associations with infections. Mamm Genome 2004;15:843–50.

79. Horin P, Sabakova K, Futas J, et al. Immunity-related gene single nucleotide polymorphisms associated with Rhodococcus equi infection in foals. Int J Immunogenet 2010;37:67–71.

80. Fraser RS, Arroyo LG, Meyer A, et al. Identification of genetic variation in equine collagenous lectins using targeted resequencing. Vet Immunol Immunopathol 2018;202:153–63.

81. Dobo J, Kocsis A, Gal P. Be on target: strategies of targeting alternative and lectin pathway components in complement-mediated diseases. Front Immunol 2018;9:1851.

82. Bronkhorst MWGA, Lomax MAZ, Vossen RHAM, et al. Risk of infection and sepsis in severely injured patients related to single nucleotide polymorphisms in the lectin pathway. Br J Surg 2013;100:1818–26.

83. Chong YP, Park K-H, Kim ES, et al. Association of mannose-binding lectin 2 gene polymorphisms with persistent Staphylococcus aureus bacteremia. PLoS One 2014;9:e89139.

84. van Kempen G, Meijvis S, Endeman H, et al. Mannose-binding lectin and l-ficolin polymorphisms in patients with community-acquired pneumonia caused by intracellular pathogens. Immunology 2017;151:81–8.

85. Wang C, Liu M, Li Q, et al. Three novel single-nucleotide polymorphisms of MBL1 gene in Chinese native cattle and their associations with milk performance traits. Vet Immunol Immunopathol 2011;139:229–36.

86. Wang X, Ju Z, Huang J, et al. The relationship between the variants of the bovine MBL2 gene and milk production traits, mastitis, serum MBL-C levels and complement activity. Vet Immunol Immunopathol 2012;148:311–9.

87. Podolsky MJ, Lasker A, Flaminio MJBF, et al. Characterization of an equine mannose-binding lectin and its roles in disease. Biochem Biophys Res Commun 2006;343:928–36.

88. Meyer D, VR CA, Bitarello BD, et al. A genomic perspective on HLA evolution. Immunogenetics 2018;70:5–27.

89. Dendrou CA, Petersen J, Rossjohn J, et al. HLA variation and disease. Nat Rev Immunol 2018;18:325–39.
90. Lazary S, Gerber H, Glatt PA, et al. Equine leucocyte antigens in sarcoid-affected horses. Equine Vet J 1985;17:283–6.
91. Meredith D, Elser AH, Wolf B, et al. Equine leukocyte antigens: relationships with sarcoid tumors and laminitis in two pure breeds. Immunogenetics 1986;23:221–5.
92. Broström H, Fahlbrink E, Dubath ML, et al. Association between equine leucocyte antigens (ELA) and equine sarcoid tumors in the population of Swedish halfbreds and some of their families. Vet Immunol Immunopathol 1988;19:215–23.
93. Lazary S, Marti E, Szalai G, et al. Studies on the frequency and associations of equine leucocyte antigens in sarcoid and summer dermatitis. Anim Genet 1994;25(Suppl 1):75–80.
94. Staiger EA, Tseng CT, Miller D, et al. Host genetic influence on papillomavirus-induced tumors in the horse. Int J Cancer 2016;139:784–92.
95. Jandova V, Klukowska-Rotzler J, Dolf G, et al. Whole genome scan identifies several chromosomal regions linked to equine sarcoids. Schweiz Arch Tierheilkd 2012;154:19–25.
96. Angelos J, Oppenheim Y, Rebhun W, et al. Evaluation of breed as a risk factor for sarcoid and uveitis in horses. Anim Genet 1988;19:417–25.
97. Antczak DF, Bailey E, Barger B, et al. Joint report of the Third International Workshop on Lymphocyte Alloantigens of the horse, Kennett Square, Pennsylvania, 25-27 April 1984. Anim Genet 1986;17:363–73.
98. Nasir L, Brandt S. Papillomavirus associated diseases of the horse. Vet Microbiol 2013;167:159–67.
99. Knottenbelt DC. The equine sarcoid: why are there so many treatment options? Vet Clin North Am Equine Pract 2019;35:243–62.
100. de Araujo Souza PS, Sichero L, Maciag PC. HPV variants and HLA polymorphisms: the role of variability on the risk of cervical cancer. Future Oncol 2009;5:359–70.
101. Alaez-Verson C, Berumen-Campos J, Munguia-Saldana A, et al. HPV-16 and HLA-DRB1 alleles are associated with cervical carcinoma in Mexican Mestizo women. Arch Med Res 2011;42:421–5.
102. Wang SS, Hildesheim A, Gao X, et al. Comprehensive analysis of human leukocyte antigen class I alleles and cervical neoplasia in 3 epidemiologic studies. J Infect Dis 2002;186:598–605.
103. Han R, Breitburd F, Marche PN, et al. Linkage of regression and malignant conversion of rabbit viral papillomas to MHC class II genes. Nature 1992;356:66–8.
104. Marti E, Gerber V, Wilson AD, et al. Report of the 3rd Havemeyer workshop on allergic diseases of the horse, Hólar, Iceland, June 2007. Vet Immunol Immunopathol 2008;126:351–61.
105. Halldorsdottir S, Lazary S, Gunnarsson E, et al. Distribution of leucocyte antigens in Icelandic horses affected with summer eczema compared to non-affected horses. Equine Vet J 1991;23:300–2.
106. Andersson LS, Swinburne JE, Meadows JRS, et al. The same ELA class II risk factors confer equine insect bite hypersensitivity in two distinct populations. Immunogenetics 2012;64:201–8.
107. Schurink A, da Silva VH, Velie BD, et al. Copy number variations in Friesian horses and genetic risk factors for insect bite hypersensitivity. BMC Genet 2018;19:49.

108. Shrestha M, Eriksson S, Schurink A, et al. Genome-wide association study of insect bite hypersensitivity in Swedish-Born Icelandic horses. J Hered 2015;106: 366–74.
109. Velie BD, Shrestha M, François L, et al. Using an inbred horse breed in a high density genome-wide scan for genetic risk factors of insect bite hypersensitivity (IBH). PLoS One 2016;11:e0152966.
110. Schurink A, Ducro BJ, Bastiaansen JWM, et al. Genome-wide association study of insect bite hypersensitivity in Dutch Shetland pony mares. Anim Genet 2013; 44:44–52.
111. Deeg CA, Marti E, Gaillard C, et al. Equine recurrent uveitis is strongly associated with the MHC class I haplotype ELA-A9. Equine Vet J 2004;36:73–5.
112. Fritz KL, Kaese HJ, Valberg SJ, et al. Genetic risk factors for insidious equine recurrent uveitis in Appaloosa horses. Anim Genet 2014;45:392–9.
113. Kulbrock M, Lehner S, Metzger J, et al. A genome-wide association study identifies risk loci to equine recurrent uveitis in German warmblood horses. PLoS One 2013;8:e71619.
114. Rockwell H, Mack M, Famula T, et al. Genetic investigation of equine recurrent uveitis in Appaloosa horses. Anim Genet 2020;51:111–6.

Genetics of Equine Orthopedic Disease

Julia Metzger, Dr. med. vet., Dr. habil*, Ottmar Distl, Dr. med. vet., Dr. habil

KEYWORDS

• Orthopedics • Genetic disposition • Osteochondrosis • Horse

KEY POINTS

- Orthopedic diseases in the horse constitute an important group of defects, particularly including developmental and degenerative joint diseases, tendon and ligament defects, and defects of the skeleton and adnexal structures.
- They frequently underlie complex genetic effects, which can be breed specific or common in specific horse types.
- Thus, selective breeding approaches can reduce the genetic risk for orthopedic issues.
- Further support of veterinarians and breeders in the future is necessary to evaluate major disease-causing genetic variants supporting targeted breeding against undesirable traits.

INTRODUCTION

The modern horse is regarded as an exceptionally specialized high-performance athlete, highly selected for conformation, pronounced movement, and endurance.[1,2] For this reason, disorders of the locomotor system have a significant impact on these specific characteristics and thus severely affect the efficient use of horses in equestrian sports.[3,4] Even more, diseases of the joints and skeleton were found to be a major cause for culling of warmblood and coldblood horses.[3] Thus, because of its economic importance to the value of a horse, prepurchase radiologic examinations are frequently performed and used for genetic selection strategies against orthopedic issues.[5,6]

Genetic dispositions for orthopedic diseases have been detected in multiple horses and were often found within specific breeds or horse types. In particular, osteochondrosis (OC) and degenerative joint diseases were reported to be frequent among sports horses.[7,8] Other defects include tendons, ligaments, bone, or adnexal structures, which underlie complex genetic effects.

Institute for Animal Breeding and Genetics, University of Veterinary Medicine Hannover, Buenteweg 17p, Hannover 30559, Germany
* Corresponding author.
E-mail address: Julia.metzger@tiho-hannover.de

Vet Clin Equine 36 (2020) 289–301
https://doi.org/10.1016/j.cveq.2020.03.008
0749-0739/20/© 2020 Elsevier Inc. All rights reserved.

The aim of this review is to give a comprehensive overview of hereditary orthopedic diseases in the horse in order to provide knowledge of its phenotypic occurrences, breed dispositions, and genetic background.

OSTEOCHONDROSIS

Diseases in the joints, including developmental, acute, and chronic disorders, are commonly observed in the horse (**Table 1**).[8–10] They continue to plague performance horses and are thus subject to intense research worldwide.[11] One of these disorders, particularly common in growing individuals, is OC.[9] OC is proposed to result from an abnormal chondrocyte development and maturation causing an altered endochondral ossification.[12] This focal persistence of growth cartilage can occur in the epiphyseal or in the physeal growth plates.[13] A thicker immature cartilage and lesions of retained cartilage adjacent to the joint surface are proposed to be more susceptible to further damage within the joint or even result in a separation of osteochondral fragments designated as osteochondrosis dissecans (OCD).[12,14] Frequently affected joints are fetlock joints, talocrural joints, femoropatellar joints as well as the metacarpophalangeal and metatarsophalangeal joints.[15] Furthermore, signs of OCD can also be found in the cervical region, associated with a generalized dysmaturation and a resulting equine cervical vertebral malformation.[16] The occurrence of OC in other joints like the shoulder and hip was also reported, but suggested to be rare.[15,17]

OC at different predilection sites can occur in various different horse breeds. Prevalence estimations in studies on OC/OCD were found to be highly variable dependent on the study population and investigated radiographic findings.[8] Estimates of as many as 64% in Holsteiner, 20.7% in Hanoverian, 21.9% in Dutch warmblood, 12.5% in Swedish warmblood, 23% in Australian thoroughbred horses, 9.2% in Italian Maremmano, and 53.9% in South German coldblood were reported.[7,18–27] The prevalence in Danish trotters, Norwegian trotters, Swedish trotters, Norwegian standardbred trotters, and French trotters ranged from 10.5% to 17.0%.[28–32]

The cause for OC/OCD is thought to be multifactorial, thus associated with a genetic predisposition, weight, rapid growth, exercise, nutritional factors, and mineral imbalances.[12,31–36] However, despite the not fully understood etiopathogenesis, genetic components are known to play an essential role in the development of the disease.[14,31,32,37] Estimates of heritability for OC are in the low to moderate range of 0.02 to 0.36 in warmblood horses (Hanoverian, Holsteiner, Dutch warmblood, Swedish warmblood), 0.11 to 0.45 in trotters, 0.04 to 0.16 in South German coldblood horses, and 0.00 to 0.16 in thoroughbred horses.[7,18–32,37] For OCD, estimated heritabilities of up to 0.46 could be reached.[26] Thus, various studies have been performed using highly repetitive DNA sequences, designated as microsatellites, as well as single nucleotide polymorphisms/variants (SNPs/SNVs), which can be found within the equine genome, in order to identify risk loci for OC.[8] So far, quantitative trait loci (QTL) are proposed to be located on *Equus caballus* autosome (ECA) 2, 4, 5, 16, 18, and 21 in the Hanoverian and on ECA5, 15, 16, 17, 23, 27, 28, and 31 in the South German coldblood.[38–45] In addition to that, further QTL were found for palmar/plantar osseous fragments at the attachment sites of the short sesamoidean ligaments to the proximal phalanx in the South German coldblood, although the correlation with OC is controversially discussed.[32,45] Genome-wide association studies on BeadChip genotyping data have led to the identification of OC/OCD-associated SNPs/SNVs on ECA3, 5, 10, 16, 18, and 21 in warmblood horses and on ECA3, 10, 13, 14, 15, 21, 27, and 28 in various trotters.[29,46–49] Significantly associated variants with different locations of OC lesions in Spanish purebred horses are proposed to be on ECA2 and 4, whereas

Table 1
Hereditary orthopedic diseases in the joints

Disease	Identified Genomic Region(s) (Study Type)	Breed/Populations Under Study	Reference
OC/OCD, palmar/plantar osseous fragments at the attachment sites of the short sesamoidean ligaments to the proximal phalanx	ECA2, 4, 5, 16, 18, 21 (QTL analysis)	Hanoverian	Dierks et al,[38,42,43] 2010; Felicetti et al,[44] 2009; Lampe et al,[39–41] 2009
	ECA5, 15, 16, 17, 23, 27, 28, 31 (QTL analysis)	South German coldblood	Wittwer et al,[45] 2007
	ECA3, 5, 10, 16, 18, 21 (GWAS)	Dutch warmblood, Hanoverian	Lampe,[49] 2009; Orr et al,[46] 2013
	ECA3, 10, 13, 14, 15, 21, 27, 28 (GWAS)	French trotter, Norwegian standardbred trotters, US standardbred	Teyssedre et al,[29] 2012; Lykkjen et al,[48] 2010; McCoy et al,[47] 2016
	—	Danish trotters, Swedish trotters, Holstein, Italian Maremmano, Swedish warmblood, thoroughbred	Schougaard et al,[30] 1990; Philipsson et al,[32] 1993; Willms,[19] 1999; Pieramati et al,[20] 2003; Jönsson et al,[25] 2011; Russell et al,[27] 2017
Podotrochlosis (navicular disease)	ECA3, 10 (QTL analysis for canales sesamoidales) ECA2, 3, 4, 26 (QTL analysis for contour) ECA4, 7, 26, 29, 30, 31 (QTL analysis for structure)	Hanoverian	Diesterbeck et al,[66] 2007; Lopes et al,[57] 2010; Lopes et al,[67] 2009
Osteoarthrosis in tarsal joints (bone spavin)	—	Dutch warmblood, German warmblood, Icelandic horse	KWPN,[18] 1994; Winter et al,[7] 1996; Arnason & Bjornsdottir,[71] 2003
Osteoarthrosis in carpal joints	—	Norwegian trotter	Dolvik & Klemetsdal,[73] 1994

Identified genomic regions and studied breeds or populations are shown.
Abbreviation: GWAS, genome-wide association analysis.

Polish sport horses are thought to harbor SNPs associated with the occurrence of OC on ECA2, 4, 16, 18, and 28.[50,51] A strong association with hock-OCD could be validated across multiple horse breeds on ECA2, 3, 4, 14, 27, and 29.[8] Despite the high number of different loci and variants identified to be associated with OC/OCD, their role in disease development remains unclear. Some key risk genes, including *insulin-like growth factor-I* (*IGF1*), *runt related transcription factor 2* (*RUNX2*), *tousled-like kinase 2* (*TLK2*), *matrix metalloproteinase-13* and *-3* (*MMP-13, MMP-3*), *platelet derived growth factor subunit A* (*PDGF-A*), *Indian hedgehog homolog* (*IHH*), and *parathyroid hormone-related protein* (*PTH-RP*) are thought to affect pathways involving cartilage maturation and ossification and are thus expected to be altered in early OC.[52–56]

DEGENERATIVE DISORDERS OF THE JOINTS

Apart from cases affected by the developmental joint disease OC/OCD, such signs of lameness and altered performance can also be a result of degenerative effects on the joints. A prevalent cause of chronic and often therapy-resistant forelimb lameness is podotrochlosis, also called navicular disease.[57] The podotrochlea is composed of the navicular bone (os sesamoideum distale), the navicular bursa (bursa podotrochlearis), the distal end of the deep flexor tendon, the 3 components that are primary affected by pathologic alterations, as well as the sesamoid ligaments (collaterale laterale/mediale, distale impar).[58–60] Lameness caused by a progressive, chronic podotrochlosis usually occurs in mature riding horses.[61] However, radiographic appearance of the navicular bones in young horses can provide evidence for a higher risk of disease development.[58] Particularly the shape of the proximal articular border of the navicular bone is thought to predispose horses for radiographic findings.[58] Furthermore, signs of branched, deep, or lollypop-shaped canales sesamoidales, increased numbers of canales sesamoidales, spurs at the margins of navicular bone, or a reduced radiographic density increase the incidence of podotrochlosis.[58–60,62,63] The reasons these radiographic variances appear and podotrochlosis can subsequently occur are still unclear. However, it is proposed that genetic factors play an important role in disease development.[58,64,65] Putatively linked genomic regions with the occurrence of deformed canales sesamoidales were identified on ECA3 and 10 in Hanoverian horses.[57,66] Furthermore, QTL on ECA2, 3, 4, 26 were associated with contour of the navicular bones and on ECA4, 7, 26, 29, 30, 31 with radiologic alterations in the structure of the navicular bones.[66,67] The heritability estimations lie in between 0.06 and 0.34 for warmblood horses.[7,68,69]

Podotrochlosis is not the only condition designated as a degenerative joint disorder, called osteoarthrosis, affected by genetic components in horses. Osteoarthrosis means degeneration of the joint and is thus considered the right term for factors leading to the process of joint cartilage "tear and wear," which stands for degeneration and noninflammatory breakdown.[70] The often-used term osteoarthritis is assumed to be misleading, because inflammation is not a primary feature of the degenerative joint disease but plays a secondary or concomitant role in this condition.[70]

Thus, another considerably frequent form of osteoarthrosis in horses is bone spavin, a chronic joint-deforming disease in the tarsal joints.[69] Studies in Dutch warmblood horses estimated heritabilities of 0.16 to 0.30, whereas further investigations in German warmblood horses showed estimations of up to 0.65.[7,18,69] In Icelandic horses, medium to high heritabilities of 0.1 and 0.33 were suggested.[71] Furthermore, it is assumed that bone spavin is not associated with trauma or overloading but with conformation of the limbs and joint architecture.[72]

In addition to bone spavin, osteoarthroses can be found in the carpal joints as reported in Norwegian trotters with a prevalence of 10% and 27%.[73] Heritability estimates, based on data of 407 horses, were 0.67 and 0.25.[73]

In general, the cause of osteoarthrosis is thought to be multifactorial.[74,75] It is a complex disease process characterized by degeneration of the cartilage, subchondral bone sclerosis, synovitis, and osteophyte formation as a sign of joint instability.[76] The periarticular structures often show fibrosis leading to pain and a decreased range of motion in affected joints.[76] Osteoarthroses are classified into 3 types: type 1, a primary osteoarthrosis, often found in carpal, distal tarsal, and distal interphalangeal joints and fetlock; type 2, usually a secondary type to other joint-damaging conditions like intraarticular fractures, OCD, or septic arthritis; and type 3, which displays incidental or nonprogressive articular cartilage damage.[76,77] The relationship of osteoarthrosis to other orthopedic diseases supports the findings of a positive genetic correlation of 0.25 to 0.77 between deforming arthropathy in hock joints with osseous fragments in fetlock joints in warmblood horses.[22] Although the cause of osteoarthrosis is unclear, it is widely agreed that an increased synthesis and activation of extracellular proteinases, mainly matrix metalloproteinases, are the reason for the degradation of cartilage matrix components.[74] In addition, a deficient stimulation of growth factors is also thought to play a role in the degenerative processes potentially affecting the synthesis of new matrix macromolecules.[74] For this reason, a gene transfer of interleukin-1 receptor antagonist is considered to be a practical treatment modality in horses, which revealed a significant improvement in clinical and histologic parameters in studied equine osteoarthrosis patients.[78] Furthermore, *metalloproteinase domain-like protein decysin-1* (*ADAMDEC1*), *glucose-regulated protein* (*GRP*) *94*, *hematopoietic cell signal transducer* (*HCST*), *Unc-93 homolog A* (*hUNC-93A*), and *ribonucleotide reductase M2 polypeptide* (*RRM2*) were found to be significantly differentially expressed in peripheral white blood cells in affected horses with experimentally induced osteoarthrosis and thus considered to be potential gene biomarkers for osteoarthrosis diagnostics.[79] For this reason, veterinarians could offer such a biomarker test for diagnostics. However, breeders should be made aware that all these chronic as well as developmental joint diseases are multifactorial and underlie complex genetic mechanisms.

TENDON AND LIGAMENT DEFECTS

The locomotor system of the horse is an intricate construction of bones, joints, ligaments, and tendons, which can be disturbed by various effects on its individual components. Fibrous connective tissues, including tendons attached to muscle and bone as well as ligaments for bone-bone attachments, play an important part in this design (**Table 2**).[80] A common problem of the stifle joint particularly found in small ponies is a lateral (sub)luxation of the patella.[81,82] Affected horses show a lateral displacement of the patella at rest or movement. This luxation can be recurrent or permanent.[83] Horses with a permanent lateral displacement display a characteristic, usually bilateral, crouched hind limb stance with a flexion of the stifle as well as the hock joint.[81] This scenario occurs because of a change of the quadriceps muscles' line of force by the lateral displacement of the patella.[81] It was demonstrated in a study of affected Shetland ponies that the height of the medial and lateral trochlear ridge of the femur is not significantly different from the height in unaffected horses.[81] However, a broadening and flattening of the distal part of the medial ridge were proposed to be a characteristic feature in affected individuals leading to luxation of the patella.[81] Such

Table 2
Hereditary tendon and ligament defects

Disease	Identified Genomic Region(s) (Study Type)	Breed/Populations Under Study	Reference
Congenital lateral luxation of the patella	—	Shetland pony, miniature horse	Hermans et al,[81] 1987; Engelbert et al,[82] 1993
	—	Morgan horse, standardbred	Rooney et al,[84] 1971
Superficial digital flexor tendon injury	—	Thoroughbred	Oki et al,[87] 2008; Welsh et al,[85] 2013
Suspensory ligament injury	—	Thoroughbred	Welsh et al,[85] 2013
DSLD	ECA6, 7, 11, 14, 26 (QTL analysis)	Peruvian Paso	Strong,[90] 2005

Identified genomic regions and studied breeds or populations are shown.

hypoplasia of the lateral ridge of the trochlea was also found to be related to a lateral patellar luxation in a Morgan horse and a standardbred.[84] Experimental matings suggested a monogenic autosomal-recessive mode of inheritance for this trait.[81]

In addition to lateral patellar luxation, a significant involvement of a genetic component is also proposed for other ligament and tendon–related defects, including superficial digital flexor tendon injury, suspensory ligament injury as well as degenerative suspensory ligament desmitis (DSLD).[85] In particular, racing thoroughbreds are known to be under high risk of musculoskeletal injuries.[86] The prevalence of suspensory ligament injury and tendon injury was reported to be 10% and 19% in a study population of thoroughbred racehorses in Hong Kong.[85] In this study, a heritability of 0.047 to 0.19 for suspensory ligament injury and 0.088 to 0.203 for tendon injury was estimated.[85,87] In addition, a positive genetic correlation of fracture with osteoarthritis and suspensory ligament injury was suggested.[85] The injury of the suspensory ligament is thought to be triggered by a subclinical degeneration of the tendon matrix, which has an ultrasonographic appearance of a clinical injury with swollen areas or a subclinical injury showing only slight edema and heat.[87]

In contrast, in DSLD, disease development is more complex. DSLD affects connective tissues of the cardiovascular system, patellar and nuchal ligaments, suspensory ligaments, patellar ligaments, superficial/deep digital flexor tendons, and the sclera of the eye.[88] It is considered a systemic disorder characterized by an accumulation of excessive amounts of proteoglycans in tissues and organs with significant connective tissue component.[88] For this reason, it was also named equine systemic proteoglycan accumulation. The result is lameness at the front legs or all 4 legs without a history of trauma.[89] The high prevalence of DSLD particularly in the Peruvian Paso breed suggests a recessive mode of inheritance for the development of connective tissue defects.[90] A genome scan of DSLD affected and unaffected Peruvian Paso horses identified a significant linkage in 5 chromosomal regions on ECA6, 7, 11, 14, and 26.[90] So far, the chondroitin sulfate proteoglycan 2 (CSPG2) gene on ECA14 was sequenced but ruled out as a potential candidate for DSLD.

DEFECTS OF THE SKELETON AND ADNEXAL STRUCTURES

A developing fetus of a horse underlies various genetically programmed mechanisms for rapid early skeletal development.[91] Thus, genetic variants can have a large effect on the architecture of the skeleton, the density of the bones, or stability in the long term (**Table 3**). In thoroughbred racing horses, disturbances in bone metabolism are assumed to underlie complex genetic influences causing nontraumatic distal limb bone fractures during racing or exercise.[92] A genome-wide association analysis revealed significantly disease-associated SNPs on ECA9, 18, 22, and 31 potentially contributing to susceptibility to fracture risk.[92] Furthermore, a risk of injury can also occur in sports horses by dorsiflexion of the fetlock with a subsequent potential effect on the proximal sesamoid bones.[93] Studies on warmblood horses estimated heritabilities of 0.11 to 0.17 for the so-called sesamoiditis, which is characterized by an inflammation of the periost and bone accompanied by secondary calcification in the ligaments.[18,94,95]

In addition to the long bones, the hoof can also be subject to genetically determined defects. Unequally distributed pressure and an incorrect exterior are thought to increase the risk of an ossification of the hoof cartilage (cartilaginous ungulae).[93] In German riding horses, the heritability for ossification of cartilaginous ungulae was estimated to be 0.18.[95] In Connemara ponies, a severe hoof wall separation disease was described, characterized by a separation of the dorsal hoof wall along the weight-bearing surface of the hoof in during the first year of life.[96] An insertion within *serpin family B member 11 (SERPINB11)* resulting in a frameshift and premature stop codon is highly associated with this disease in Connemara ponies.[96]

In addition, causative variants are also known for more complex malformations of the horse's body. An abnormal growth of the ulna and fibula causing instability in the tarsocrural and antebrachiocarpal joints is considered skeletal atavism. In affected Shetland ponies, 2 large deletions associated with this trait were found in the region of short stature homeobox (SHOX).[97] Furthermore, an extreme lordosis (swayback) was observed to be frequent in American saddlebred horses.[98] The results of genome-wide association analysis show a promising association signal on ECA20, but no causative variant is known so far.[98]

Table 3				
Skeletal defects and disorders at adnexal structures				
Disease	Affected Gene(s)	Identified Variants or Genomic Region(s) (Study Type)	Breed/Populations Under Study	Reference
Bone fracture	—	ECA9, 18, 22, 31 (GWAS)	Thoroughbred	Blott et al,[92] 2014
Sesamoiditis	—		Dutch warmblood, German sports horse	KWPN,[18] 1994; Winter et al,[7] 1996
Hoof wall separation disease	SERPINB11	c.504_505insC, frameshift	Connemara pony	Finno et al,[96] 2015
Extreme lordosis (swayback)	—	ECA20 (GWAS)	American saddlebred horses	Cook et al,[98] 2010
Skeletal atavism	SHOX	2 large deletions	Miniature horse	Rafati et al,[97] 2016

Affected genes, identified genomic regions, and studied breeds or populations are shown.

SUMMARY

Orthopedic diseases in the horse constitute an important group of defects, particularly including developmental and degenerative joint diseases, tendon and ligament defects, and defects of the skeleton and adnexal structures. They frequently underlie complex genetic effects, which can be breed specific or common in specific horse types. Thus, selective breeding approaches can reduce the genetic risk for orthopedic issues. Further support of veterinarians and breeders in the future is necessary to evaluate major disease-causing genetic variants supporting targeted breeding against undesirable traits.

REFERENCES

1. Poole DC, Erickson HH. Highly athletic terrestrial mammals: horses and dogs. Compr Physiol 2011;1(1):1–37.
2. Koenen EPC, Aldridge LI, Philipsson J. An overview of breeding objectives for warmblood sport horses. Livest Prod Sci 2004;88:77–84.
3. Wallin L, Strandberg E, Philipsson J, et al. Estimates of longevity and causes of culling and death in Swedish warmblood and coldblood horses. Livest Prod Sci 2000;63(3):275–89.
4. van Oldruitenborgh-Oosterbaan MMS, Genzel W, van Weeren PR. A pilot study on factors influencing the career of Dutch sport horses. Equine Vet J 2010;42: 28–32.
5. van Hoogmoed LM, Snyder JR, Thomas HL, et al. Retrospective evaluation of equine prepurchase examinations performed 1991-2000. Equine Vet J 2003; 35(4):375–81.
6. Stock KF, Hamann H, Distl O. Estimation of genetic parameters for the prevalence of osseous fragments in limb joints of Hanoverian warmblood horses. J Anim Breed Genet 2005;122(4):271–80.
7. Winter D, Bruns E, Glodek P, et al. Genetic disposition of bone diseases in sport horses. Zuchtungskunde 1996;68(2):92–108.
8. Naccache F, Metzger J. Genetic risk factors for osteochondrosis in various horse breeds. Equine Vet J 2018;50(5):556–63.
9. Serteyn D, Piquemal D, Vanderheyden L, et al. Gene expression profiling from leukocytes of horses affected by osteochondrosis. J Orthop Res 2010;28(7): 965–70.
10. Hilla D, Distl O. Prevalence of osteochondral fragments, osteochondrosis dissecans and palmar/plantar osteochondral fragments in Hanoverian warmblood horses. Berl Munch Tierarztl Wochenschr 2013;126(5–6):236–44.
11. Caron JP, Genovese RL. Principles and practices of joint disease treatment. In: Penny Rudolph, editor. Diagnosis and management of lameness in the horse. St. Louis, Missouri: Elsevier; 2003. p. 746–64.
12. Jeffcott LB, Henson FM. Studies on growth cartilage in the horse and their application to aetiopathogenesis of dyschondroplasia (osteochondrosis). Vet J 1998; 156(3):177–92.
13. Olsson SE. General and local [corrected] aetiologic factors in canine osteochondrosis. Vet Q 1987;9(3):268–78.
14. Laverty S, Girard C. Pathogenesis of epiphyseal osteochondrosis. Vet J 2013; 197(1):3–12.
15. van Weeren PR. Etiology, diagnosis, and treatment of OC (D). Clin Tech Equ P 2006;5(4):248–58.

16. Trostle S, Dubielzig R, Beck K. Examination of frozen cross sections of cervical spinal intersegments in nine horses with cervical vertebral malformation: lesions associated with spinal cord compression. J Vet Diagn Invest 1993;5(3):423–31.

17. Nyack B, Morgan JP, Pool R, et al. Osteochondrosis of the shoulder joint of the horse. Cornell Vet 1981;71(2):149–63.

18. KWPN. The frequency and heredity of navicular disease, sesamoidosis, fetlock joint arthrosis, bone spavin, osteochondrosis of the hock. A radiographic progeny study. Zeist: KWPN (Koninklijke Vereniging Warmbloed Paardenstamboek Nederland); 1994.

19. Willms F. Genetische Analyse von Merkmalskomplexen der Reitpferdezucht unter Berucksichtigung von Gliedmassenveranderungen. Züchtungskunde 1999;71: 330–45.

20. Pieramati C, Pepe M, Silvestrelli M, et al. Heritability estimation of osteochondrosis dissecans in Maremmano horses. Livest Prod Sci 2003;79(2–3):249–55.

21. Stock KF, Hamann H, Distl O. Prevalence of osseous fragments in distal and proximal interphalangeal, metacarpo- and metatarsophalangeal and tarsocrural joints of Hanoverian warmblood horses. J Vet Med A Physiol Pathol Clin Med 2005; 52(8):388–94.

22. Stock KF, Distl O. Genetic correlations between osseous fragments in fetlock and hock joints, deforming arthropathy in hock joints and pathologic changes in the navicular bones of warmblood riding horses. Livest Sci 2006;105(1–3):35–43.

23. Wittwer C, Hamann H, Rosenberger E, et al. Genetic parameters for the prevalence of osteochondrosis in the limb joints of South German coldblood horses. J Anim Breed Genet 2007;124(5):302–7.

24. van Grevenhof EM, Schurink A, Ducro BJ, et al. Genetic variables of various manifestations of osteochondrosis and their correlations between and within joints in Dutch warmblood horses. J Anim Sci 2009;87(6):1906–12.

25. Jönsson L, Dalin G, Egenvall A, et al. Equine hospital data as a source for study of prevalence and heritability of osteochondrosis and palmar/plantar osseous fragments of Swedish warmblood horses. Equine Vet J 2011;43(6):695–700.

26. Hilla D, Distl O. Heritabilities and genetic correlations between fetlock, hock and stifle osteochondrosis and fetlock osteochondral fragments in Hanoverian warmblood horses. J Anim Breed Genet 2014;131(1):71–81.

27. Russell J, Matika O, Russell T, et al. Heritability and prevalence of selected osteochondrosis lesions in yearling thoroughbred horses. Pferdeheilkunde 2017; 33(4):396.

28. Lykkjen S, Olsen H, Dolvik N, et al. Heritability estimates of tarsocrural osteochondrosis and palmar/plantar first phalanx osteochondral fragments in standardbred trotters. Equine Vet J 2014;46(1):32–7.

29. Teyssedre S, Dupuis MC, Guerin G, et al. Genome-wide association studies for osteochondrosis in French trotter horses. J Anim Sci 2012;90(1):45–53.

30. Schougaard H, Ronne JF, Phillipson J. A radiographic survey of tibiotarsal osteochondrosis in a selected population of trotting horses in Denmark and its possible genetic significance. Equine Vet J 1990;22(4):288–9.

31. Grondahl AM, Dolvik NI. Heritability estimations of osteochondrosis in the tibiotarsal joint and of bony fragments in the palmar plantar portion of the metacarpophalangeal and metatarsophalangeal joints of horses. J Am Vet Med Assoc 1993;203(1):101–4.

32. Philipsson J, Andreasson E, Sandgren B, et al. Osteochondrosis in the tarsocrural joint and osteochondral fragments in the fetlock joints in standardbred trotters. II. Heritability 1993;25(S16):38–41.

33. van Weeren P, Sloet van Oldruitenborgh-Oosterbaan MM, Barneveld A. The influence of birth weight, rate of weight gain and final achieved height and sex on the development of osteochondrotic lesions in a population of genetically predisposed Warmblood foals. Equine Vet J 1999;31(S31):26–30.

34. Lepeule J, Bareille N, Robert C, et al. Association of growth, feeding practices and exercise conditions with the prevalence of developmental orthopaedic disease in limbs of French foals at weaning. Prev Vet Med 2009;89(3–4):167–77.

35. Vervuert I, Coenen M, Winkelsett S, et al. Growth rates in Hanoverian warmblood foals and the development of osteochondrosis. EAAP Scientific Series 2004; 114:85–9.

36. Lepeule J, Bareille N, Robert C, et al. Association of growth, feeding practices and exercise conditions with the severity of the osteoarticular status of limbs in French foals. Vet J 2013;197(1):65–71.

37. Schober M. Schätzung von genetischen Effekten beim Auftreten von Osteochondrosis dissecans beim Warmblutpferd. Cuvillier. Göttingen: Georg-August-University of Göttingen; 2003.

38. Dierks C, Lohring K, Lampe V, et al. Genome-wide search for markers associated with osteochondrosis in Hanoverian warmblood horses. Mamm Genome 2007; 18(10):739–47.

39. Lampe V, Dierks C, Komm K, et al. Identification of a new quantitative trait locus on equine chromosome 18 responsible for osteochondrosis in Hanoverian warmblood horses. J Anim Sci 2009;87(11):3477–81.

40. Lampe V, Dierks C, Distl O. Refinement of a quantitative gene locus on equine chromosome 16 responsible for osteochondrosis in Hanoverian warmblood horses. Animal 2009;3(9):1224–31.

41. Lampe V, Dierks C, Distl O. Refinement of a quantitative trait locus on equine chromosome 5 responsible for fetlock osteochondrosis in Hanoverian warmblood horses. Anim Genet 2009;40(4):553–5.

42. Dierks C, Komm K, Lampe V, et al. Fine mapping of a quantitative trait locus for osteochondrosis on horse chromosome 2. Anim Genet 2010;41(Suppl 2):87–90.

43. Dierks C, Komm K, Lampe V, et al. Fine mapping of quantitative trait loci on equine chromosome 4 responsible for osteochondrosis in Hanoverian warmblood horses. Hannover (Germany): University of Veterinary Medicine Hannover; 2010.

44. Felicetti M, Lampe V, Ehrhardt S, et al. Mapping of a quantitative trait locus on equine chromosome 21 responsible for osteochondrosis in hock joints of Hanoverian warmblood horses. Hannover (Germany): University of Veterinary Medicine Hannover; 2009.

45. Wittwer C, Lohring K, Drogemuller C, et al. Mapping quantitative trait loci for osteochondrosis in fetlock and hock joints and palmar/plantar osseus fragments in fetlock joints of South German coldblood horses. Anim Genet 2007;38(4):350–7.

46. Orr N, Hill EW, Gu J, et al. Genome-wide association study of osteochondrosis in the tarsocrural joint of Dutch warmblood horses identifies susceptibility loci on chromosomes 3 and 10. Anim Genet 2013;44(4):408–12.

47. McCoy AM, Beeson SK, Splan RK, et al. Identification and validation of risk loci for osteochondrosis in standardbreds. BMC Genomics 2016;17:41.

48. Lykkjen S, Dolvik NI, McCue ME, et al. Genome-wide association analysis of osteochondrosis of the tibiotarsal joint in Norwegian standardbred trotters. Anim Genet 2010;41(Suppl 2):111–20.

49. Lampe V. Fine mapping of quantitative trait loci (QTL) for osteochondrosis in Hanoverian warmblood horses. Hannover (Germany): University of Veterinary Medicine Hannover; 2009.

50. Sevane N, Dunner S, Boado A, et al. Candidate gene analysis of osteochondrosis in Spanish purebred horses. Anim Genet 2016;47(5):570–8.

51. Wypchlo M, Korwin-Kossakowska A, Bereznowski A, et al. Polymorphisms in selected genes and analysis of their relationship with osteochondrosis in Polish sport horse breeds. Anim Genet 2018;49(6):623–7.

52. Kemper AM, Drnevich J, McCue ME, et al. Differential gene expression in articular cartilage and subchondral bone of neonatal and adult horses. Genes (Basel) 2019;10(10) [pii:E745].

53. Riddick TL, Duesterdieck-Zellmer K, Semevolos SA. Gene and protein expression of cartilage canal and osteochondral junction chondrocytes and full-thickness cartilage in early equine osteochondrosis. Vet J 2012;194(3):319–25.

54. Austbo L, Roed KH, Dolvik NI, et al. Identification of differentially expressed genes associated with osteochondrosis in standardbred horses using RNA arbitrarily primed PCR. Anim Biotechnol 2010;21(2):135–9.

55. Mirams M, Tatarczuch L, Ahmed YA, et al. Altered gene expression in early osteochondrosis lesions. J Orthop Res 2009;27(4):452–7.

56. Verwilghen DR, Vanderheyden L, Franck T, et al. Variations of plasmatic concentrations of insulin-like growth factor-I in post-pubescent horses affected with developmental osteochondral lesions. Vet Res Commun 2009;33(7):701–9.

57. Lopes MS, Diesterbeck U, Machado Ada C, et al. Refinement of quantitative trait loci on equine chromosome 10 for radiological signs of navicular disease in Hanoverian warmblood horses. Anim Genet 2010;41(Suppl 2):36–40.

58. Dik KJ, Vandenbroek J. Role of navicular bone shape in the pathogenesis of navicular disease–a radiological study. Equine Vet J 1995;27(5):390–3.

59. Macgregor CM. Radiographic assessment of navicular bones, based on changes in the distal nutrient foramina. Equine Vet J 1986;18(3):203–6.

60. Brunken E. Röntgenologische Verlaufsuntersuchungen am Strahbein des Pferdes. Hannover: University of Veterinary Medicine Hannover; 1986.

61. Dyson S, Murray R, Blunden T, et al. Current concepts of navicular disease. Equine Vet Educ 2006;18(1):45–56.

62. Kaser-Hotz B, Ueltschi G. Radiographic appearance of the navicular bone in sound horses. Vet Radiol Ultrasound 1992;33(1):9–17.

63. Wright IM. A study of 118 cases of navicular disease: radiological features. Equine Vet J 1993;25(6):493–500.

64. Stock KF, Hamann H, Distl O. Variance component estimation on the frequency of pathologic changes in the navicular bones of Hanoverian warmblood horses. J Anim Breed Genet 2004;121(5):289–301.

65. Bos H, van der Meij GJ, Dik KJ. Heredity of navicular disease. Vet Q 1986;8(1): 68–72.

66. Diesterbeck US, Hertsch B, Distl O. Genome-wide search for microsatellite markers associated with radiologic alterations in the navicular bone of Hanoverian warmblood horses. Mamm Genome 2007;18(5):373–81.

67. Lopes MS, Diesterbeck U, da Camara Machado A, et al. Fine mapping a quantitative trait locus on horse chromosome 2 associated with radiological signs of navicular disease in Hanoverian warmblood horses. Anim Genet 2009;40(6): 955–7.

68. Stock KF, Distl O. Genetic analyses of the radiographic appearance of the distal sesamoid bones in Hanoverian warmblood horses. Am J Vet Res 2006;67(6): 1013–9.

69. Willms F, Roehe R, Kalm EJZ. Genetic analysis of different traits in horse breeding by considering radiographic findings. 1: importance of radiographic findings in breeding sport horses. Zuchtungskunde 1999;71(5):330–45.

70. Tanchev P. Osteoarthritis or osteoarthrosis: commentary on misuse of terms. Reconstr Rev 2017;7(1):45.

71. Arnason T, Bjornsdottir S. Heritability of age-at-onset of bone spavin in Icelandic horses estimated by survival analysis. Livest Prod Sci 2003;79(2–3):285–93.

72. Bjornsdottir S, Ekman S, Eksell R, et al. High detail radiography and histology of the centrodistal tarsal joint of Icelandic horses age 6 months to 6 years. Equine Vet J 2004;36(1):5–11.

73. Dolvik NI, Klemetsdal G. Arthritis in the carpal joints of Norwegian trotter–heritability, effects of inbreeding and conformation. Livest Prod Sci 1994;39(3):283–90.

74. Hedbom E, Hauselmann HJ. Molecular aspects of pathogenesis in osteoarthritis: the role of inflammation. Cell Mol Life Sci 2002;59(1):45–53.

75. Peterson B, Szabo RM. Carpal osteoarthrosis. Hand Clin 2006;22(4):517–28.

76. Kidd JA, Fuller C, Barr ARS. Osteoarthritis in the horse. Equine Vet Educ 2001; 13(3):160–8.

77. McIlwraith CW. General pathobiology of the joint and response to injury. Joint disease in the horse, vol. 1. St. Louis, Missouri: Elsevier; 1996. p. 40–63.

78. Frisbie DD, McIlwraith CW. Evaluation of gene therapy as a treatment for equine traumatic arthritis and osteoarthritis. Clin Orthop 2000;379:S273–87.

79. Kamm JL, Frisbie DD, McIlwraith CW, et al. Gene biomarkers in peripheral white blood cells of horses with experimentally induced osteoarthritis. Am J Vet Res 2013;74(1):115–21.

80. Pilliner S, Elmhurst S, Davies Z. The horse in motion: the anatomy and physiology of equine locomotion. Oxford, UK: John Wiley & Sons; 2009.

81. Hermans WA, Kersjes AW, Vandermey GJW, et al. Investigation into the heredity of congenital lateral patellar (sub)luxation in the Shetland pony. Vet Q 1987; 9(1):1–8.

82. Engelbert TA, Tate LP, Richardson DC, et al. Lateral patellar luxation in miniature horses. Vet Surg 1993;22(4):293–7.

83. Rathor SS. Clinical aspects of the functional disorders of the equine and bovine femoro-patellar articulation with some remarks on its biomechanics. Utrecht: Hoeijenbos; 1968.

84. Rooney JR, Raker CW, Harmany KJ. Congenital lateral luxation of the patella in the horse. Cornell Vet 1971;61(4):670–3.

85. Welsh CE, Lewis TW, Blott SC, et al. Preliminary genetic analyses of important musculoskeletal conditions of thoroughbred racehorses in Hong Kong. Vet J 2013;198(3):611–5.

86. Goodship A. The pathophysiology of flexor tendon injury in the horse. Equine Vet Educ 1993;5(1):23–9.

87. Oki H, Miyake T, Kasashima Y, et al. Estimation of heritability for superficial digital flexor tendon injury by Gibbs sampling in the thoroughbred racehorse. J Anim Breed Genet 2008;125(6):413–6.

88. Halper J, Kim B, Khan A, et al. Degenerative suspensory ligament desmitis as a systemic disorder characterized by proteoglycan accumulation. BMC Vet Res 2006;2(1):12.

89. Dyson SJ, Arthur RM, Palmer SE, et al. Suspensory ligament desmitis. Vet Clin North Am Equine Pract 1995;11(2):177–215.

90. Strong DI. The use of a whole genome scan to find a genetic marker for degenerative suspensory ligament desmitis in the Peruvian Paso horse. KY: University of Kentucky Master's Kentucky: Theses, University of Kentucky; 2005.

91. Firth EC. The response of bone, articular cartilage and tendon to exercise in the horse. J Anat 2006;208(4):513–26.

92. Blott SC, Swinburne JE, Sibbons C, et al. A genome-wide association study demonstrates significant genetic variation for fracture risk in thoroughbred racehorses. BMC Genomics 2014;15:147.

93. Stashak TS. Adams' lameness in horses. Alfeld (Leine), Germany: Verlag M. & H. Schaper; 2008.

94. O'Brien T, Morgan J, Wheat J, et al. Sesamoiditis in the thoroughbred: a radiographic study 1. Vet Radiol 1971;12(1):75–87.

95. Winter D. Genetische disposition von Gliedmaßenerkrankungen in der Reitpferdezucht. Göttingen, Germany: University of Göttingen; 1995.

96. Finno CJ, Stevens C, Young A, et al. SERPINB11 frameshift variant associated with novel hoof specific phenotype in Connemara ponies. PLoS Genet 2015; 11(4):e1005122.

97. Rafati N, Andersson LS, Mikko S, et al. Large deletions at the SHOX locus in the pseudoautosomal region are associated with skeletal atavism in Shetland ponies. G3 (Bethesda) 2016;6(7):2213–23.

98. Cook D, Gallagher PC, Bailey E. Genetics of swayback in American saddlebred horses. Anim Genet 2010;41(Suppl 2):64–71.

Genetics of Equine Ocular Disease

Rebecca R. Bellone, PhD

KEYWORDS

- Genetics • Ocular diseases • Night blindness • Recurrent uveitis
- Ocular squamous cell carcinoma • Multiple congenital ocular anomalies • Horses

KEY POINTS

- Advances in equine genetics tools and resources are enabling discoveries that can assist in clinical management of ocular disorders.
- Genetic testing is available to identify horses with multiple congenital ocular anomalies in a variety of breeds and congenital stationary night blindness in the Appaloosa and related breeds.
- Genetic testing can also help identify horses at risk for developing ocular disorders, including equine recurrent uveitis in the Appaloosa and squamous cell carcinoma in the Haflinger, Belgian, and Rocky Mountain horse breeds.

INTRODUCTION

The vision of horses has been adapted to survival as a prey animal with a substantial field of view, up to 350°. Adaptations to enhance vision during dim light include a large elongated cornea and large horizontal rectangular pupil that enables more light to enter the eye and wider lateral vision, respectively. A reflective fibrous tapetum also provides additional opportunities for photoreceptors to capture each photon. Adaptations for enhanced vision in bright light include yellow filtering pigments in the lens to reduce glare and improve contrast. In addition, to further reduce glare, the corpora nigra functions to shield excess light entering from above the eye. Horses also have one of the largest eyes among terrestrial vertebrates, providing extensive retinal surface and a large number of photoreceptor cells that enable quick adaptation to variation in light intensities.[1] Horses perform in a variety of disciplines that are visually demanding. Therefore, any ocular disorder that has the potential to threaten these adapted structures, and thus, vision can affect the utility of the horse. Understanding inherited ocular disorders and their impact on vision can assist in both clinical management and breeding decisions.

Department of Population Health and Reproduction, Veterinary Genetics Laboratory, School of Veterinary Medicine, University of California–Davis, One Shields Avenue, Davis, CA 95616, USA
E-mail address: rbellone@ucdavis.edu

Vet Clin Equine 36 (2020) 303–322
https://doi.org/10.1016/j.cveq.2020.03.009
0749-0739/20/© 2020 Elsevier Inc. All rights reserved.

The availability of the horse genome sequence allowed for development of tools and resources to study inherited ocular disease. Associated or causal variants have been identified for multiple congenital ocular anomalies (MCOA) in horse breeds with the silver coat color dilution mutation, congenital stationary night blindness (CSNB), and equine recurrent uveitis (ERU) in the Appaloosa and related breeds with the appaloosa spotting patterns, and ocular squamous cell carcinoma (SCC) in the Haflinger, Belgian, and Rocky Mountain horse breeds[2–8] (**Table 1**). Ocular manifestations have also been reported for 5 additional disorders, and genetic tests are available for 4 of these (**Table 2**). Genetic testing has the potential to help clinicians identify causes of ocular anomalies and can greatly aid in the identification of those horses at highest risk of developing diseases, such as ERU and SCC. Careful screening of horses at highest risk may allow for early detection and better prognosis. Utilization of genetic tests can advise breeding decisions. Genotyping for the variants known to cause or be associated with ocular disease are now routinely performed by several academic and commercial laboratories. For more information on genetic testing, see Rebecca R. Bellone and Felipe Avila's article, "Genetic Testing in the Horse," in this issue. The focus of this report is to provide clinicians with a comprehensive description of known inherited ocular disorders and manifestations and to discuss the inherited ocular diseases for which studies are underway (**Table 3**).

MULTIPLE CONGENITAL OCULAR ANOMALIES

MCOA was the first disorder in which genetic studies enabled the development of a DNA test for an inherited ocular disease. MCOA was first described in Rocky Mountain horses and was initially referred to as anterior segment dysgenesis.[9,10] Subsequent studies identified the same clinical manifestations in other breeds, including the Kentucky Mountain saddle and pleasure horses, the Icelandic horse, the Shetland pony, the American Miniature horse, the Morgan horse, and the Comtois.[11–16] Clinically, there are 2 phenotypes of ocular findings related to this disease: (1) cysts only, and (2) cysts with additional anomalies (MCOA phenotype). The cysts typically are translucent, ranging up to a centimeter in size, and represent spherical bubble-shaped projections of nonpigmented epithelium in the posterior iris, ciliary body, or the peripheral retina. The more severe MCOA phenotype is characterized by other abnormalities, including retinal dysplasia, iris hypoplasia, corneal globosa, megaloblepharon, pectinate ligament hypoplasia, immature nuclear cataracts, and iridocorneal hypoplasia,[10,11,17] in addition to the described intraocular cysts (**Fig. 1**).

Several studies investigating pedigrees of affected horses determined that the mode of inheritance was incompletely dominant with horses heterozygous for the condition having the cyst-only phenotype and those homozygous generally having the MCOA phenotype.[9,11] Investigating pedigrees of 2 large half-sibling families also supports incomplete penetrance of disease, meaning horses could have the mutation but not express the phenotype.[11] Subsequent molecular studies determined that MCOA results from a pleiotropic effect of the silver color dilution mutation (Z), a missense mutation (ECA6g.74569773C > T, p.R625C) in premelanosome protein (*PMEL*).[2,18,19] Silver dilutes black (eumelanin) pigment most notably in the mane and the tail of bay and black horses (see **Fig. 1**) and can also cause dappling to appear in the coat. In terms of pigmentation, PMEL is essential for forming amyloid fibrils for melanin pigments to polymerize within the melanosome.[20,21] Cross-species comparisons have shown that mutation in PMEL regulates hypopigmentation with concurrent ocular anomalies in dogs and zebrafish, but in mice and chicken no ocular anomalies have been

Table 1
Inherited ocular diseases with DNA tests available

Ocular Disease	Alias Names/Acronym	Breeds	Mode of Inheritance/Gene	Reported Allele	Important Clinical Considerations
Multiple congenital ocular anomalies	Anterior segment dysgenesis/MCOA	Rocky Mountain horse, Kentucky Mountain saddle horse, Kentucky Mountain pleasure horse, Icelandic horse, Shetland pony, American miniature horse, Comtois, American quarter horse, and Morgan	Incomplete dominance/*PMEL*	Z	*Z/Z* horses typically have a more severe phenotype than *Z/N* and should be evaluated for blindness
Congenital stationary night blindness	CSNB	Appaloosa, American miniature horse, Knabstrupper, Noriker, pony of the America	Recessive/*TRPM1*	LP	*LP/LP* horses are night blind and management decisions for safety of horse and handler should be discussed with owners
Equine recurrent uveitis	Moon blindness/ERU	Appaloosa	Additive/*TRPM1*	LP	Risk for ERU is defined as *LP/LP > LP/N > N/N*. *LP/LP* horses should be frequently examined for evidence of inflammation
Squamous cell carcinoma	Ocular SCC	Haflinger, Belgian, Rocky Mountain horse	Recessive/*DDB2*	R	*R/R* horses are at highest risk of developing ocular SCC; these horses should have frequent ocular examinations and wear UV protective fly masks

Table 2
Ocular manifestations of other equine disorders

Disorder	Ocular Manifestations	Breeds	Mode of Inheritance/ Gene Involved	DNA Test Available
Hyperkalemic periodic paralysis (HYPP)	Third eyelid prolapse	Quarter horse and quarter horse–related breeds	Dominant with variable expression/ SCN4A	Yes
HERDA	Thin corneas and increased incidence of corneal ulcers	Quarter horse and quarter horse–related breeds	Recessive/PPIB	Yes
JEB1	Corneal ulcers	Draft breeds	Recessive/ LAMC2	Yes
JEB2	Corneal ulcers	American saddlebreds	Recessive/ LAMA3	Yes
Incontinentia pigmenti (IP)	Developmental ocular anomalies	Quarter horse	X-linked dominant/ IKBKG	Yes
eNAD/equine degenerative myeloencephalopathy	Pigment retinopathy	Warmbloods	Unknown	No

Table 3
Inherited ocular disease under investigation

Ocular Disease	Breeds	Proposed Mode of Inheritance
SCC	Quarter Horse, American Paint Horse, Appaloosa	Unknown
ERU	Knabstrupper, Pony of the America, Icelandic Horse, Warmblood	Unknown but likely complex
CSNB	Thoroughbred, Paso Fino, and likely others	Unknown
Cataracts	Exmoor Pony, American Quarter Horse, Arabian, Thoroughbred, and Morgan	Dominant in Morgan and sex-linked in Exmoor
Aniridia	Belgian and American Quarter Horse	Dominant
Corneal dystrophy/ bilateral corneal stroma loss	Friesian	Multigenic with a potential X-linked gene
Distichiasis	Friesian	Unknown

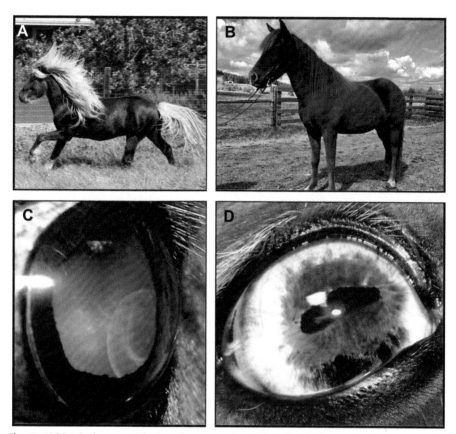

Fig. 1. MCOA in horses with the silver mutation. (*A*) Icelandic horse displaying the silver phenotype as noted by the slightly dilute body of a black base coat color and the lighter mane and tail. (*B*) In this chestnut Icelandic horse, it is not possible to know by appearance if this horse has the silver allele (Z) because silver does not dilute chestnut-based coat colors. (*C*) The cyst-only phenotype as evidenced by large temporal ciliary cysts. This phenotype is found in horses heterozygous for the silver allele (Z/N). (*D*) MOCA phenotype (Z/Z) that most often includes cysts and other ocular anomalies as those depicted here includes iridial hypoplasia and dyscoric pupil. (*Courtesy of* Lucy Nold and Dr. Ann Dwyer.)

reported for the PMEL mutations that cause hypopigmentation.[22–25] The precise role of this variant in ocular defects in horses remains to be determined.

Several commercial laboratories offer a DNA test for silver/MCOA, and this test can help to identify horses whose vision should be further evaluated by ocular examination. Horses homozygous for the silver mutation (*Z/Z*) are noted to have impaired vision or are blind. The extent to which the cyst-only phenotype (*Z/N*) affects vision is not fully known.[16,19] However, a study in Comtois and Rocky Mountain horses suggested that vision is also impaired in heterozygotes because deeper anterior chambers were noted in both homozygotes and heterozygotes (*Z/Z* and *Z/N*), compared with wild-type horses (*N/N*).[26]

Horses heterozygous for the *PMEL* mutation (*Z/N*) are most often reported to have the cyst-only phenotype; however, a study from 2017 noted 8 out of 71 heterozygotes (*Z/N*) had mild cornea globosa in one or both eyes and one also had bilateral miotic pupils and abnormal pupillary reflexes in both eyes, thus illustrating the need to have the horses with the Z mutation evaluated by an ocular specialist.[26] That same study also detected cysts in only 32% of the heterozygotes. As noted by the Grahn and colleagues[11] study in 2007, it is possible that the incomplete penetrance may explain some of the cases of heterozygotes without cysts. It is also possible that the detection methods used in that study were not sensitive enough to detect all cysts, because ultrasonography was previously shown to identify cysts in 70% of (Z/N) horses that were not detected with direct ophthalmoscopy.[16] One study that measured refractive index in Icelandic horses noted that horses heterozygous for silver (Z/N), that were older than 16 years of age, were more likely to be myopic than non-silver horses (N/N), suggesting a progressive nature to this disease.[26]

Horses from breeds with the silver mutation should be considered candidates for genetic testing for silver and screening for clinical symptoms of disease. The reported cases of incomplete penetrance make genetic screening important to determine which animals should be evaluated for ocular anomalies more closely. The genetic test can also assist in breeding decisions because breeding heterozygotes results in a 25% chance of producing horses with the most severe phenotype and visual deficits (Z/Z). Furthermore, the silver mutation does not dilute red pigment; therefore, chestnut horses (or chestnut dilute horses such as palominos) with the Z allele (Z/Z or Z/N) will not show a dilute phenotype and thus should be DNA tested for silver to help inform breeding and clinical decisions.

CONGENITAL STATIONARY NIGHT BLINDNESS

The second ocular disease to have its genetic basis solved is CSNB. CSNB is a nonprogressive condition, present at birth, and characterized by impaired vision in dark conditions. Clinical diagnosis is determined by electroretinography (ERG) under scotopic conditions with an absent "negative" b-wave and an a-wave with increased amplitude indicative of disease (**Fig. 2**).[27] This condition has been reported in the Appaloosa, American Miniature Horse, and Knabstrupper.[3,28–34] There has also been a case report describing 1 Paso Fino and 1 Thoroughbred with a similar presentation.[35]

Appaloosa, Knabstrupper, and American Miniature Horse are all breeds with white coat spotting patterns, known as leopard complex spotting (see **Fig. 2**). This white patterning is typically symmetric, centered over the hips, and can occur with and without pigmented spots in the white patterned area. Additional characteristics include visible sclera, stripes of pigment on an otherwise unpigmented hoof, mottled skin around the muzzle, anus, and genitalia, and progressive increase in the number of white hairs in the coat as the animal ages (known as varnish roaning). The extent of the white patterning and level of roaning with age can vary extensively between animals. White pattern level can range from a few white flecks on the rump to nearly completely white from birth (see **Fig. 2**). Leopard complex spotting is thought to be a polygenic trait with the presence of the coat pattern and associated characteristics inherited by an incompletely dominant form of a gene known as LP, for leopard complex spotting. The extent of the white patterning is thought to be caused by additional genes, known as modifiers. Only one of these modifiers has been identified at the molecular level. Horses homozygous for LP (LP/LP) tend to have few to no oval spots of pigment in their white patterned area as compared with heterozygotes (LP/N) that typically have many, although the size and number of these pigmented spots are also variable. Genotype with respect to LP is not always easily distinguished by appearance of the horse.

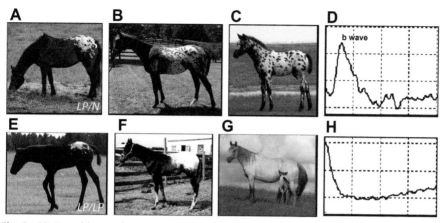

Fig. 2. CSNB and leopard complex spotting patterns. The white spotting pattern of Appaloosas and related breeds has been directly tied to CSNB. This leopard complex spotting coat patterning can range on a continuum from a few white flecks on the rump (*A, E*) to a horse almost completely white, known as a few spot (*G*). Horses that are heterozygous (*LP/N*) have pigmented spots in the white patterned area (*A–C*) and are not night blind as evidenced by an a-wave followed by the b-wave of a normal ERG (*D*). Horses that are homozygous for LP (*E–G*) have few to no spots of pigment in the white patterned area and have CSNB, as evidenced by the negative ERG, which shows increased amplitude a-wave and the absence of the b-wave (*H*). The variability in pigmentation phenotype (*A–C* and *E–G*) is thought to be controlled by other loci. Thus, it is not always evident based on appearance to know what the genotype of the horse is with respect to *LP* (panels *A, E*, and *G*, for example). Genotyping for the *LP* mutation is recommended to determine if horses have or are carriers for CSNB. (*Courtesy of* Sheila Archer, Martha Mitchell, Cheryl Woods, and Lynne Sandmeyer.)

Several molecular genetic studies have identified the genetic cause for *LP* and CSNB as an insertion of 1378 bp in the first intron of the calcium ion channel gene, *Transient receptor potential cation channel subfamily M Member 1 (TRPM1)*.[3,36] Homozygosity for *LP* was perfectly concordant with CSNB and was documented in several studies in 3 breeds with LP spotting patterns (Appaloosas, Miniature Horse, and Knabstrupper).[3,32,33] This insertion disrupts the normal transcription of *TRPM1*. Horses homozygous for *LP* have reduced expression of *TRPM1* and are proposed to have little to no functional protein.[3,36] Work in humans and mice has demonstrated that a reduction in glutamate released by retinal rod cells occurs upon detection of light, and this in turn signals the opening of the TRPM1 channels in the ON bipolar cells. Calcium signaling thru TRPM1 results in depolarization of the ON bipolar cells, which is identified on ERG as the b-wave.[37,38] Absence of TRPM1 in *LP* homozygous horses explains the "negative ERG" because without TRPM1, bipolar cells are unable to respond to changes in glutamate release by the retinal rod cells. Approximately 30 different loss-of-function mutations in TRPM1 have been shown to cause complete CSNB in humans but with no known pigmentation defects.[39] However, similar to horses, humans with mutations in *TRPM1* are also reported to have strabismus and nystagmus.[32,40] Nonetheless, not every CSNB horse has strabismus and nystagmus, and thus, more work is needed to investigate the connection between these ocular anomalies.

CSNB is a pleiotropic effect of the *LP* mutation. The spotting pattern is inherited in an incompletely dominant fashion, and the disease is inherited as a recessive trait.

Horses homozygous for *LP* are night blind. One way to diagnose horses with CSNB is by DNA testing for the *LP* mutation because the lack of pigmented spots within the white patterned area is not always indicative of *LP* genotype (see **Fig. 2**). Similarly, genetic testing is recommended for horses with minimal white LP patterning. For horses that test homozygous for *LP*, a complete ophthalmic examination should be performed, including an ERG under scotopic conditions to confirm genetic diagnosis. Given that the mutation causing the white coat pattern is the same as the one causing the ocular disease, it is not possible to breed away from CSNB in breeds with leopard complex spotting. Therefore, owners of horses that test as *LP/LP* should be advised on handling, training, and riding these animals in low light or dark conditions and be counseled on breeding decisions.

Genetic testing for CSNB is not necessary for horses that show many obvious pigmented spots in their white patterned area, because these horses are heterozygous for LP (*LP/N*) and are not night blind. However, *LP/N* horses are an elevated risk for developing ERU (see later discussion).

EQUINE RECURRENT UVEITIS

ERU, also known as moon blindness, is a disease syndrome that affects many horse breeds. ERU is the leading cause of blindness in horses and is characterized by repeated or persistent inflammatory episodes of the uveal tract of the eye, including the iris, ciliary body, and choroid. The cumulative effects of the immune-mediated process lead to blindness resulting from glaucoma, cataracts, retinal detachment, and phthisis bulbi (**Fig. 3**).

ERU has been subclassified clinically into 3 syndromes: classic, insidious, and posterior ERU. Classic ERU is characterized by periods of active painful inflammation in one or both eyes followed by a quiescent phase. Insidious ERU is distinguished by a persistent low-grade intraocular inflammation, most often bilateral, with gradual and cumulative destruction of ocular tissue that does not typically manifest in outwardly painful episodes.[41] Posterior ERU is characterized by inflammation primarily present in the vitreous, retina, and choroid. Retinal degeneration is commonly present with this form of ERU. It is most often observed in warmbloods and draft breeds[42] and can be unilateral or bilateral.

Although the pathogenesis of ERU is complex and not entirely elucidated, all 3 subclassifications of ERU are thought to have an autoimmune component with environmental factors and genetics contributing to risk and severity of disease. It is unknown how or if the immune mechanisms differ for the 3 subclassifications of ERU, and the precise inciting cause has not been fully determined. Some evidence supports that inflammation and breakdown of the blood ocular barrier is triggered by a cross-reactive microbial antigen, whereas other evidence suggests that autoantigens derived from ocular tissue may trigger the immune reaction.[43] In some cases, intraocular antibodies to *Leptospira* maybe the inciting cause for ERU.[44–47] Furthermore, horses testing positive for *Leptospira* antibodies to pathogenic serovars (*Leptospira pomona* or *Leptospira grippotyphosa*) were more likely to go blind from ERU than those testing negative.[48] How these pathogenic variants of leptospira cause either recurring bouts or persistent inflammation is not understood. One hypothesis is that infection with a pathogenic serovar of *Leptospira* leads to autoimmunity with autoantigens presented by class II molecules to the CD4$^+$ T cells in the uveal tract.[49,50] Better understanding of the T-cell phenotype would help to further test this hypothesis and may lead to better treatment strategies. For example, in a recent study investigating lymphocyte phenotypes between ERU affected and control horses, greater

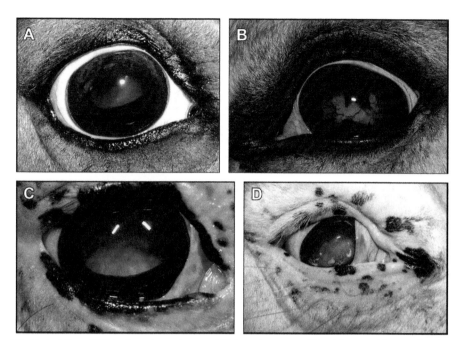

Fig. 3. Insidious ERU in Appaloosa horses. (*A*) Appaloosa eye OD with no evidence of active uveitis or evidence of previous inflammation. (*B*) OS chronic uveitis evidenced by hyperpigmented iris and mature cataract (white opacity in center of eye) and posterior synechia causing an irregular pupil. (*C*) OD evidence of chronic severe ERU with secondary glaucoma. The globe is buphthalmic with vitreous degeneration, cataract, and a posterior lens luxation. (*D*) OD severe chronic ERU, including conjunctival hyperemia, epiphora, corneal fibrosis, cataract, and a yellowed vitreous. Previous intraocular inflammation has led to adhesions between the iris and the lens, seen as irregularities of the pupil. The globe has become shrunken consistent with phthisis bulbi. As the disease progresses, cumulative damage leads to cataract development (as in *B–D*), glaucoma (as in *C*), or phthisis bulbi (as in *D*) leading to blindness. (*Courtesy of* Ann Dwyer and Mary Lassaline.)

expression of interferon-gamma in CD4+ T cells from horses with ERU indicated a proinflammatory T helper type-1 ERU response phenotype.[51] Interestingly, when coincubated with mesenchymal stem cells, CD4+ T cells had decreased activation, and thus, mesenchymal stem cells may serve as a promising treatment of some cases of ERU.[51]

Not all ERU cases can be explained by the presence of *Leptospira*,[42,48,52] so identifying other risk factors is essential to elucidating the cause of this complex disease. The breeds with the highest occurrence of ERU reported in the United States include the Appaloosa, Quarter Horse, Thoroughbred, Warmblood, Hanoverian, and the American Paint Horse.[48] Of these, Appaloosas are most often clinically diagnosed with the insidious form and have been reported to be 8 times more likely to develop ERU and 4 times more likely to go blind as a result of the inflammatory process in one or both eyes than any other breed.[49] Several retrospective studies have been performed, the most recent indicating that 62.5% of the horses diagnosed with ERU were Appaloosas.[53] A recent prospective study examining 145 Appaloosa horses in western Canada over a 12-year period determined the prevalence of ERU to be 14%, with 90% of the cases having bilateral disease and 80% eventually becoming blind.[54] The most common clinical manifestations observed were aqueous flare, conjunctival hyperemia, miosis, and iris hyperpigmentation. This study also identified a common ancestor within 6 generations in 78% of the cases. Given the high prevalence of ERU in the Appaloosa, the severity and bilateral nature of disease, combined with a common ancestor among many of the affected horses, supports genetics as a major contributing factor in this breed.

Genetic risks for both insidious and posterior ERU have been documented in the Appaloosa and German Warmblood, respectively.[4,55] Associations with different markers in the region of the major histocompatibility complex (MHC) in horses known as the equine leukocyte antigen (ELA) have been identified in both of these breeds.[4,55] The homologous region in humans, the HLA has been associated with several different types of uveitis, and these have become important tests for inherited risk for ocular and other inflammatory diseases.[56,57] German warmblood horses carrying the ELA-A9 haplotype had the highest risk of ERU. This haplotype was absent in the controls but found in 41% of the cases.[58] Further studies in German Warmbloods using a genome-wide association study (GWAS) identified 2 loci significantly associated with ERU risk and disease severity.[55] A SNP (single nucleotide polymorphism) located near 2 interleukin genes, IL-17A and IL-17F, on horse chromosome 20 (ECA20) was significantly associated with disease status. An SNP on ECA 18 was also associated with disease severity. Causal variants for the associated loci on ECA18 or ECA20 have not been reported, and no genetic tests for ELA type or these associated variants are currently being offered for warmbloods.

In the Appaloosa, a candidate gene approach was used to investigate the LP spotting locus (described above as the cause of CSNB) as well as the MHC locus.[4] Significant associations, based on an additive model, with a maker linked with LP as well as 2 microsatellites on ECA20 (microsatellite 472–260 located in the MHC class I region and microsatellite EqMHC1 located in intron 1 of the class II DRA gene) were detected. Genotypes from these associated loci accurately predicted ERU risk with approximately 80% accuracy in a second population of Appaloosas.[4] To develop a more robust risk model, a GWAS was performed. Loci on ECA1, 12, and 29 were associated based on an initial population of 91 horses.[59] However, the only risk locus that has been consistently replicated across multiple Appaloosa populations is LP, with homozygotes (LP/LP) being at the highest risk (**Fig. 4**).[54,59] At this time, it is unknown if LP is the causal risk variant or is simply tagging another nearby variant. More work is needed to characterize the LP loci and to evaluate if the other loci on ECA1, 12, and 20 represent true genetic risk loci or false positives.

It has been suggested that the amount of white and/or depigmentation that occurs as a horse ages (varnish roaning) may be a risk factor for ERU. The variability in Appaloosa pattern levels was thought to be dependent on modifier genes (see **Fig. 2**). One such modifier gene that has been investigated at the molecular level is known as PATN1, for first pattern modifier. PATN1 behaves in a dominant fashion, and an SNP in the RING finger and WD repeat domain 3 gene (RFWD3 ECA3g.24352525T > G) has been associated with high amounts of white patterning in Appaloosas and related breeds.[60] Modeling ERU disease risk did not support varnish roaning as an indicator of risk.[59] However, modeling disease risk in a population of 98 horses genotyped for both LP and PATN1 provided further support of an additive effect of LP and suggested an additive effect of PATN1 on ERU risk. Based on this study, horses homozygous for LP appear to be at the greatest risk of ERU, whereas horses that do not carry LP or PATN1 have the lowest probability of being affected with ERU. Therefore, genotyping for LP and PATN1 in the Appaloosa can be used to identify which horses to frequently evaluate and treat for signs of ocular

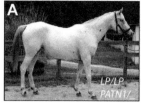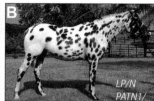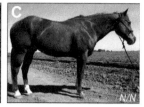

Fig. 4. Genetic risk for insidious ERU in Appaloosa horses. Leopard complex spotting *LP* is a risk factor for ERU. Homozygotes (*LP/LP*) (*A*) are at the highest risk for ERU (*LP/LP*) followed by heterozygotes (*LP/N*) (*B*) and then solid non-leopard complex spotted horses (*N/N*) (*C*). Recent work suggests that the modifier that contributes to large amounts of white patterning in breeds with leopard complex spotting (shown in *A* and *B*) may also contribute to ERU disease risk. Horses that do not have the *LP* or the *PATN1* alleles (in other words *N/N* at both loci) are at the lowest risk of developing the disease in the Appaloosa breed (*C*). (*Courtesy of* Martha Mitchell and Jocelyn Tanaka.)

inflammation as they age. Careful management of "at-risk" horses should be considered to include practices that decrease the risk of injury or inflammatory stimuli. More work is needed to investigate the specific role of *PATN1* in ERU risk in the Appaloosa, and genomic studies are ongoing to identify additional loci that explain the inherited risk component. Investigating *LP* and *PATN1* as risk factors in other breeds with leopard complex spotting remains to be performed.

OCULAR SQUAMOUS CELL CARCINOMA

Another common equine ocular disease across breeds is SCC. SCC is the most common cancer of the equine eye.[61] Ocular SCC can originate on the limbus of the cornea, or within the conjunctiva of the nictitans, or the conjunctiva or skin of the upper or lower haired eyelids. Tumors starting at or spreading to the cornea can lead to visual impairment and destruction of the eye.[13] The cause of SCC is not entirely understood, but recent work has connected the environmental factor of increased UV exposure to the genetic risk caused by a variant in a gene known to repair UV light damage to DNA.[5,62]

The involvement of genetics in ocular SCC was first supported by reports of bilateral disease and breed predispositions with the Appaloosa, American Paint Horse, Thoroughbred, Quarter Horse, Haflinger, and various draft breeds among those overrepresented.[62–65] The first genetic studies investigated SCC originating on the limbus in Haflingers (**Fig. 5**). These studies identified a prevalence of 35% in the breed and an autosomal-recessive mode of inheritance.[64,65] Using a GWAS approach, a 1.5-Mb associated locus on ECA12 was identified.[5] Sequencing a candidate gene from this locus, *damage-specific DNA binding protein 2* (*DDB2*) identified a missense mutation (c.1013C > T p.Thr338Met) strongly associated with limbal SCC status. Threonine 338 is part of the B-loop that inserts and interacts with the UV-damaged DNA to then recruit other proteins to repair the damage.[66] This risk allele is predicted to impair the ability of DDB2 to recognize and bind to UV-damaged DNA, thus leading to accumulation of mutations that connect genetic and environmental risks that can result in cancer. Five mutations in the same exon in DDB2 in humans have been shown to cause xeroderma pigmentosum complementation group E, which is clinically defined as sensitivity to UV light and increased risk for basal cell carcinoma, melanoma, and SCC of the epidermis.[67] Interestingly, none of these mutations have been linked directly to increased risk for ocular SCC in humans, and to date, this equine *DDB2*

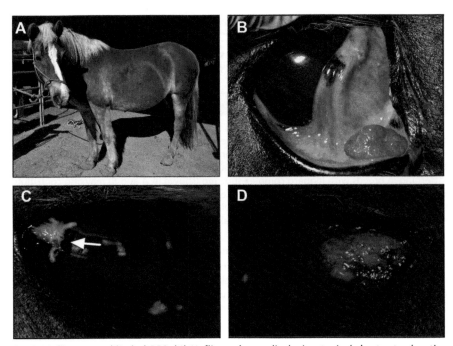

Fig. 5. Haflingers and limbal SCC. (*A*) Haflinger horse displaying typical chestnut coloration with flaxen mane and tail that are breed-defining characteristics. (*B*) Pink, raised tissue on the nictitans OD consistent with SCC. (*C*) Pink, slightly raised tissue OD consistent with lateral limbal mass (*arrow*). (*D*) More advanced OS limbal SCC that has spread over a portion of the cornea. (*Courtesy of* Rebecca Bellone, Kelly Knickelbein, and Mary Lassaline.)

variant has not been linked to SCC of other epidermal origins (specifically oral and urogenital SCCs) in horses.[68] Therefore, the role of DDB2 in DNA repair may differ between mammals.

In the initial study in Haflingers, homozygosity for the risk allele (the T allele is the risk allele and genetic tests denote this as R for risk) explained 77% of the limbal SCC cases.[5] Subsequent studies determined that homozygosity for this risk allele also explained a higher percentage of SCC of the conjunctiva of the nictitans (third eyelid) cases in the Haflinger breed (88%),[6] demonstrating that this risk allele is not restricted to the limbus. Furthermore, 76% of cases of all ocular SCC, including SCC of the limbus, nictitans, and other areas of ocular conjunctiva in the Belgian breed, were also explained by homozygosity for this allele.[7] Evaluating data from 166 Haflinger and Belgians showed horses homozygous for the *DDB2* risk allele were significantly younger than those with ocular SCC who were heterozygous (R/N) or wild type (N/N).[68] A recent limbal SCC case in a Rocky Mountain horse was also homozygous for the ocular SCC risk factor.[8] The allele frequency in the Rocky Mountain horse breed (0.20) is similar to that of the Haflinger and Belgian breed, which supports the use of this ocular SCC genetic test in Rocky Mountain horses. Given the distribution of this allele in multiple breeds, its role as a risk factor for ocular SCC in other breeds is warranted. Recently, this *DDB2* risk variant was shown to not be associated with ocular SCC in Appaloosas or Arabians.[68] Work is ongoing to investigate this variant in several additional breeds.

It is possible that other risk factors, both genetic and environmental, may contribute to ocular SCC in the horse. Several studies have implicated an increased risk of ocular SCC with chestnut coat color and gray coat depigmentation pattern across breeds.[63,69,70] The chestnut coat color results from a recessive mutation in the *melanocortin 1 receptor* (*MC1R c.248C > T, p.S83F*), allowing only for the production of pheomelanin, or red pigment. Research studies in people have shown that pheomelanin may be less photoprotective than eumelanin.[71] People with *MC1R* mutations tend to have red hair and fair skin and are generally photosensitive, prone to sunburn when exposed to UV light, and have an increased risk of melanomas tied to UV associated somatic C > T transitions.[72] All Haflinger and Belgian horses evaluated to date have been chestnut (see **Fig. 5**), so exploring the direct link with this equine variant has not yet been possible. In evaluating the Haflinger data set, geldings were more likely to be affected than stallions, which supports previous claims that hormonal differences between geldings and stallions are an additional risk factor.[68–70,73]

The *DDB2* risk allele is not perfectly concordant with disease status, as 20/84 affected Haflingers and Belgians were not homozygous (*R/R*). In addition, 1 control out of 80 unaffected Haflinger and Belgians was *R/R* but showed no clinical signs of disease by 20 years of age. Analyzing high-throughput sequencing data to further interrogate the 1.5-Mb associated locus on ECA12 did not identify another variant that was more concordant with phenotype.[68] These data provide further support that the *DDB2* variant is the functional risk allele.[68] It is possible that additional genetic risk loci, such as the *MC1R* locus that causes the chestnut coat color, may help to explain those Haflinger and Belgian cases not explained by the *DDB2* variant. Genomic investigations are underway.

In summary, genetic testing (https://www.vgl.ucdavis.edu/services/HaflingerSCC.php) can help to identify horses at risk for ocular SCC in the Haflinger, Belgian, and Rocky Mountain horse breeds. This test can be used to inform clinical and breeding decisions. Horses with the *R/R* genotype are more likely to develop SCC than *R/N* or *N/N*. Horses whose genotype is *R/R* should be examined frequently for early detection of dysplastic or neoplastic tissue, and excision of suspicious lesions should be carefully considered. Horses with ocular lesions that test *R/R* likely have a higher risk for recurrence; these horses should also be examined frequently. Because many of the risks for ocular SCC are tied to UV radiation, exposure should be minimized by the use of UV protective fly masks or keeping at-risk horses in stalls during peak hours. Breeding decisions should include avoidance of mating *R/R* or *R/N* horses with each other.

OCULAR MANIFESTATIONS OF EQUINE DISEASES CAUSED BY KNOWN GENETIC MUTATIONS

Inherited equine disorders impacting other systems can result in ocular manifestations. These diseases are covered at length in other articles of this equine genetics issue (Rebecca R. Bellone and Felipe Avila's article, "Genetic Testing in the Horse"; Lisa Edwards and Carrie J. Finno's article, "Genetics of Equine Neurologic Disease"; Gabriella Lindgren and colleagues' article, "Genetics of Skin Disease in Horses"; Stephanie Valberg's article, "Genetics of Equine Muscle Disease," in this issue). For diseases whereby the causal mutation is known, genetic test results can assist with clinical diagnosis (see **Table 2**). Hyperkalemic periodic paralysis is an example of an autosomal disorder that impacts skeletal muscles,[74] and ocular manifestations resulting from muscle weakness include third eyelid prolapse secondary to globe retraction.[75] Hereditary equine regional dermal asthenia (HERDA) is an example of an autosomal-recessive disorder characterized by hyperextensible skin and caused by a mutation in the *cyclophilin B gene* (*PPIB*).[76] PPIB is thought to play a role in collagen fibrillogenesis, and this can impact corneal development because horses with HERDA have abnormally thin corneas and are at an increased risk for corneal ulcers.[77] A second recessive condition causing mechanical stress–induced skin lesions is known as junctional epidermolysis bullosa (JEB). Mutations in 2 genes have been described for this condition in the horse, and each has been associated with corneal ulcers.[78] In the Belgian draft breed, an insertion of 1 nucleotide in the laminin gene *LAMC2* causes JEB, whereas in American saddlebreds a large deletion in the laminin gene *LAMA3* causes this disorder.[79,80] An X-linked trait, incontinentia pigmenti, can cause skin lesions that evolve over time; the family reported to have this condition was also noted to have teeth, hoof, and ocular developmental abnormalities.[81] A pigment retinopathy characterized by granular dark pigment was observed in 4 warmblood horses with equine neuroaxonal dystrophy (eNAD), but this ocular manifestation has not been reported in other breeds with eNAD.[82,83] Causal genetic variants for this disorder are not yet known, and the precise link of the pigment retinopathy to warmblood-specific eNAD has not been determined.

INHERITED OCULAR DISEASE WITH UNKNOWN GENETIC CAUSES

ERU, SCC, and CSNB occur in additional breeds for which a causal variant has yet to be identified (see **Table 3**). Although at this time it is not possible to genetically test for these disorders, knowing the breeds that are most likely affected by these and other ocular disorders can help to identify additional cases that will eventually make genetic discoveries possible. For example, a Thoroughbred and a Paso Fino were reported to have CSNB; it is unlikely that CSNB in these breeds are caused by the *LP* mutation. Given the number of genes causing human CSNB, it is plausible that this disease is present in other non-Appaloosa breeds, and mutations in additional genes will be discovered.

Further identification of causal risk variants for ERU, particularly in Appaloosas and other breeds with leopard complex spotting and in warmbloods, is needed because this condition is the leading cause of blindness in horses around the world. Robust genetic prediction for this complex trait is an active area of research. Concerning ocular SCC, identifying additional variants that explain risk for this cancer in Haflinger and Belgian breeds is underway as is investigating genetic risk factors in the Quarter Horse, American Paint Horse, and Appaloosa breeds.

Several additional ocular disorders are thought to be inherited, but the investigations have been mostly limited to studying the modes of inheritance, and therefore, causal mutations have not been determined (see **Table 3**). Evidence that an ocular disease has a genetic basis often comes from breed predilection and bilateral presentation. For example, developmental and congenital bilateral cataracts have been reported in the American Quarter Horse, Arabian, Thoroughbred, Morgan, and Exmoor breeds; however, to date no causal mutations have been found. Pedigree analysis suggests different modes of inheritance by breed; thus, multiple genetic mechanisms are likely. In Morgan horses, pedigree analysis of congenital nuclear cataracts suggested a dominant mode of inheritance that is sex influenced, with females being more severely affected.[84] In Exmoor ponies, a sex-linked mode of inheritance has been proposed.[85] Aniridia and iridial hypoplasia have been documented as dominantly inherited in Belgians and American Quarter Horses, but to date, no molecular studies have been performed.[86,87] Given the dominant mode of inheritance, offspring of affected horses should be carefully evaluated for disease.

Friesian horses have several reported inherited collagen disorders, including mega-esophagus, aortic rupture, dwarfism, and hydrocephalus. These disorders may be related to 2 ocular disorders reported to be prevalent in the breed, corneal dystrophy and distichiasis.[88–90] Corneal dystrophy, also referred to as bilateral corneal stromal loss (BCSL), is characterized by focal, symmetric thinning of the inferior peripheral corneal stroma unaccompanied by inflammation. BCSL has been reported to have a higher occurrence in male Friesians, making an inherited X-linked recessive hypothesis likely,[89] and additional pedigree analysis of 15 cases identified a common ancestor that further supports an X-linked recessive trait. However, sequencing *biglycan*, a candidate gene involved in collagen fibrogenesis located on the X-chromosome, did not identify a causal variant that could explain a simple X-linked trait.[91] Distichiasis is a condition whereby cilia emerge aberrantly from the meibomian gland openings along the eyelid margin. When the aberrant hairs point toward the cornea, they can cause corneal irritation or ulceration.[90] The breed predisposition implies a genetic cause. A dominant mode of inheritance has been proposed for a similar disorder in humans,[92] but the mode of inheritance has not been reported for the horse. The genetics of both BCSL and distichiasis is an active area of research, and causal mutations will likely be identified in the near future.

SUMMARY

Genetic testing for ocular disorders can complement ocular examinations and assist with clinical diagnosis. Currently, genetic tests to identify horses are available for MCOA in several breeds and for CSNB in breeds with leopard complex spotting. Genetic testing is also available to identify horses at risk for developing ERU in the Appaloosa breed and ocular SCC in Haflinger, Belgian, and Rocky Mountain horses. Screening horses for genetic mutations helps inform management decisions and provides evidence for clinicians to advocate frequent screening of at-risk patients, permitting early diagnosis and treatment of progressive ocular disorders and an opportunity to improve the prognosis of some conditions. Genetic testing also identifies horses with increased chances of producing offspring that will develop serious ocular disease or anomalies, allowing for selective breeding to reduce these problems. With continued advances in the knowledge of the equine genome, along with reduction in costs for experiments involving whole-genome sequencing, and assistance of clinicians contributing relevant case samples and phenotypes, additional causal variants for ocular disease will soon be discovered.

ACKNOWLEDGMENTS

The author thanks Nicole Kingsley and Jocelyn Tanaka for their assistance in preparing the figures and acknowledges Drs Ann Dwyer, Lynne Sandmeyer, and Mike Mienaltowski for edits that improved the article.

DISCLOSURE

R.R. Bellone is affiliated with the Veterinary Genetics Laboratory, a genetic testing laboratory offering diagnostic tests in horses and other species. Genetic investigation of ERU in the Appaloosa was supported by the Morris Animal Foundation Grant D16EQ-028. The mission of the Morris Animal Foundation is to bridge science and resources to advance the health of animals. Investigation of the inherited risk for ocular SCC was supported by Morris Animal Foundation Grant D13EQ-808 and by UC Davis Center for

Equine Health Grants with funds provided by the State of California Pari-Mutuel Fund and contributions by private donors.

REFERENCES

1. Miller P, Murphy CJ. Equine vision. Equine ophthalmology. 3rd edition. Hoboken, New Jersey: John Wiley & Sons, Inc; 2017. p. 508–44.
2. Brunberg E, Andersson L, Cothran G, et al. A missense mutation in PMEL17 is associated with the silver coat color in the horse. BMC Genet 2006;7:46.
3. Bellone RR, Holl H, Setaluri V, et al. Evidence for a retroviral insertion in TRPM1 as the cause of congenital stationary night blindness and leopard complex spotting in the horse. PLoS One 2013;8:e78280.
4. Fritz KL, Kaese HJ, Valberg SJ, et al. Genetic risk factors for insidious equine recurrent uveitis in Appaloosa horses. Anim Genet 2014;45:392–9.
5. Bellone RR, Liu J, Petersen JL, et al. A missense mutation in damage-specific DNA binding protein 2 is a genetic risk factor for limbal squamous cell carcinoma in horses. Int J Cancer 2017;141:342–53.
6. Singer-Berk M, Knickelbein KE, Vig S, et al. Genetic risk for squamous cell carcinoma of the nictitating membrane parallels that of the limbus in Haflinger horses. Anim Genet 2018;49:457–60.
7. Knickelbein KE, Lassaline ME, Singer-Berk M, et al. A missense mutation in damage-specific DNA binding protein 2 is a genetic risk factor for ocular squamous cell carcinoma in Belgian horses. Equine Vet J 2020;52(1):34–40.
8. Knickelbein KE, Lassaline ME, Bellone RR. Limbal squamous cell carcinoma in a Rocky Mountain horse: case report and investigation of genetic contribution. Vet Ophthalmol 2019;22:201–5.
9. Ewart SL, Ramsey DT, Xu J, et al. The horse homolog of congenital aniridia conforms to codominant inheritance. J Hered 2000;91:93–8.
10. Ramsey DT, Ewart SL, Render JA, et al. Congenital ocular abnormalities of Rocky Mountain horses. Vet Ophthalmol 1999;2:47–59.
11. Grahn BH, Pinard C, Archer S, et al. Congenital ocular anomalies in purebred and crossbred Rocky and Kentucky Mountain horses in Canada. Can Vet J 2008;49: 675–81.
12. Andersson LS, Axelsson J, Dubielzig RR, et al. Multiple congenital ocular anomalies in Icelandic horses. BMC Vet Res 2011;7:21.
13. Kaps S, Richter M, Philipp M, et al. Primary invasive ocular squamous cell carcinoma in a horse. Vet Ophthalmol 2005;8:193–7.
14. Komaromy AM, Rowlan JS, La Croix NC, et al. Equine multiple congenital ocular anomalies (MCOA) syndrome in PMEL17 (silver) mutant ponies: five cases. Vet Ophthalmol 2011;14:313–20.
15. Plummer CE, Ramsey DT. A survey of ocular abnormalities in miniature horses. Vet Ophthalmol 2011;14:239–43.
16. Segard EM, Depecker MC, Lang J, et al. Ultrasonographic features of PMEL17 (silver) mutant gene-associated multiple congenital ocular anomalies (MCOA) in Comtois and Rocky Mountain horses. Vet Ophthalmol 2013;16:429–35.
17. Ramsey DT, Hauptman JG, Petersen-Jones SM. Corneal thickness, intraocular pressure, and optical corneal diameter in Rocky Mountain horses with cornea globosa or clinically normal corneas. Am J Vet Res 1999;60:1317–21.
18. Andersson LS, Lyberg K, Cothran G, et al. Targeted analysis of four breeds narrows equine multiple congenital ocular anomalies locus to 208 kilobases. Mamm Genome 2011;22:353–60.

19. Andersson LS, Wilbe M, Viluma A, et al. Equine multiple congenital ocular anomalies and silver coat colour result from the pleiotropic effects of mutant PMEL. PLoS One 2013;8:e75639.

20. Berson JF, Harper DC, Tenza D, et al. Pmel17 initiates premelanosome morphogenesis within multivesicular bodies. Mol Biol Cell 2001;12:3451–64.

21. Theos AC, Berson JF, Theos SC, et al. Dual loss of ER export and endocytic signals with altered melanosome morphology in the silver mutation of Pmel17. Mol Biol Cell 2006;17:3598–612.

22. Gelatt KN, Powell NG, Huston K. Inheritance of microphthalmia with coloboma in the Australian shepherd dog. Am J Vet Res 1981;42:1686–90.

23. Schonthaler HB, Lampert JM, von Lintig J, et al. A mutation in the silver gene leads to defects in melanosome biogenesis and alterations in the visual system in the zebrafish mutant fading vision. Dev Biol 2005;284:421–36.

24. Watt B, Tenza D, Lemmon MA, et al. Mutations in or near the transmembrane domain alter PMEL amyloid formation from functional to pathogenic. PLoS Genet 2011;7:e1002286.

25. Hellstrom AR, Watt B, Fard SS, et al. Inactivation of Pmel alters melanosome shape but has only a subtle effect on visible pigmentation. PLoS Genet 2011;7: e1002285.

26. Johansson MK, Jaderkvist Fegraeus K, Lindgren G, et al. The refractive state of the eye in Icelandic horses with the silver mutation. BMC Vet Res 2017;13:153.

27. Sandmeyer LS, Grahn BH, Breaux CB. Diagnostic ophthalmology. Congenital stationary night blindness (CSNB). Can Vet J 2006;47:1131–3.

28. Witzel DA, Joyce JR, Smith EL. Electroretinography of congenital night blindness in an Appaloosa filly. J Equine Med Surg 1977;1:226–9.

29. Witzel DA, Riis RC, Rebhun WC, et al. Night blindness in Appaloosa–sibling occurrence. J Equine Med Surg 1977;1:383–6.

30. Witzel DA, Smith EL, Wilson RD, et al. Congenital stationary night blindness: an animal model. Invest Ophthalmol Vis Sci 1978;17:788–95.

31. Rebhun WC, Loew ER, Riis RC, et al. Clinical manifestations of night blindness in the Appaloosa horse. Comp Cont Educ Pract 1984;6:S103.

32. Sandmeyer LS, Breaux CB, Archer S, et al. Clinical and electroretinographic characteristics of congenital stationary night blindness in the Appaloosa and the association with the leopard complex. Vet Ophthalmol 2007;10:368–75.

33. Sandmeyer LS, Bellone RR, Archer S, et al. Congenital stationary night blindness is associated with the leopard complex in the miniature horse. Vet Ophthalmol 2012;15:18–22.

34. de Linde Henriksen M, Blaabjerg K, Baptiste KE, et al. Congenital stationary night blindness (CSNB) in the Danish Knabstrupper horse. Vet Ophthalmol 2007; 10:326.

35. Nunnery C, Pickett JP, Zimmerman KL. Congenital stationary night blindness in a thoroughbred and a Paso Fino. Vet Ophthalmol 2005;8:415–9.

36. Bellone RR, Brooks SA, Sandmeyer L, et al. Differential gene expression of TRPM1, the potential cause of congenital stationary night blindness and coat spotting patterns (LP) in the Appaloosa horse (Equus caballus). Genetics 2008;179:1861–70.

37. Morgans CW, Brown RL, Duvoisin RM. TRPM1: the endpoint of the mGluR6 signal transduction cascade in retinal ON-bipolar cells. Bioessays 2010;32:609–14.

38. Morgans CW, Zhang J, Jeffrey BG, et al. TRPM1 is required for the depolarizing light response in retinal ON-bipolar cells. Proc Natl Acad Sci U S A 2009;106: 19174–8.

39. Zeitz C, Robson AG, Audo I. Congenital stationary night blindness: an analysis and update of genotype-phenotype correlations and pathogenic mechanisms. Prog Retin Eye Res 2015;45:58–110.

40. Miraldi Utz V, Pfeifer W, Longmuir SQ, et al. Presentation of TRPM1-associated congenital stationary night blindness in children. JAMA Ophthalmol 2018;136: 389–98.

41. Gilger BC. Equine recurrent uveitis: the viewpoint from the USA. Equine Vet J Suppl 2010;(37):57–61.

42. Kulbrock M, von Borstel M, Rohn K, et al. Occurrence and severity of equine recurrent uveitis in warmblood horses–a comparative study. Pferdeheilkunde 2013;29:27–36.

43. Deeg CA, Kaspers B, Gerhards H, et al. Immune responses to retinal autoantigens and peptides in equine recurrent uveitis. Invest Ophthalmol Vis Sci 2001; 42:393–8.

44. Davidson MG, Nasisse MP, Roberts SM. Immunodiagnosis of leptospiral uveitis in two horses. Equine Vet J 1987;19:155–7.

45. Brem S, Gerhards H, Wollanke B, et al. Demonstration of intraocular leptospira in 4 horses suffering from equine recurrent uveitis (ERU). Berl Munch Tierarztl Wochenschr 1998;111:415–7 [in German].

46. Brem S, Gerhards H, Wollanke B, et al. 35 leptospira isolated from the vitreous body of 32 horses with recurrent uveitis (ERU). Berl Munch Tierarztl Wochenschr 1999;112:390–3 [in German].

47. Brandes K, Wollanke B, Niedermaier G, et al. Recurrent uveitis in horses: vitreal examinations with ultrastructural detection of leptospires. J Vet Med A Physiol Pathol Clin Med 2007;54:270–5.

48. Gerding JC, Gilger BC. Prognosis and impact of equine recurrent uveitis. Equine Vet J 2016;48:290–8.

49. Dwyer AE, Crockett RS, Kalsow CM. Association of leptospiral seroreactivity and breed with uveitis and blindness in horses: 372 cases (1986-1993). J Am Vet Med Assoc 1995;207:1327–31.

50. Pearce JW, Galle LE, Kleiboeker SB, et al. Detection of Leptospira interrogans DNA and antigen in fixed equine eyes affected with end-stage equine recurrent uveitis. J Vet Diagn Invest 2007;19:686–90.

51. Saldinger LK, Nelson SG, Bellone RR, et al. Horses with equine recurrent uveitis have an activated CD4+ T-cell phenotype that can be modulated by mesenchymal stem cells in vitro. Vet Ophthalmol 2020;23(1):160–70.

52. Gilger BC, Salmon JH, Yi NY, et al. Role of bacteria in the pathogenesis of recurrent uveitis in horses from the southeastern United States. Am J Vet Res 2008;69: 1329–35.

53. Sandmeyer LS, Bauer BS, Feng CX, et al. Equine recurrent uveitis in western Canadian prairie provinces: a retrospective study (2002-2015). Can Vet J 2017;58: 717–22.

54. Sandmeyer LS, Kingsley NB, Waldner CL, et al. Risk factors for equine recurrent uveitis in a population of Appaloosa horses in western Canada. Vet Ophthalmol 2020. https://doi.org/10.1111/vop.12749.

55. Kulbrock M, Lehner S, Metzger J, et al. A genome-wide association study identifies risk loci to equine recurrent uveitis in German warmblood horses. PLoS One 2013;8:e71619.

56. Feltkamp TE. HLA and uveitis. Int Ophthalmol 1990;14:327–33.

57. Zamecki KJ, Jabs DA. HLA typing in uveitis: use and misuse. Am J Ophthalmol 2010;149:189–93.e2.

58. Deeg CA, Marti E, Gaillard C, et al. Equine recurrent uveitis is strongly associated with the MHC class I haplotype ELA-A9. Equine Vet J 2004;36:73–5.

59. Rockwell H, Mack M, Famula TR, et al. Genetic investigation of equine recurrent uveitis in Appaloosa horses. Anim Genet 2020;51:111–6.

60. Holl HM, Brooks SA, Archer S, et al. Variant in the RFWD3 gene associated with PATN1, a modifier of leopard complex spotting. Anim Genet 2016;47:91–101.

61. Strafuss AC. Squamous cell carcinoma in horses. J Am Vet Med Assoc 1976; 168:61–2.

62. Dugan S, Curtis C, Roberts S, et al. Epidemiologic study of ocular/adnexal squamous cell carcinoma in horses. J Am Vet Med Assoc 1991;198:251–6.

63. Plummer CE, Smith S, Andrew SE, et al. Combined keratectomy, strontium-90 irradiation and permanent bulbar conjunctival grafts for corneolimbal squamous cell carcinomas in horses (1990–2002): 38 horses. Vet Ophthalmol 2007;10: 37–42.

64. Bosch G, Klein WR. Superficial keratectomy and cryosurgery as therapy for limbal neoplasms in 13 horses. Vet Ophthalmol 2005;8:241–6.

65. Lassaline M, Cranford TL, Latimer CA, et al. Limbal squamous cell carcinoma in Haflinger horses. Vet Ophthalmol 2015;18:404–8.

66. Yeh JI, Levine AS, Du S, et al. Damaged DNA induced UV-damaged DNA-binding protein (UV-DDB) dimerization and its roles in chromatinized DNA repair. Proc Natl Acad Sci U S A 2012;109:E2737–46.

67. Oh KS, Emmert S, Tamura D, et al. Multiple skin cancers in adults with mutations in the XP-E (DDB2) DNA repair gene. J Invest Dermatol 2011;131:785–8.

68. Singer-Berk MH, Knickelbein KE, Lounsberry ZT, et al. Additional evidence for DDB2 T338M as a genetic risk factor for ocular squamous cell carcinoma in horses. Int J Genomics 2019;2019:10.

69. Mosunic CB, Moore PA, Carmicheal KP, et al. Effects of treatment with and without adjuvant radiation therapy on recurrence of ocular and adnexal squamous cell carcinoma in horses: 157 cases (1985-2002). J Am Vet Med Assoc 2004;225:1733–8.

70. Michau TM, Davidson MG, Gilger BC. Carbon dioxide laser photoablation adjunctive therapy following superficial lamellar keratectomy and bulbar conjunctivectomy for the treatment of corneolimbal squamous cell carcinoma in horses: a review of 24 cases. Vet Ophthalmol 2012;15:245–53.

71. Marklund L, Moller MJ, Sandberg K, et al. A missense mutation in the gene for melanocyte-stimulating hormone receptor (MC1R) is associated with the chestnut coat color in horses. Mamm Genome 1996;7:895–9.

72. Robles-Espinoza CD, Roberts ND, Chen S, et al. Germline MC1R status influences somatic mutation burden in melanoma. Nat Commun 2016;7:12064.

73. Kafarnik C, Rawlings M, Dubielzig RR. Corneal stromal invasive squamous cell carcinoma: a retrospective morphological description in 10 horses. Vet Ophthalmol 2009;12:6–12.

74. Rudolph JA, Spier SJ, Byrns G, et al. Periodic paralysis in quarter horses: a sodium channel mutation disseminated by selective breeding. Nat Genet 1992;2: 144–7.

75. Cullen CL, Webb AA. Ocular manifestations of systemic disease. Part 3: the horse. In: Gelatt KN, Gilger BC, Kern TJ, editors. Veterinary Ophthalmology. 5th edition. Ames (IA): John Wiley and Sons, Inc; 2013. p. 2037–70.

76. Tryon RC, White SD, Bannasch DL. Homozygosity mapping approach identifies a missense mutation in equine cyclophilin B (PPIB) associated with HERDA in the American quarter horse. Genomics 2007;90:93–102.

77. Mochal CA, Miller WW, Cooley AJ, et al. Ocular findings in quarter horses with hereditary equine regional dermal asthenia. J Am Vet Med Assoc 2010;237:304–10.
78. Kohn CW, Johnson GC, Garry F, et al. Mechanobullous disease in two Belgian foals. Equine Vet J 1989;21:297–301.
79. Milenkovic D, Chaffaux S, Taourit S, et al. A mutation in the LAMC2 gene causes the Herlitz junctional epidermolysis bullosa (H-JEB) in two French draft horse breeds. Genet Sel Evol 2003;35:249–56.
80. Graves KT, Henney PJ, Ennis RB. Partial deletion of the LAMA3 gene is responsible for hereditary junctional epidermolysis bullosa in the American saddlebred horse. Anim Genet 2009;40:35–41.
81. Towers RE, Murgiano L, Millar DS, et al. A nonsense mutation in the IKBKG gene in mares with incontinentia pigmenti. PLoS One 2013;8:e81625.
82. Finno CJ, Aleman M, Ofri R, et al. Electrophysiological studies in American Quarter horses with neuroaxonal dystrophy. Vet Ophthalmol 2012;15(Suppl 2):3–7.
83. Finno CJ, Kaese HJ, Miller AD, et al. Pigment retinopathy in warmblood horses with equine degenerative myeloencephalopathy and equine motor neuron disease. Vet Ophthalmol 2017;20:304–9.
84. Beech J, Irby N. Inherited nuclear cataracts in the Morgan horse. J Hered 1985; 76:371–2.
85. Pinard CL, Basrur PK. Ocular anomalies in a herd of Exmoor ponies in Canada. Vet Ophthalmol 2011;14:100–8.
86. Eriksson K. Hereditary aniridia with secondary cataract in horses. Nord Vet Med 1955;7:773–93.
87. Joyce JR, Martin JE, Storts RW, et al. Iridial hypoplasia (aniridia) accompanied by limbic dermoids and cataracts in a group of related quarterhorses. Equine Vet J Suppl 1990;(10):26–8.
88. Boerma S, Back W, Sloet van Oldruitenborgh-Oossterbaan MM. The Friesian horse breed: a clinical challenge to the equine veterinarian? Equine Vet Education 2012;24:66–71.
89. Lassaline-Utter M, Gemensky-Metzler AJ, Scherrer NM, et al. Corneal dystrophy in Friesian horses may represent a variant of pellucid marginal degeneration. Vet Ophthalmol 2014;17:186–94.
90. Hermans H, Ensink JM. Treatment and long-term follow-up of distichiasis, with special reference to the Friesian horse: a case series. Equine Vet J 2014;46: 458–62.
91. Alberi C, Hisey E, Lassaline M, et al. Ruling out BGN variants as simple X-linked causative mutations for bilateral corneal stromal loss in Friesian horses. Anim Genet 2018;49(6):656–7.
92. Samlaska CP. Congenital lymphedema and distichiasis. Pediatr Dermatol 2002; 19:139–41.

Genetics of Skin Disease in Horses

Gabriella Lindgren, PhD[a,b], Rakan Naboulsi, PhD[a], Rebecka Frey, DVM[c],
Marina Solé, PhD[a,*]

KEYWORDS

- Genetics • Hereditary skin disorders • Horses • Insect bite hypersensitivity
- Melanoma • Ehlers-Danlos syndrome • Chronic progressive lymphedema

KEY POINTS

- Genetic testing can be used as an instrument for breeding against hereditary genetic skin diseases in horses.
- Genetic tests are available for hereditary equine regional dermal asthenia, warmblood fragile foal syndrome, junctional epidermolysis bullosa, incontinentia pigmenti, and hypotrichosis.
- Insect bite hypersensitivity is a common complex disease affected by several genes (polygenic inheritance) and environmental factors.
- Genomic technologies emerge as a useful tool to understand the genetics behind common complex skin diseases.
- Horse can serve as an animal model for the human skin conditions.

INTRODUCTION
Structure and Function of the Skin

Skin displays an astonishing diverse set of phenotypes and physiologic functions ranging from skin and hair color to immune function. Acting as a primary barrier between the body and its environment, its key functions are (1) to prevent environmental compounds from permeating into the epidermal and dermal layers, giving rise to an immune response and (2) to restrain excessive water passage from one side to the other of the epidermis, in particular providing an effective barrier to the loss of water. Skin functions as an immunologic barrier and is often the first organ to connect to adverse allergens. It is an immunologic organ, nominated as a peripheral lymphoid organ that contains several important types of immunocompetent cells in both epidermis and dermis.[1–3] The immune competence in epidermis is mainly mediated

[a] Department of Animal Breeding and Genetics, Swedish University of Agricultural Sciences, Almas Allé 8, Uppsala 75007, Sweden; [b] Livestock Genetics, Department of Biosystems, KU Leuven Leuven, KasteelparkArenberg 30, Leuven 3001, Belgium; [c] AniCura Norsholms Djursjukhus, Norsholm 61791, Sweden
* Corresponding author.
E-mail address: marina.sole@slu.se

Vet Clin Equine 36 (2020) 323–339
https://doi.org/10.1016/j.cveq.2020.03.010
0749-0739/20/© 2020 The Author(s). Published by Elsevier Inc. This is an open access article under the CC BY-NC-ND license (http://creativecommons.org/licenses/by-nc-nd/4.0/).
vetequine.theclinics.com

by keratinocytes secreting immunoregulatory compounds and antigen-presenting Langerhans cells, whereas in the deeper layer dermis cells such as assorted dendritic cells, mast cells, and T-cell subsets play a crucial role.[1] As a group, these well-organized cells mediate cutaneous immunosurveillance. It can be expected that immune reactions in the skin are equally important to those occurring within classical lymphoid organs in protection from harmful foreign substances. Further, skin provides sensory perception for touch and pain, temperature regulation, and pigmentation and produces structures such as hair and hoof.

Mammal skin is a multicellular organ, and its *morphogenesis* includes expression of multiple genes in a coordinated fashion. The anatomic structures of equine skin have been reported in multiple studies[4–7] (**Fig. 1**). Skin is generally composed of 2 layers, the outer nonvascular epidermis and the inner vascular and sensitive dermis. In horses, the epidermis consists of 5 to 7 cell layers, excluding the horny layer in haired body skin, that are constantly multiplying from its deeper layers and eventually drop off at the surface.[6,8] The most abundant cell type of the epidermis is keratinocytes (about 85%).[6,9] The dermis is mostly composed of connective tissue and account for most of the strength and elasticity of the skin. It composes an interconnected mesh of elastin and collagenous fibers, produced by fibroblasts. Normally the dermis is sparsely populated with cells; however, fibroblasts, dermal dendrocytes, and mast cells are present throughout with varying density.[5,8,10] Melanocytes are most commonly present in the basal layer of epidermis; however, these cells can also be present in the superficial layers of dermis in strongly pigmented skin. The dermis also supports and maintains many other structures, such as blood and lymph vessels, hair follicles, muscles, nerves, and glands (sweat and sebaceous). In horses, the general skin thickness varies over the body (eg, thickest on the forehead, dorsal neck, dorsal thorax, rump, and base of the tail),[8] with the average thickness of the mane and tail epidermis being 91 μm versus 53 μm for the epidermis of the general body skin under the coat.[8]

Under normal circumstances, hair growth occurs in a cycle, rather than continuous growth.[11] Hair follicles are the structures that contain the roots of the hair and consist of 5 major components: the dermal hair papilla, the hair matrix, the inner root sheath, the outer root sheath, and the hair shaft itself.[12] There are 3 main phases of the hair growth cycle: anagen, catagen, and telogen. Anagen is the growing stage where

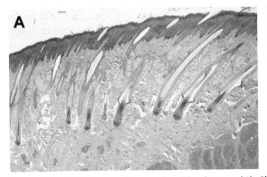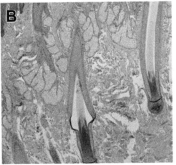

Fig. 1. Lip skin biopsy from a healthy horse. (*A*) Skin structure: epidermis and dermis including hair follicles (light microscopy X1). (*B*) Zoom of the dermis hair follicles (light microscopy X4). (*Courtesy of* Eva Hellmén, DVM, Professor, Dipl. ECVP. Swedish University of Agricultural Sciences, Department of Anatomy, Physiology and Biochemistry, Uppsala, Sweden.)

hair is produced by mitosis in cells of the dermal papilla. Catagen is the transition stage where a constriction of the hair bulb takes place and the distal follicle becomes broad and presses the hair outward. Telogen is the resting stage where a secondary germ is formed. The hair growth continues until it attains its predetermined length, a mechanism that is under genetic regulation. Knowledge of the genetic factors that regulate the hair cycle is limited. Equine mane hairs are similar to human scalp hairs because they grow to a greater length than the body hairs, that is, mane hairs have a long anagen growth phase. Periodic molting of hairs allows the pelage to adapt to seasonal changes. Shedding is predominantly influenced by photoperiod and affects the hairs of the body, whereas hairs of the mane, tail, and fetlock are basically exempt from such regulation.[12]

Role of Genetics in Skin Morphogenesis and Disease

The process of generating the anatomic structures of the equine skin has, to the authors' knowledge, not been reported. However, information on skin morphogenesis in other domestic mammals and human is available.[12] In mammals, distinct signaling patterns specify different developmental stages that ensure correct morphogenesis of skin and its associated structures such as hair and hoof.[13,14] The whole process requires a tightly controlled sequence of signaling events. Because genetics regulate organ development, and adult phenotypes are usually defined during development, investigations on differences in gene expression, contribution of new genes, changes in alternative splicing, and role of regulatory RNAs (long noncoding RNA [lncRNA] and microRNA [miRNA] [**Box 1**]) are important to understand phenotypic diversity such as disease. Genetic regulation of mammalian organ development/ morphogenesis is only partly understood.[15–17] For instance, the contribution of lncRNAs to organ development remains vastly unexplored in mammals, including horses.

Since the onset of domestication, horses have been strongly selected for speed, strength, gaits, and endurance-exercise traits. The development of specific horse breeds has resulted in the selection for athletic phenotypes that enable the use of horses for riding, racing, and recreation, with clear differences in morphology and behavior. The breed formation process has also enriched different horse breeds for

---

Box 1
Definitions of biological terminologies

Morphogenesis: the developmental process of the shape/morphology of an organism.

lncRNA: long (200 bp) nonconding RNAs are molecules that are not translated to proteins. They play a role in *the regulation of gene expression.*

miRNA: micro (~20 bp) RNA are shorter than lncRNA but also function in regulating gene expression.

Genome-to-phenome research: the study of the link between the DNA sequence (genome) and the different phenotypic characteristics (phenome) of an organism.

GWAS: a genome-wide association study is an approach used to investigate the association of a specific trait (a phenotype such as a shape or disease) to its causative genetic variants.

SNP: a single nucleotide that is polymorphic in a population.

Epistasis: is when the effect of one gene depends on the effect of another gene.

Breeding value: the value of an individual animal in a breeding program for a specific trait. An animal's expected breeding value is the sum of the halves of the breeding values of each parent.

disease mutations, and sometimes these mutations are breed specific. Disease mutations in horses offer the advantages of spontaneous disease models.

This review on equine genetic skin disease aims to present some of the latest advances in *genome-to-phenome research* in a nonmodel species of both medical and agricultural interest. It will summarize equine skin disease for which genetic tests are available and discuss their potential role as a complementing diagnostic tool. Genetic testing as an instrument for breeding against genetic skin diseases in horses will also be outlined. The review ends with perspectives on future studies in relation to these skin diseases.

Insect Bite Hypersensitivity

Insect bite hypersensitivity (IBH) is the most common allergic skin diseases in horses worldwide. The allergic reaction is toward the biting midges *Culicoidesspp*, but other insects can also be involved or be cross-reactive.[18] The acute stage of the disease involves an immunoglobulin E (IgE)-mediated type I hypersensitivity reaction, but a delayed type IV hypersensitivity reaction is likely present during the chronic stages of the disease. The clinical signs are gradual in onset and seasonally recurrent because the insects only live during the warm period from spring to autumn. The symptoms are severe pruritus in the mane and tail, leading to self-excoriations and secondary changes in the skin including crusted papules, hyperkeratosis, lichenification with thickening of the skin, diffuse to complete alopecia, and ulcerations (**Fig. 2**). The lesions can also be seen in the face and ears, at the chest and/or ventrum, in the axillae, and at the hips.[19]

All breeds can develop IBH and the prevalence has been calculated as a wide range, between 3% and 60% in different studies.[20–23] The Icelandic horse is particularly affected because the midges do not exist in Iceland and the horses get sensitized when exported abroad. The higher prevalence for Icelandic horses exported to the continent has been demonstrated in several studies and shows that the exposure to the midges is essential for development of IBH. It also shows that the prevalence for Icelandic horses born outside Iceland does not differ very much from other breeds, with figures between 6.7% and 8%.[20,22] The heritability in various breeds ranges from 0.16 to 0.30.[24] Heritability was estimated to be 0.16 in Friesian horses, 0.24 in Dutch Shetland ponies, and 0.27 in Icelandic horses.[24–26] When severity was taken into account in the Swedish study of Icelandic horses, heritability was estimated at 0.30. In the same study, offspring from mares with IBH demonstrated a higher risk of developing the disease. The prevalence was in the range of 0% to 30% in different paternal half-sib groups, which clearly shows the difference on an individual level in the heritability of the disease.[24]

At this time, there are no validated tests for the diagnosis of IBH. Therefore, the diagnosis is clinical and involves ruling out other pruritic diseases such as parasites, together with the typical clinical presentation of seasonal recurrent pruritus in the mane and tail. Intradermal skin tests or serology tests for antigen-specific IgE have been used to identify allergens involved in the allergic reaction, but several studies have shown that the available tests have low sensitivity and/or specificity and are not standardized.[27,28]

In the 1990s, it was determined using serology that certain major histocompatibility complexes (MHC), that is, equine leukocyte antigen (ELA) specificities, were linked to IBH susceptibility.[20,29,30] Later, DNA genotyping, as a substitute for ELA serology, showed that the ELA class II region in horses was associated with IBH susceptibility.[31] The same ELA class II risk factors were shown to contribute to equine IBH in 2 distinct horse breeds, Icelandic horses and Exmoorponies.[31] Yet another study found

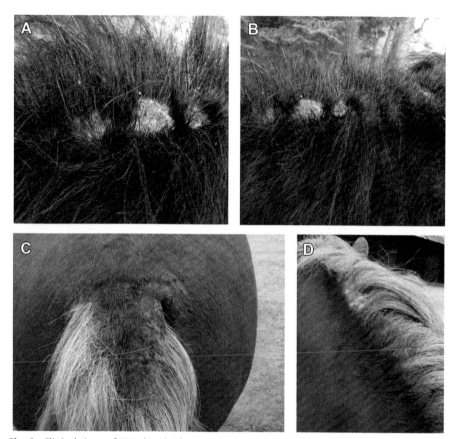

Fig. 2. Clinical signs of IBH. (*A, B*) Alopecia, broken hairs, and focal ulcerations in the mane. (*C, D*) Alopecia, hyperpigmentation, and lichenification at the base of the tail and in the mane. (*Courtesy of* Rebecka Frey, DVM, AniCura Norsholms Djursjukhus, Norsholm, Sweden.)

associations between genetic markers in ELA class II region and IBH susceptibility in Icelandic horses.[32] However, this study also identified susceptibility to IBH in 4 candidate allergy-related genes: CD14 receptor (*CD14*), interleukin 23 receptor (*IL23R*), thymic stromal lymphopoietin (*TSLP*), and transforming growth factor beta 3 (*TGFB3*).[32] Because the genomic structure of the horse MHC class II region has been resolved,[33,34] it may now be possible to fine map the responsible susceptibility risk factors. The MHC haplotype diversity was recently determined in Icelandic horses, which should further facilitate gene mapping within the region in this particular breed.[35]

With the overall goal to both breed against IBH and improve the health and welfare of IBH-affected horses via development of new treatments, several studies had the aim to scan the whole equine genome to identify susceptibility genes. *Genome-wide association studies (GWAS)* using large numbers of *single nucleotide polymorphisms (SNPs)* in cases and control animals have most frequently been used for this purpose. The first GWAS on IBH in horses was performed on Shetland pony mares living in the Netherlands.[36] Significant associations to IBH were detected on 12 chromosomes, including ECA20, where ELA is located. Subsequently, several GWAS for IBH have been performed within Icelandic horses, Exmoor ponies, Friesian horses, and Belgian Warmbloodhorses[37–42] (**Table 1**). One of these GWAS was performed using both

Table 1
Summary of genomic regions identified in genome-wide association studies on insect bite hypersensitivity

Method (Array)	Breed	GWAS Windows Hits	Overlapping Windows Hits[a]	ELA	References
Case-control GWAS (70K)	Icelandic horse	20	9	Yes	Schurink et al,[36] 2012
Case-control GWAS (50K)	Icelandic horse	29	6	No	Shrestha et al,[38] 2015
Case-control GWAS (50K & 70K)	Icelandic horse	30	12	No	Shrestha et al,[42] 2019
GWAS IgE levels (70K)	Icelandic horse	35	8	Yes	François et al,[41] 2019
Case-control GWAS (70K)	Shetland pony	20	8	Yes	Schurink et al,[36] 2012
Case-control GWAS (50K)	Shetland pony	18	5	No	Schurink et al,[37] 2013
GWAS IgE levels (70K)	Shetland pony	35	5	Yes	François et al,[41] 2019
Case-control GWAS (670K)	Exmoor pony	24	4	Yes	Velie et al,[39] 2016
Chi-square test (TaqMan assay)	Exmoor pony	2	2	No	Shrestha et al,[42] 2019
Case-control SNP- & CNV-based GWAS (670K)	Friesian horse	23	6	Yes	Schurink et al,[40] 2018
GWAS IgE levels (670K)	Belgian Warmblood horse	35	5	No	François et al,[41] 2019

[a] Comparison with recent bibliography up to 2019.[36–42]

copy number variants (one type of structural variation) and SNPs in the analysis, and both types of genetic markers were able to identify a clear association between the ELA region and IBH susceptibility in Friesian horses.[40] Recently, in an attempt to improve the power to identify underlying genetic variants for IBH, an objective diagnosis of horses with and without IBH was performed using IgE levels against several recombinant *Culicoides* spp. allergens.[41] The study was performed in Shetland ponies, Icelandic horses, and Belgian Warmblood horses. Several chromosome regions could be detected that confirmed previously IBH-associated regions, but novel regions were also identified. The use of allergen-specific IgE levels as a quantitative phenotype had an added value because a larger number of associations were obtained, as compared with a binary case-control design using the same horse material.

In summary, breed differences in susceptibility to IBH exist, although a common genetic background is present to some extent among certain breeds. The overall conclusions from these genomic studies are that IBH is a complex disease that involves the additive effects of many genes and the interplay between genetic and environmental factors (see **Table 1**).

Melanoma and Vitiligo

Melanomas in horses appear as black lumps or nodules most commonly near hairless areas, such as under the tail, around the anus, or in the sheath of geldings. They can develop anywhere and, even if most of the tumors are benign, they tend to become malignant by aging. The melanomas occur in higher frequency in gray-colored horses, and around 80% of all greying horses will get melanomas by 15 years of age. The diagnosis is made by fine-needle aspiration or biopsy of the nodules. Vitiligo is a disease that leads to depigmentation of the skin due to destruction of melanocytes and as a result the hairs turn white. It presents as small, focal, and often well-circumscribed white spots in the coat or at mucocutaneous junctions. Arabian fading syndrome is a form of vitiligo that develops in young Arabians by 1 to 2 years of age. All colors in the breed can have vitiligo, but it is more common in horses with gray hair coat. It is characterized by round depigmented macules that coalesce to patches, around the eyelids, lips, and muzzle and occasionally around the genitalia. There is no visible inflammation of the skin, and the horse has no other symptoms. The depigmentation can wax and wane in intensity but is usually permanent. The diagnosis is done by clinical picture and biopsy for histopathology.

Melanoma and vitiligo-like depigmentation are among the most common skin diseases in gray horses and they can reach a prevalence between 10% and 80%, depending on the horse's age or breed.[43–46] Malignancy of melanomas in solid colored horses is more severe than in gray horses,[47] although metastases in the lymph nodes, liver, spleen, skeletal muscle, lungs, and surrounding or within blood vessels may occur in gray horses.[48] In 2008, a 4.6 kb duplication in the STX17 (syntaxin 17) gene was identified as the cause of gray phenotype.[49] This duplication, therefore, was proposed to be involved in the promotion of melanocyte proliferation by upregulating the expression of STX17 and/or NR4A3 (nuclear receptor subfamily 4, group A, member 3) genes. The region contains regulatory elements with melanocyte-specific effects (microphthalmia-associated transcription factors), and higher copy number of the STX17 duplication is present in aggressive tumors of gray horses.[50,51] However, the mechanistic features of the duplication remain unknown. Moreover, RACK1 (receptor for activated C kinase 1) protein stands as a candidate molecular marker for the veterinary diagnosis of malignant melanocytic tumors in horses.[52]

Recent studies in Spanish Purebred horses and derived breeds such as the Old Kladrubers or the Lipizzaners indicate that there is a genetic link between melanoma and vitiligo.[45,53,54] Although varying between breeds, the heritability of vitiligo (h2 = 0.20–0.63) is higher than melanoma (h2 = 0.07–0.37).[45,53,54] Either melanoma or vitiligo predisposition is known to have complex inheritance patterns with polygenic and pleiotropic effects involved. In this sense, Curik and colleagues[53] (2013) demonstrated that these diseases are influenced by few genes of moderate-to-large effects (eg, STX17 and ASIP [agouti signaling protein]), as well as a large number of genes with small additive effects, influenced by genes of moderate-to-large effects. However, the study has been limited to investigate the patterns of inheritance and therefore causal mutations have not been yet determined.

The availability of whole genome sequences within the emerged "genomic era" has afforded the opportunity to develop a next-generation high-density SNP array for the domestic horse in 2017.[55] Numerous genome studies have been performed in large sample designs on many different traits; however, none of the studies reported novel insights into the underlying molecular processes of melanoma and vitiligo diseases in horses. However, a recent study in the Lipizzaner horse identified a common long overlapping homozygous region on ECA14:34.05–35.18 Mb (EquCab2.0), which contains several genes involved in melanoma metastasis and survival rate of melanoma patients in humans (eg, SPRY4 [sprouty RTK signaling antagonist 4] and HSP90AB1 [heat shock protein 90 alpha family class B member 1]).[56] Overall, this approach allowed the identification of potential novel genomic regions that may play a role in equine melanoma. Further studies including larger cohorts and careful clinical classification of cases are required to better understand the complex genetic and molecular mechanisms leading to skin diseases.

Ehlers-Danlos Syndrome Subtypes: Hereditary Equine Regional Dermal Asthenia and Warmblood Fragile Faol Syndrome

Ehlers-Danlos syndrome (EDS) comprises a group of genetically heterogeneous connective tissue disorders linked with genetic defects affecting collagen or other extracellular matrix proteins.[57] In horses, EDS subtypes include different inherited connective tissue disorders clinically characterized by skin fragility and hyperextensibility.[58] To date, 2 EDS subtypes have been described based on causative genetic mutations, hereditary equine regional dermal asthenia (HERDA),[59,60] and Warmblood fragile foal syndrome (WFFS).[61,62]

Hereditary Equine Regional Dermal Asthenia

HERDA, also known as hyperelastosis cutis, is a subtype of EDS disorder classified as degenerative skin disease with an autosomal recessive inheritance predominantly observed in the American Quarter Horses.[59] The defect is in the collagen fibers in the skin and leads to a separation between the epidermis and dermis. The symptoms often start when the horse is broken in to a saddle at around 2 years of age. The pressure from the saddle causes the skin to tear and can lead to wounds with prolonged healing time, which may develop into disfiguring scars. The skin is loose and hyperelastic in affected horses.[63]

The disease has a prevalence of 3.5% within the general Quarter Horse population, but it is much more prevalent within the cutting horse industry (up to 28%) or within pleasure/working-cow horses (carrier frequency rates of 12.8% and 11.5%, respectively).[64] A whole-genome scan approach was used to identify a homozygous missense mutation in exon 1 of $PPIB$ (peptidylprolyl isomerase B) gene (c.115G > A) in affected HERDA horses.[59] The gene acts as a chaperon involved in proper folding of collagens, and the mutation affects collagen folding and secretion by a decrease in hydroxylysine and glucosyl-galactosylhydroxylysine in affected horse fibroblasts.[60] However, not all horses displaying an EDS phenotype have a mutation in the $PPIB$ gene, suggesting genetic heterogeneity of EDS disorders.[65,66]

Warmblood Fragile Foal Syndrome Type 1

WWFS is another subtype of EDS disorder of autosomal recessive inheritance characterized as a fatal defect of the connective tissue involving severe skin malformations in neonatal foals, prominobly observed in Warmblood horses and related breeds.[61,62] The disease has a carrier frequency in normal adult Warmblood population around ~11%.[62,67] WFFS is caused by a mutation in the $PLOD1$ (procollagen-lysine, 2-oxoglutarate 5-dioxygenase 1) gene (c.2032G > A), which codes for an enzyme important for collagen biosynthesis.[62]

In summary, 2 different genetic tests are available for the diagnosis of HERDA and WFFS EDS subtypes (**Table 2**). However, a new case of EDS observed in a Mangalarga–Campolina crossbreed mare with $PPIB$ and $PLOD1$ mutations tested negative, indicating that another gene involved in the collagen biosynthesis may be responsible for other EDS subtypes.[58]

Chronic Progressive Lymphedema

Chronic progressive lymphedema (CPL) is a disabling skin disorder in draft horse breeds such as Clydesdales, Shire, and Belgian draft horses.[68,69] It starts at an early

Table 2
Summary of mode of inheritance and genetic tests available for equine skin diseases

Disease	Breeds	Mode of Inheritance	DNA Test Available
Insect bite hypersensitivity	Multiple breeds (see **Table 1**). Higher prevalence in Icelandic horse	Complex	No
Melanoma and vitiligo	Gray horses. Higher prevalence in Iberian horses and related breeds	Complex	No
Hereditary equine regional dermal asthenia	Quarter horse and related breeds	Recessive	Yes
Warmblood fragile foal syndrome type 1	Warmblood horses and related breeds	Recessive	Yes
Chronic progressive lymphedema	Draft breeds	Complex	No
Junctional epidermolysis bullosa	Draft breeds, American Saddlebreds	Recessive	Yes
Incontinentia pigmenti	Quarter horse	X-linked dominant	Yes
Hypotrichosis	American Bashkir Curly horse, Missouri Fox trotter, Percheron draft horse	Complex	Yes

age and leads to progressive swelling of the legs and development of severe chronic skin changes such as hyperkeratosis and dermal fibrosis with thick skin folds and nodules. Secondary infections contribute to the chronic changes, and the condition gives rise to severe discomfort to the horse and commonly leads to euthanasia. There seems to be a genetic predisposition to altered elastin metabolism and impaired function of the lymphatic system in the extremities.[69] The diagnosis is made by clinical picture and by ruling out primary causes to the skin changes such as *Chorioptes*.

CPL has been classified as a multifactorial disorder with a prevalence of 96% within Belgian and some German breeds.[70] Heritability coefficients for the occurrence of clinical CPL lesions in Belgian Draught Horses have been estimated to be 0.26 for horses older than 3 years.[71] Genetic components are therefore likely to play a role in this disease. However, none of the potential candidate genes known to affect lymphedema-distichiasis syndrome and Darier-White disease (Keratosis follicularis) in humans (eg, *FOXC2* [Forkhead box C2] and *ATP2A2* [ATPase sarcoplasmic/endoplasmic reticulum Ca2+ transporting 2]) are associated to CPL in horses.[72,73]

A whole-genome scan performed across several draft horse breeds affected by CPL identified significant quantitative trait loci on ECA1, 10, and 17.[74] The study proposed several potential candidate genes involved in the regulation of inflammatory autoimmune responses (eg, *UBE3A* [ubiquitin protein ligase E3A], *CD109* [CD109 molecule], and *MTMR6* [myotubularin-related protein 6]), which will require further functional analysis to confirm whether any of these genes are truly associated with clinical signs observed with CPL. Another GWAS for CPL in Friesian horses did not achieve any genome-wide significance.[75] However, recent findings in the Belgian Draught horse identified several regions surpassing nominal significance with candidate genes described in previous studies on CPL (eg, *FOXC2*, *UBE3A*, or *CD109*). The study confirms the involvement of several processes of the immune response, thereby supporting the hypothesis to consider CPL as an inflammatory autoimmune response.[76] Further functional research is needed to identify the genetic cause underlying CPL and the involvement of the immune response.

Junctional Epidermolysis Bullosa

Junctional epidermolysis bullosa (JEB) is a severe skin blistering disease of genetic origin that affects newborn foals. It has an autosomal recessive mode of inheritance and has been found in the Belgian, Italian, and French draft horses and in American Saddlebred horses (see **Table 2**).[77–84] It is a mechanobullous disease that leads to the development of ulcers and blisters in the skin, most commonly at pressure points including the hocks or the stifle and at mucocutaneous junctions such as the mouth and anus. The defect leads to a separation between the skin layers, and only minor trauma leads to severe detachment of the skin and even sloughing of the hoof wall. The foals can also have oral abnormalities with premature eruption of the teeth and loss of enamel that cause bleeding in the mouth. This disease was first called epitheliogenesis imperfecta, but when it was shown that it involved a defect in the lamina propria, it was renamed as JEB. The pathologic signs of JEB closely match what can be observed in Herlitz junctional epidermolysis bullosa in humans, although in horses, the dense hair may act as a protection against trauma.[79] There is no treatment of JEB, and the foals are euthanized because of animal welfare reasons. The diagnosis can be made from biopsy of intact blisters (macroscopic, histologic, and ultrastructural) or genetic testing in draft and American Saddlebred horses.

Two mutations that affect the dermal-epidermal junction have been identified in horses: one large deletion in *LAMA3* (laminin subunit alpha 3) in American Saddlebred horses and an insertion (1368insC) *in LAMC2* (laminin subunit gamma 2) in Belgians and other draft horse breeds.[79,80,84] The deletion in American Saddlebred horses is 6589 base pairs and span exons 24 to 27 in *LAMA3*. The mutations affect the anchoring fibril laminin 5 protein located in the basement membrane in the dermal-epidermal junction. Laminin 5 is a heterotrimeric basement membrane protein that consists of 3 glycoprotein subunits—the $\alpha 3$, $\beta 3$, and $\gamma 2$ chains—that are encoded by the *LAMA3* (laminin subunit alpha 3), *LAMB3* (laminin subunit beta 3), and *LAMC2* (laminin subunit gamma 2) genes, respectively.[84] Identification of healthy carriers is important to prevent the spread of this disease.

Incontinentia Pigmenti

Incontinentia pigmenti (IP) is a congenital skin disorder characterized by abnormalities in the skin but also other structures of ectodermal origin as the teeth and eyes. Based on a single pedigree consisting of 23 horses, the disorder follows an X-linked dominant inheritance pattern, where affected males are aborted and only affected females survive (see **Table 2**). The foals develop exudative and pruritic skin lesions soon after birth. These develop to wartlike lesions, and healing is seen as alopecia or occasional wooly hair regrowth. Additional symptoms include dental, hoof, and ocular developmental anomalies.[85] Horses with IP in this pedigree display many similarities to human IP.[85]

Human familial IP also segregates as an X-linked dominant disorder and is usually lethal prenatally in males. The condition predominantly affects the skin. Cells expressing the mutated X chromosome are eliminated selectively around the time of birth, so females with IP exhibit extremely skewed X-inactivation.[86] Infants usually have a blistering rash that heals and develops into wartlike skin growths. Hyperpigmentation in a swirled pattern occur in early childhood. In humans, dental, eye, hair, and nail abnormalities can occur.[86]

In human, IP is caused by a mutation in the *IKBKG* (inhibitor of nuclear factor kappa B [NFkB] kinase subunit gamma) gene. The gene is found on the X chromosome (Xq28) and codes for the protein NFkB's essential modulator (IKK-gamma, formerly called NEMO) found in almost all cells of the body. The function of the IKK-gamma protein is to activate the protein NFkB inside the cell. NFkB then migrates into the cell nucleus and in turn activates genes that are important for, among other things, fetal development and the function of the immune system.

The IKK-gamma protein is needed for the organism to develop properly, control cell growth and death, and protect cells from infection. This is important, for example, in the early fetal development of ectodermal tissues such as skin, nails, and hair, as well as parts of the central nervous system and the immune system. The most common mutation that causes IP implies a complete loss of function of the protein.

In horses, a nonsense mutation (c.184C > T, p.Arg62*) in *IKBKG* has been identified in mares with IP.[85] This was achieved by whole-genome resequencing (WGS) of one affected mare and comparison with WGS data from 44 control horses from 11 breeds. The variant is predicted to result in a premature stop codon and truncates approximately 85% of the protein.[85] Since a homologous mutation (p.Arg62*) has been observed in a human IP patient, horses with the same variant can serve as an animal model for the human condition.

Hypotrichosis

Hypotrichosis implies a less than normal amount of hair. The condition results in alopecia that is apparent at birth or develops during the neonatal period and can be associated with defects in other ectodermal structures such as teeth, hooves, eyes, or sweat glands. It is a genetic disease seen predominantly in the curly coated breeds American Bashkir Curly horses and Missouri Fox trotters. The breeds have normal shedding periods, but, in some individuals, there are permanent hair loss of the mane and tail. It is seen as diffuse to complete alopecia due to dysplasia of hair follicles. Horses with incomplete hypotrichosis are presented with broken hairs and shedding of hairs at the lateral upper tail and at the forelock.

Congenital progressive hypotrichosis has been reported in a blue roan Percheron draught horse.[87] This horse was born with patchy alopecia of the trunk and legs and at 5 years of age the body hair was almost absent (mane and tail hairs were present, but sparse). There were no abnormalities of the teeth and hoof. Histopathology revealed follicular hypoplasia and hyperkeratosis, as well as an excess of catagen and telogen hair follicles.

Curly coated horse breeds present an exceptional coat that vary in curliness of the body, mane, tail, and ear hairs. Both autosomal recessive and dominant inheritance patterns have been suggested to explain the diversity of the curly phenotype.[88,89] A GWAS study of 70 curly and straight-haired North American and French horses hypothesized to carry the dominant curly hair trait has been performed.[90] By using WGS, the study identified a missense variant (g.21891160G > A, p.R89H) in the coil 1A domain of the *KRT25* (keratin 25) gene to be associated with the dominant curly phenotype. The variant was confirmed by genotyping additional 150 curly and 203 randomly chosen straight-haired animals from 35 different breeds. Five discordant curly horses were observed, and sequencing 2 of those horses suggests locus heterogeneity for the dominant curly phenotype within North American Curly horses.[90]

Hypotrichosis is not observed in all curly coated horses. Therefore, a research team aimed at investigating the genetic component of curly coat with and without hypotrichosis.[91] A GWAS analysis identified significant signals on chromosome 11. WGS data detected 2 variants in the region within *KRT25* and *SP6* (transcription factor Sp6) that could explain all hair phenotypes. Curly coat with no hypotrichosis was present in horses carrying only the *SP6* variant. However, a variant allele of the *KRT25* gene was found to be *epistatic* to *SP6*, where horses carrying the *KRT25* variant (heterozygous or homozygous state), regardless of their *SP6* genotype, exhibited a curly hair phenotype with incomplete or complete hypotrichosis, respectively.

Future Directions

Understanding the molecular basis of mammalian phenotypic traits is a fundamental biological goal and is primarily important for understanding the development of diseases. Equine skin diseases are common, and the interest in equine dermatology is therefore increasing.[92] For instance, 80% of gray coat horses will develop melanoma after 15 years of age, and up to 60% of horses are susceptible to IBH. Often, there is a genetic component involved in skin disease development, as presented in this article. Notably for monogenic traits where the causative mutation has been identified, genetic testing can serve as a complementing diagnostic tool and could also, when relevant, guide early treatment. However, in domestic animals, genetic testing is of particular value for informed breeding decisions. For instance, genetic testing of a monogenic trait enables identification of healthy carriers of recessive disease alleles (eg, the EDS subtypes HERDA or WFFS).

For complex traits, genomic selection is a more suitable approach. Genomic selection, a form of marker-assisted selection in which genetic markers covering the entire genome are used, is rapidly increasing in importance in other species.[61,72] The basic concept of genomic selection is to combine whole-genome molecular markers with phenotypic and pedigree data in an attempt to increase the accuracy of prediction for *breeding values*. Genomic selection can be especially valuable for traits that are difficult to measure in large scale, and for lower-heritability traits, such as IBH.

Genomic selection using only significantly disease-associated markers or all markers could increase the efficiency of breeding for decreased IBH disease prevalence.[36] This would be of particular value because it can be applied at a young age of the horse, before any mating occurs, as well as because the occurrence of IBH in individual horses highly depends on the exposure to *Culicoides spp*.

Disease mutations may reside either within the coding part of a gene or in a unit that regulates the disease-associated gene. The regulation of gene activity may disrupt protein production and cell processes and result in disease. Therefore, it is important to link variations in the expression of certain genes to the development of each genetic skin disease. A continued focus is to develop and apply genome-based strategies for the early detection, diagnosis, and treatment of equine skin disease. Breeding against genetic disease is an efficient and cost-effective strategy for the management of the disease severity levels, with particular interest in complex traits such as IBH, CPL, or melanoma.

DISCLOSURE

The authors have nothing to disclose.

REFERENCES

1. Matejuk A. Skin immunity. Arch ImmunolTherExp (Warsz) 2018;66(1):45–54.
2. Egawa G, Kabashima K. Skin as a peripheral lymphoid organ: revisiting the concept of skin-associated lymphoid tissues. J Invest Dermatol 2011;131(11): 2178–85.
3. Ono S, Kabashima K. Proposal of inducible skin-associated lymphoid tissue (iSALT). ExpDermatol 2015;24(8):630–1.
4. Dunstan RW. A pathomechanistic approach to diseases of the hair follicle. Br Vet DermatolStudy Group 1995;17:37.

5. Scott DW. Large animal dermatology. Philadelphia: WB Saunders company; 1988.
6. Smith F. Histology of the skin of the horse. J AnatPhysiol 1888;22(Pt 2):142.
7. Sokolov VE, Sokolov VE. Mammal skin. Oakland, CA: Univ of California Press; 1982.
8. Talukdar A, Calhoun M, Stinson A. Microscopic anatomy of the skin of the horse. Am J Vet Res 1972;33(12):2365–90.
9. Trautmann A. Fundamentals of the histology of domestic animals. Ithaca, NY: Comstock Pub. Associates; 1957.
10. Goldsmith LA, Strauss J, Downing D, et al. Physiology, Biochemistry and Molecular Biology of the Skin. In: New York,: Oxford University Press, Inc; 1991.
11. Silver A, Chase H. An in vivo method for studying the hair cycle. Nature 1966; 210(5040):1051.
12. Scott DW, Miller WH. Structure and Function of the Skin. In: Equine Dermatology. Elsevier Saunders, Maryland Heights, Missouri; 2003. 63043.
13. Duan C, Liu M, Zhang Z, et al. Radiofrequency ablation versus hepatic resection for the treatment of early-stage hepatocellular carcinoma meeting Milan criteria: a systematic review and meta-analysis. World journal of surgical oncology. 2013; 11(1):190.
14. Duan Y-C, Ma Y-C, Zhang E, et al. Design and synthesis of novel 1, 2, 3-triazole-dithiocarbamate hybrids as potential anticancer agents. European journal of medicinal chemistry 2013;62:11–9.
15. Cardoso-Moreira M, Halbert J, Valloton D, et al. Gene expression across mammalian organ development. Nature 2019;571:505–9.
16. Cardoso-Moreira M, Velten B, Mort M, et al. Developmental gene expression differences between humans and mammalian models. bioRxiv 2019;747782. https://doi.org/10.1101/747782.
17. Sarropoulos I, Marin R, Cardoso-Moreira M, et al. Developmental dynamics of lncRNAs across mammalian organs and species. Nature 2019;571:510–4.
18. Schaffartzik A, Hamza E, Janda J, et al. Equine insect bite hypersensitivity: what do we know? Veterinary immunology and immunopathology 2012;147(3–4): 113–26.
19. Miller JE, Mann S, Fettelschoss-Gabriel A, et al. Comparison of three clinical scoring systems for Culicoides hypersensitivity in a herd of Icelandic horses. Vet Dermatol 2019;30(6):536–e163.
20. Halldórsdóttir S, Larsen H. An epidemiological study of summer eczema in Icelandic horses in Norway. Equine Vet J 1991;23(4):296–9.
21. Anderson GS, Belton P, Kleider N. The hypersensitivity of horses to Culicoides bites in British Columbia. Can Vet J 1988;29(9):718.
22. Björnsdóttir S, Sigvaldadóttir J, Broström H, et al. Summer eczema in exported Icelandic horses: influence of environmental and genetic factors. Acta Veterinaria Scandinavica 2006;48(1):3.
23. Broström H, Larsson Å, Troedsson M. Allergic dermatitis (sweet itch) of Icelandic horses in Sweden: an epidemiological study. Equine Vet J 1987;19(3):229–36.
24. Eriksson S, Grandinson K, Fikse W, et al. Genetic analysis of insect bite hypersensitivity (summer eczema) in Icelandic horses. Animal 2008;2(3):360–5.
25. Schurink A, Ducro B, Heuven H, et al. Genetic parameters of insect bite hypersensitivity in Dutch Friesian broodmares. Journal of animal science 2011;89(5): 1286–93.

26. Schurink A, Van Grevenhof E, Ducro B, et al. Heritability and repeatability of insect bite hypersensitivity in Dutch Shetland breeding mares. Journal of animal science 2009;87(2):484–90.

27. Frey R, Bergvall K, Egenvall A. Allergen-specific IgE in Icelandic horses with insect bite hypersensitivity and healthy controls, assessed by FcεR1α-based serology. Vet ImmunolImmunopathol 2008;126(1–2):102–9.

28. Wilkołek P, Szczepanik M, Sitkowski W, et al. A Comparison of Intradermal Skin Testing and Serum Insect Allergen-specific IgE Determination in Horses With Insect Bite Hypersensitivity From 2008 to 2016. Journal of equine veterinary science 2019;75:65–8.

29. Marti E, Gerber H, Lazary S. On the genetic basis of equine allergic diseases: II. Insect bite dermal hypersensitivity. Equine Vet J 1992;24(2):113–7.

30. Lazary S, Marti E, Szalai G, et al. Studies on the frequency and associations of equine leucocyte antigens in sarcoid and summer dermatitis. Animal genetics 1994;25(S1):75–80.

31. Andersson LS, Swinbune JE, Meadows JR, et al. The same ELA class II risk factors confer equine insect bite hypersensitivity in two distinct populations. Immunogenetics 2012;64(3):201–8.

32. Klumplerova M, Vychodilova L, Bobrova O, et al. Major histocompatibility complex and other allergy-related candidate genes associated with insect bite hypersensitivity in Icelandic horses. Molecular biology reports 2013;40(4):3333–40.

33. Viļuma A, Mikko S, Hahn D, et al. Genomic structure of the horse major histocompatibility complex class II region resolved using PacBio long-read sequencing technology. Scientific reports 2017;7:45518.

34. Skow LC, Brinkmeyer-Langford CL. Unexpected Structural Features of the Equine Major Histocompatibility Complex 93. In: Equine Genomics. Chowdhary BP. Hoboken, NJ: Wiley-Blackwell; 2013.

35. Holmes CM, Violette N, Miller D, et al. MHC haplotype diversity in Icelandic horses determined by polymorphic microsatellites. Genes Immun 2019;20:660–70.

36. Schurink A, Wolc A, Ducro BJ, et al. Genome-wide association study of insect bite hypersensitivity in two horse populations in the Netherlands. Genetics Selection Evolution 2012;44(1):31.

37. Schurink A, Podesta SC, Ducro BJ, et al. Risk factors for insect bite hypersensitivity in Friesian horses and Shetland ponies in The Netherlands. Vet J 2013;195(3):382–4.

38. Shrestha M, Eriksson S, Schurink A, et al. Genome-wide association study of insect bite hypersensitivity in Swedish-born Icelandic horses. Journal of Heredity 2015;106(4):366–74.

39. Velie B, Shrestha M, Francois L, et al. A high density genome-wide scan for genetic risk factors of insect bite hypersensitivity (IBH): A Horsegene Project Initiative. Journal of Animal Science 2016;94:156–7.

40. Schurink A, da Silva VH, Velie BD, et al. Copy number variations in Friesian horses and genetic risk factors for insect bite hypersensitivity. BMC genetics 2018;19(1):49.

41. François L, Hoskens H, Velie BD, et al. Genomic regions associated with IgE levels against culicoides spp. Antigens in three horse breeds. Genes 2019;10(8):597.

42. Shrestha M, Solé M, Ducro B J, et al. Genome-wide association study for insect bite hypersensitivity susceptibility in horses revealed novel associated loci on chromosome 1. J Anim Breed Genet 2020;137(2):223–33.

43. Valentine BA. Equine melanocytic tumors: a retrospective study of 53 horses (1988 to 1991). Journal of Veterinary Internal Medicine 1995;9(5):291–7.
44. Johnson PJ. Dermatologic tumors (excluding sarcoids). Veterinary clinics of North America: equine practice 1998;14(3):625–58.
45. Sánchez-Guerrero MJ, Solé M, Azor PJ, et al. Genetic and environmental risk factors for vitiligo and melanoma in Pura Raza Español horses. Equine Vet J 2019; 51(5):606–11.
46. Teixeira R, Rendahl A, Anderson S, et al. Coat color genotypes and risk and severity of melanoma in gray quarter horses. Journal of veterinary internal medicine 2013;27(5):1201–8.
47. Seltenhammer M, Simhofer H, Scherzer S, et al. Equine melanoma in a population of 296 grey Lipizzaner horses. Equine veterinary journal 2003;35(2):153–7.
48. MacGillivray KC, Sweeney RW, Piero FD. Metastatic melanoma in horses. J Vet Intern Med 2002;16(4):452–6.
49. Pielberg GR, Golovko A, Sundström E, et al. A cis-acting regulatory mutation causes premature hair graying and susceptibility to melanoma in the horse. Nature genetics 2008;40(8):1004.
50. Sundström E, Imsland F, Mikko S, et al. Copy number expansion of the STX17 duplication in melanoma tissue from Grey horses. BMC genomics 2012; 13(1):365.
51. Sundström E, Komisarczuk AZ, Jiang L, et al. Identification of a melanocyte-specific, microphthalmia-associated transcription factor-dependent regulatory element in the intronic duplication causing hair greying and melanoma in horses. Pigment cell & melanoma research 2012;25(1):28–36.
52. Campagne C, Julé S, Bernex F, et al. RACK1, a clue to the diagnosis of cutaneous melanomas in horses. BMC veterinary research 2012;8(1):95.
53. Curik I, Druml T, Seltenhammer M, et al. Complex inheritance of melanoma and pigmentation of coat and skin in Grey horses. PLoS genetics 2013;9(2): e1003248.
54. Hofmanová B, Vostrý L, Majzlík I, et al. Characterization of greying, melanoma, and vitiligo quantitative inheritance in Old Kladruber horses. Czech Journal of Animal Science 2015;60(10):443–51.
55. Schaefer RJ, Schubert M, Bailey E, et al. Developing a 670k genotyping array to tag~ 2MSNPs across 24 horse breeds. BMC genomics 2017;18(1):565.
56. Grilz-Seger G, Druml T, Neuditschko M, et al. High-resolution population structure and runs of homozygosity reveal the genetic architecture of complex traits in the Lipizzan horse. BMC genomics 2019;20(1):174.
57. Rashmir-Raven A, Spier S. Hereditary equine regional dermal asthenia (HERDA) in Quarter Horses: a review of clinical signs, genetics and research. Equine Vet Education 2015;27(11):604–11.
58. Oliveira-Filho JP, Badial PR, Liboreiro RM, et al. Ehlers-Danlos Syndrome in a Mangalarga-Campolina Crossbreed Mare. Journal of equine veterinary science 2017;57:95–9.
59. Tryon RC, White SD, Bannasch DL. Homozygosity mapping approach identifies a missense mutation in equine cyclophilin B (PPIB) associated with HERDA in the American Quarter Horse. Genomics 2007;90(1):93–102.
60. Ishikawa Y, Vranka JA, Boudko SP, et al. Mutation in cyclophilin B that causes hyperelastosis cutis in American Quarter Horse does not affect peptidylprolyl cis-trans isomerase activity but shows altered cyclophilin B-protein interactions and affects collagen folding. Journal of Biological Chemistry 2012;287(26): 22253–65.

61. Winand NJ. Identification of the causative mutation for inherited connective tissue disorders in equines and methods for testing for same. Google Patents; 2014.
62. Monthoux C, de Brot S, Jackson M, et al. Skin malformations in a neonatal foal tested homozygous positive for Warmblood Fragile Foal Syndrome. BMC veterinary research 2015;11(1):12.
63. White SD, Affolter VK, Bannasch DL, et al. Hereditary equine regional dermal asthenia ('hyperelastosis cutis') in 50 horses: clinical, histological, immunohistological and ultrastructural findings. Veterinary dermatology 2004;15(4):207–17.
64. Rashmir-Raven A. Heritable equine regional dermal asthenia. Vet Clin Equine Pract 2013;29(3):689–702.
65. Rüfenacht S, Straub R, Steinmann B, et al. Swiss warmblood horse with symptoms of hereditary equine regional dermal asthenia without mutation in the cyclophylin B gene (PPIB). Schweizer Archiv fur Tierheilkunde 2010;152(4):188–92.
66. Steelman SM, Jackson ND, Conant E, et al. Ehlers-Danlos syndrome in a Quarter horse gelding: a case report of PPIB-independent Hereditary Equine Regional Dermal Asthenia. Journal of Equine Veterinary Science 2014;34(4):565–8.
67. Dias NM, de Andrade DGA, Teixeira-Neto AR, et al. Warmblood Fragile Foal Syndrome causative single nucleotide polymorphism frequency in Warmblood horses in Brazil. Veterinary Journal 2019;248:101–2.
68. Cheville A, McGarvey CL, Petrek JA, et al. Lymphedema management. Seminars in Radiation Oncology 2003;13(3):290–301.
69. Affolter VK. Chronic progressive lymphedema in draft horses. Vet Clin Equine Pract 2013;29(3):589–605.
70. De Keyser K, Janssens S, Buys N. Chronic progressive lymphoedema in draught horses. Equine Vet J 2015;47(3):260–6.
71. De Keyser K, Janssens S, Peeters L, et al. Genetic parameters for chronic progressive lymphedema in Belgian Draught Horses. Journal of animal breeding and genetics 2014;131(6):522–8.
72. Young AE, Bower LP, Affolter VK, et al. Evaluation of FOXC2 as a candidate gene for chronic progressive lymphedema in draft horses. The Veterinary Journal 2007; 174(2):397–9.
73. Mömke S, Distl O. Molecular genetic analysis of the ATP2A2 gene as candidate for chronic pastern dermatitis in German draft horses. J Hered 2007;98(3): 267–71.
74. Mittmann EH, Mömke S, Distl O. Whole-genome scan identifies quantitative trait loci for chronic pastern dermatitis in German draft horses. Mamm Genome 2010; 21(1–2):95–103.
75. Dalley BC. Genome-wide association study of chronic progressive lymphedema in Friesian horses. University of California, Davis; 2016.
76. François L. Conservation genomics of living heritage breeds. KU Leuven, Belgium; 2018. Available at: https://lirias.kuleuven.be/1717252?limo=0.
77. Johnson GC, Kohn CW, Johnson CW, et al. Ultrastructure of junctional epidermolysis bullosa in Belgian foals. Journal of comparative pathology 1988;99(3): 329–36.
78. Frame S, Harrington D, Fessler J, et al. Hereditary junctional mechanobullous disease in a foal. Journal of the American Veterinary Medical Association 1988; 193(11):1420–4.
79. Spirito F, Charlesworth A, Ortonne J-P, et al. Animal models for skin blistering conditions: absence of laminin 5 causes hereditary junctional mechanobullous disease in the Belgian horse. Journal of Investigative Dermatology 2002;119(3): 684–91.

80. Milenkovic D, Chaffaux S, Taourit S, et al. A mutation in the LAMC2 gene causes the Herlitz junctional epidermolysis bullosa (H-JEB) in two French draft horse breeds. Genetics Selection Evolution. 2003;35(2):249.

81. Cappelli K, Brachelente C, Passamonti F, et al. First report of junctional epidermolysis bullosa (JEB) in the Italian draft horse. BMC veterinary research 2015; 11(1):55.

82. Lieto L, Swerczek T, Cothran E. Equine epitheliogenesisimperfecta in two American Saddlebred foals is a lamina lucida defect. Vet Pathol 2002;39(5):576–80.

83. Lieto L, Cothran E. The epitheliogenesisimperfecta locus maps to equine chromosome 8 in American Saddlebred horses. Cytogenet Genome Res 2003;102(1–4): 207–10.

84. Graves K, Henney P, Ennis R. Partial deletion of the LAMA3 gene is responsible for hereditary junctionalepidermolysisbullosa in the American Saddlebred Horse. Anim Genet 2009;40(1):35–41.

85. Towers RE, Murgiano L, Millar DS, et al. A nonsense mutation in the IKBKG gene in mares with incontinentia pigmenti. PLoS One 2013;8(12):e81625.

86. Smahi A, Courtois G, Vabres P, et al. Genomic rearrangement in NEMO impairs NF-[kappa] B activation and is a cause of incontinentia pigmenti. Nature 2000; 405(6785):466–73.

87. Valentine BA, Hedstrom OR, Miller JRWH, et al. Congenital hypotrichosis in a Percheron draught horse. Veterinary dermatology 2001;12(4):215–7.

88. Sponenberg D. Dominant curly coat in horses. Genet SelEvol 1990;22(2):257.

89. Blakeslee LH, Hudson R, Hunt H. Curly coat of horses. J Hered 1943;34(4): 115–8.

90. Morgenthaler C, Diribarne M, Capitan A, et al. A missense variant in the coil1A domain of the keratin 25 gene is associated with the dominant curly hair coat trait (Crd) in horse. Genetics Selection Evolution 2017;49(1):85.

91. Thomer A, Gottschalk M, Christmann A, et al. An epistatic effect of KRT25 on SP6 is involved in curly coat in horses. Scientific reports 2018;8(1):6374.

92. Kaneene JB, Ross WA, Miller R. The Michigan equine monitoring system. II. Frequencies and impact of selected health problems. Prev Vet Med 1997;29(4): 277–92.

Genetics of Equine Endocrine and Metabolic Disease

Elaine Norton, DVM, MS, PhD*, Molly E. McCue, DVM, MS, PhD

KEYWORDS

- Genetics • Equine metabolic syndrome • Pars pituitary intermedia dysfunction
- Heritability • Risk factors • Genome-wide association analysis

KEY POINTS

- Equine metabolic syndrome (EMS) is a complex, polygenic trait.
- A genetic contribution to pars pituitary intermedia dysfunction (PPID) in suspected but has not yet been proven.
- Continued research for the specific genetic risk factors for both EMS and PPID is crucial for gaining a better understanding of the pathophysiology of both conditions and allowing development of genetic test.

ANIMAL MODELS IN COMPLEX DISEASE GENETICS

Complex diseases are diseases in which both the environment and genetics contribute to the phenotype. The identification of the specific alleles underlying complex traits will allow for a better understanding of the fundamental pathogenesis across species. Moreover, the promise of precision medicine, or tailored treatment and management regimens based on an individual's unique combination of genetic and environmental risk factors, has instigated a drive toward identifying the genetic risk factors of many complex diseases.[1] However, unlike Mendelian (simple) traits in which the genetic variation can be explained by a single gene with a well-defined mode of inheritance, complex traits are the result of the combination of dozens to hundreds of genetic alleles with variable allele frequencies, penetrance, environmental influences, and gene-by-environment interaction. Further, although Mendelian diseases are often the consequence of high-impact variants within protein-coding genes, alleles contributing to complex traits have variable effect sizes and are often noncoding variants that presumably affect gene regulatory elements.[2–4] Therefore, the identification of the genetic variants of complex traits requires large genetic and phenotypic data sets ("big data") and statistical approaches that can account for the numerous variables influencing these traits. Recent advances in sequencing

Veterinary Population Medicine Department, University of Minnesota, 225 Veterinary Medical Center, 1365 Gortner Avenue, St Paul, MN 55108, USA
* Corresponding author.
E-mail address: norto253@umn.edu

Vet Clin Equine 36 (2020) 341–352
https://doi.org/10.1016/j.cveq.2020.03.011
0749-0739/20/© 2020 Elsevier Inc. All rights reserved.

technology have provided researchers the cost-effective, high-throughput means required to collect genomics data in a large number of individuals.

METABOLIC SYNDROME

The term equine metabolic syndrome (EMS) was coined in 2002 when the parallels between human metabolic syndrome (MetS) and what was being observed clinically in hyperinsulinemic, obese, laminitic horses was recognized.[5] Over the past few decades, the working understanding of EMS has become more refined and the clinical overlap between species more pronounced. In both species, metabolic syndrome can manifest as baseline hyperinsulinemia, an exaggerated or prolonged insulin or glucose response post carbohydrate challenge, tissue insulin resistance, dyslipidemia, and alterations in adipokines and inflammatory cytokines. Further, metabolic syndrome can lead to serious medical issues that have a major economic impact and both EMS and MetS have been characterized as a clustering of risk factors for these conditions.[6,7] EMS is considered the leading cause of laminitis,[7] and humans with MetS are 2 and 4 times more likely to develop cardiovascular disease and diabetes mellitus, respectively.[6]

Genetics of Metabolic Syndrome Theories

In horses, it has been well recognized that specific breeds have a higher prevalence of EMS, including Standardbred horses, Morgan horses, Tennessee walking horses, Andalusians, Paso Finos, and Arabians, with pony breeds being considered at the highest risk.[5,8] Although most breed predilections have been determined anecdotally through clinical observation, several scientific reports have supported differences in metabolic profiles between breeds. By as early as the 1980s, published reports concluded[9,10] that ponies were more insulin insensitive than large-breed horses[9,10] and that there were distinct breed differences in lipid and glucose profiles.[11] Further, ponies and Andalusians have been found to be more insulin insensitive when compared with Standardbreds, and Andalusians had a lower disposition index, indicating that the breed was less compensated for insulin resistance then ponies.[12] Thus, population predilections and familial incidence provided the initial evidence that EMS is a complex trait with a strong genetic basis.

A metabolically thrifty genotype has been hypothesized that proposes genetic variations in metabolism allowed for an advantageous adaptation for survival during periods of scarce feed and harsh climate conditions in undomesticated horses.[13] However, after the agricultural revolution, horses were presented with consistent feed, abundant soluble carbohydrates, and a more sedentary lifestyle, leading to derangements in metabolism associated with EMS and obesity. This theory was based on the thrifty genotype hypothesis in humans, stating that obesity and metabolic syndrome are the result of genetic variants that allowed for our ancestors to survive during periods of poor nutrition by increasing adipose stores during the reciprocal period of food abundance.[14] Extension of this hypothesis includes the thrifty epigenotype hypothesis, which advances the notion that all individuals have a thrifty genotype but that variations in phenotype expression are due to in utero epigenetic modifications resulting from the influence of environmental risk factors.[15] In contrast, the drifty gene hypothesis suggests that genetic predisposition to obesity is due to random genetic drift based on current population prevalence of obesity and MetS.[16] Based on the complexity of mammalian evolution, it is likely that the genetic origins of metabolic syndrome are the manifestation of a combination of these hypotheses and additional factors, including gene-by-environment interactions, pleiotropic effects, and microbial influences.[17]

Heritability of Metabolic Syndrome

One of the first studies evaluating the genetic basis of EMS was published in 2002 by Treiber and colleagues.[18] In this study, the investigators estimated the genetic contribution of pasture-associated laminitis using pedigree data from a single herd of 160 pure and crossbred Welsh and Dartmoor ponies. The investigators grouped ponies based on whether they had a previous diagnosis of laminitis, were clinically laminitic, or nonlaminitic. A total of 34% of ponies had a diagnosis of laminitis, of which there was an eightfold lower prevalence in mature stallions versus females. The investigators concluded that the observed prevalence of laminitis was consistent with the action of dominantly expressed gene(s) but with reduced penetrance due to sex-mediated factors, age of onset, and epigenetics.[18]

In humans, the heritability of MetS has been extensively studied using pedigree data. Heritability was primarily estimated by calculating narrow sense heritability (h2), which is the proportion of additive genetic variance over the total phenotypic variance.[19] Across studies, the range of h2 estimates for MetS as a binary trait (typically defined as the presence of 3 or more components of MetS) was low to moderately heritable,[20–23] and components of metabolic syndrome (biochemical measurements, proxies for insulin resistance, blood pressure, or measurements of obesity) were estimated to be low, moderate, or highly heritable (**Table 1**), with a large range of heritability estimates between studies.[20–31] Notably, h2 estimates can vary greatly between populations[32] and the large range between h2 estimates across studies is in part due to differences in the represented populations, as well as due to differences in study design, diagnostic criteria, and environmental factors.

It is important to note that although pedigree analysis has been historically used for calculating h2, the estimates have been shown to overestimate h2 as a consequence of (1) small populations of highly related individuals often confounded by a shared environment; (2) assortative mating (nonrandom mating due to selection of pairs based on phenotype); (3) pedigree errors; and (4) ascertainment bias (selection of pedigrees that have a high proportion of affected individuals).[33] Furthermore, to achieve an unbiased estimate of genetic variance, the data must be representative of the general population and include all potential confounders.[19] The availability of algorithms to calculate h2 using single nucleotide polymorphism (SNP) genotype data (h^2_{SNP}) has allowed for a more precise estimate of h2 by using data from a large group of unrelated individuals across multiple environments.[34] This approach was used to estimate the h^2_{SNP} of MetS using data from the Atherosclerosis Risk in Communities and Framingham Heart Study. As can be seen in **Table 1**, these results were consistent with the h2 estimates from the pedigree analyses, albeit at the lower end of the range for most traits.[35]

We estimated the heritability of EMS using approximately 1.2 million SNP markers in 264 Welsh ponies and 286 Morgan horses, 2 breeds known to be at high risk for EMS.[36] A restricted estimated maximum likelihood statistic was used to estimate the h^2_{SNP} of biochemical measurements associated with EMS, including basal insulin, glucose, nonesterified fatty acids, triglycerides, adiponectin, leptin, and insulin and glucose after oral sugar test. Statistically significant h^2_{SNP} estimates were consistent with traits that were moderately to highly heritable (see **Table 1**). As with the human h2 estimates, several estimates were similar across traits between breeds (such as basal insulin and glucose after an oral sugar test); whereas, for other traits, there was a large difference between breeds (such as with triglycerides and leptin). These larger ranges likely reflect differences in the genetic risk factors between breeds. This study provided the first concrete evidence that genetics was contributing to a large portion of the phenotypic variation for EMS.[36]

Table 1
Comparison of narrow-sense heritability estimates for metabolic syndrome in humans and horses using a pedigree-based (h2) or SNP-based (h²$_{SNP}$) analysis

Response Variable	Human h2 Estimates	Human h²$_{SNP}$ Estimates	Welsh Ponies h²$_{SNP}$ Estimates	Morgan Horses h²$_{SNP}$ Estimates
Glucose	0.14–0.81	0.33	0.41	0.21
Insulin	0.43–0.51	0.23	0.81	0.59
Insulin sensitivity				
Glucose-OST	0.17–0.24	—	0.23	0.57
Insulin-OST	—	—	0.44	0.36
HOMA-IR	0.38–0.48	—	—	—
Dyslipidemia				
NEFA	—	—	0.43	0.68
Triglycerides	0.17–0.60	0.47	0.31	0.27
Total cholesterol	0.42–0.62	—	—	—
HDL	0.42–0.63	0.48	—	—
LDL	0.58	—	—	—
Measures obesity				
BMI	0.39–0.68	0.34	—	—
WC	0.27–0.46	—	—	—
Adipokines				
Leptin	0.28–0.55	—	0.55	0.49
Adiponectin	0.51	—	0.49	0.91
Other				
MetS	0.11–0.38	—	—	—
MetS Score	0.15–0.34	0.24–0.25	—	—
Systolic BP	0.16–0.28	0.30	—	—
Diastolic BP	0.12–0.38	—	—	—

Abbreviations: BMI, body mass index; BP, blood pressure; HDL, high-density lipoproteins; HOMA-IR, homeostatic models assessment of insulin resistance; LDL, low-density lipoproteins; MetS, metabolic syndrome as a binary trait and typically defined as the presence of 3 or more components of MetS; NEFA, nonesterified fatty acids; OST, oral sugar test; SNP, single nucleotide polymorphism; WC, waste circumference.

Direct comparisons across studies and species must be taken with caution given that heritability estimates are highly dependent on the represented population because the effects of environmental variance and additive and nonadditive genetic variances are population-specific, and each study represented differences in ethnic group, study design, diagnostic criteria, and pedigree versus SNP-based analysis. However, key points that can be extrapolated are that (1) within study populations, several phenotypes were under considerable genetic influence (moderately to highly heritable), whereas other phenotypes seemed to be affected by unmeasured nongenetic factors such as the environment (low heritability); (2) differences in heritability estimates between populations in both horses and humans likely represents differences in the genetic risk factors and metabolic profiles between these groups; and (3) metabolic syndrome is a complex trait with a large portion of the phenotypic variance being explained by genetics.

Importantly, SNP-based heritability estimates represent the genetic variability that can be explained by the common SNPs present on the genotyping arrays, but cannot account for causal variants that are not inherited together (in linkage disequilibrium) with these SNPs; nor can it include other genetic variations contributing to the phenotype such as insertions, deletions, or copy number variants.[37–40] Further, although heritability estimates provide valuable information on how much genetics is contributing to a trait, they do not provide information on the number of genes involved, the interaction or penetrance of these genes, or the mode by which these genes are inherited. Therefore, additional analyses are required to identify the specific alleles contributing to metabolic syndrome.

Genome-Wide Association Analyses for Metabolic Syndrome

Over the past few decades, genome-wide association analyses (GWA) have started to identify the genetic contribution of MetS across multiple populations and environments. As with heritability, studies have defined their outcome variable for metabolic syndrome as a binary trait or components of MetS as quantitative traits. Key findings across MetS GWA studies indicate (1) that both common and rare variants contribute to MetS, (2) different populations have both shared and unique loci, and (3) a large number of variants are related to lipid metabolism.

We used GWA to identify hundreds of regions of the genome contributing to EMS in 264 Welsh ponies and 286 Morgan horses across 12 EMS traits.[41] Meta-analysis demonstrated that 65 of these regions were shared across breeds, indicating that a large percentage were unique to each breed. Regions were prioritized to identify those that were shared between breeds or shared between traits, resulting in 56 high-priority regions in the Welsh ponies and 39 high-priority regions in the Morgan horses. Functional enrichment analysis of protein coding genes within the prioritized regions identified pathways associated with inflammation, glucose metabolism, and lipid metabolism. These data demonstrated that EMS is a polygenic trait with risk alleles both unique and shared across breeds and was an important first step in the identification of the specific variants contributing to EMS. In addition, this study indicated that a single variant genetic test would not be sufficient to explain an individual's genetic risk for EMS.[41]

Two studies have used GWA and fine-mapping for the identification of candidate genes for EMS. We recently identified a pleiotropic effect of a missense variant in the high-mobility group AT-hook (*HMGA2*) gene on height and metabolic traits in Welsh ponies.[42] In this study, the Pearson correlation coefficient identified an inverse relationship between height and baseline insulin (-0.26) in a cohort of 264 Welsh ponies. GWA analyses of height and insulin revealed the same approximately 1.3-Mb region on chromosome 6, which was also identified using a di statistic for genomic signatures of selection. Haplotype analysis confirmed that there was a shared ancestral haplotype between height and insulin. This region contributed approximately 40% of the heritability for height and approximately 20% of the heritability for insulin. *HMGA2* was identified as a candidate gene, and sequencing identified a single a c.83G> A variant (p.G28E) in *HMGA2*, previously described in other small-stature horse breeds.[43] In the EMS cohort of ponies, the A allele had a frequency of 0.76, was strongly correlated with height (-0.75) and was low to moderately correlated with metabolic traits, including insulin (0.32), insulin after an oral sugar test (0.25), nonesterified fatty acids (0.19), and triglyceride (0.22) concentrations. For this allele, model analysis suggested an additive mode of inheritance with height and a recessive mode of inheritance with the metabolic traits. This was the first report of a gene with a pleotropic effect for EMS and provided evidence for the underlying cause of the unique metabolic profiles and increased EMS susceptibility in ponies.[42]

Lewis and colleagues[44] proposed a candidate allele in the 3′ untranslated region (UTR) of *FAM174A* for EMS and endocrinopathic laminitis in Arabian horses. In this study, the investigators identified a significant association on chromosome 14 in 64 Arabian horses diagnosed with laminitis secondary to EMS. The top marker for this region, SNP BIEC2-263522 (T > C), correlated with baseline insulin levels and laminitis status in this population, and increased modified insulin to glucose ratio (MIRG; a proxy for insulin resistance) and body condition score (BCS) in a second population of Arabians (n = 50), with a suspected dominant mode of inheritance. *FAM174A* was identified to be candidate gene and sequencing resulted in the identification of a polymorphic guanine homopolymer region in the 3'UTR. The 11G allele was in linkage disequilibrium with the top marker SNP and was correlated with elevated insulin concentrations in the first population, and BCS and MIRG in the second population. In addition, the 11G allele was found to be present in Welsh ponies and Tennessee walking horses, but absent in draft, standardbred, and thoroughbred horses.[44] In a population of Polish Arabian horses, the genotype frequency of the BIEC2-263522 SNP was found to be 51.6% for heterozygotes and 16.8% for homozygotes with the variant allele.[45] However, EMS phenotype data were unavailable for both the cross-breed and Polish Arabian populations, preventing the validation of genotype to phenotype correlations in these cohorts. Further, in a large, cross-breed analysis of the *FAM174A* allele in a population of Arabian horses (n = 64), Tennessee walking horses (n = 49), quarter horses (n = 59), Morgan horses (n = 292), and ponies (n = 301), we found a positive association in ponies between the *FAM174A* 11G allele and plasma adiponectin concentrations, indicating a protective effect of this allele and questioning whether *FAM174A* 11G is the true causative allele behind the locus identified by Lewis and colleagues[44] on GWA[46].

Thus, there is concrete evidence that EMS has a strong genetic component, but the identification of specific loci or genetic risk factors for EMS are in its infancy. It is imperative to continue to investigate the specific genes and genetic risk factors for EMS to gain a better understanding of the root causes of these metabolic abnormalities. More importantly, knowledge of the genetics contributing to EMS will allow for the development of genetic tests that would enable veterinarians to evaluate a patient's risk for developing EMS by assessing the number of genetic and environmental risk factors for each individual. Understanding of a horse's risk of EMS will ultimately allow veterinarians to know which horses need frequent monitoring and would benefit from early environmental modification, as well as provide advice on responsible breed decisions. Importantly, as a complex disease, dozens to hundreds or risk alleles contribute to the genetic variation. Therefore, single gene tests will not accurately determine a horse's risk of developing EMS, but instead this will require a genetic panel that represents both cross-breed and within-breed genetic risk variants. Further, an important consideration when assessing the validity of a risk allele is replication of results within independent populations, and due diligence must be met by validating the proposed risk alleles before including them in genetic testing. Finally, unraveling the genes underlying thousands of loci identified on GWA for MetS remains one of the principal challenges in complex trait genetics and is an area in which the horses as an animal model of metabolic syndrome can be used to identify the specific risk alleles across species.

DOPAMINERGIC NEURODEGENERATION

Both equine pars pituitary intermedia dysfunction (PPID) and Parkinson disease in humans are diseases of dopaminergic neurodegeneration in aged individuals. In horses, loss of periventricular dopamine inhibitory control of the melanocytes within the pars intermedia portion of the pituitary gland results in an unchecked proliferative production of proopiomelanocortin (POMC) and POMC-derived peptides, including corticotropinlike intermediate lobe peptide, α-melanocyte stimulating hormone, adrenocorticotropic hormone (ACTH), and β-endorphin, with subsequent hyperplasia, hypertrophy, or adenoma formation of the pars intermedia.[48] Excessive production of these hormones leads to the clinical signs associated with PPID, including muscle atrophy and frailty, immunosuppression, changes in mentation, and failure to shed. In addition, approximately one-third of horses with PPID exhibit regional adiposity and insulin dysregulation, and develop endocrinopathic laminitis.[48] Parkinson disease is characterized by a targeted loss of dopaminergic neurons in the substantia nigra and locus coeruleus, which is accompanied by the accumulation of intracellular inclusions of aggregated α-synuclein, termed Lewy bodies.[49] Often the initial presenting complaint in these patients is motor impairment (resting tremors, bradykinesia, rigidity, and postural instability), which is the result of depletion of striatal dopamine.[50] Thus, although the location and clinical features of PPID and Parkinson disease differ, evidence for similarities in early pathogenesis including evidence of misfolded neuronal α-synuclein, failure of autophagy, oxidative damage, and mitochondrial impairment suggest that the horse is a naturally occurring model of early dopaminergic neurodegeneration.[47]

Genetics of Parkinson Disease

Parkinson disease has been categorized into 2 forms, including the sporadic and familial form, which is often associated with an early onset of clinical signs. Heritability estimates of both forms of Parkinson disease are consistent with a disease that is moderately heritable,[51,52] and the genetic evaluation of familial Parkinson disease has led to the discovery of several genetic variants that account for approximately 30% of the familial form and 3% to 5% of the sporadic form. These mutations occur in one of several genes, including *parkin*, *α-synuclein*, *SNCA*, *PINK1*, *LRRK2*, *ATP13A2*, *PLA2G6*, *DNAJC6*, and *DJ-1*.[53] Further, genetic variants in a large number of genes have been associated with increased risk of developing Parkinson disease, including *UCHL1*, *LRRK2*, *PARK16*, *GAK*, *MAPT*, *GBA*, *NAT2*, *INOS2A*, *GAK*, *HLA-DRA*, and *APOE*.[53] Regardless of these discoveries, only a small portion of the genetic variation has been explained by known risk loci for both familial and sporadic forms of Parkinson disease.[54,55]

Genetic and Expression Analyses of Pars Pituitary Intermedia Dysfunction

Although PPID affects horses of all breeds, Morgan horses and ponies are thought to be at a higher risk.[56] Therefore, breed predilection and similarities with Parkinson disease has given rise to the hypothesis that genetics plays a role in the development of PPID; however, specific genetic variants for PPID have not yet been discovered. Several studies have used gene expression data to gain a better understanding of the underlying pathophysiology and potential genetic mechanisms of PPID.

Aleman and Nieto[57] evaluated the differential expression of proteolytic systems and negative growth regulators of skeletal muscle using gluteus medius muscle biopsies from 7 control horses and 14 horses with PPID and muscle atrophy. The investigators identified an overexpression of m-calpains, a calcium-dependent proteolytic enzyme, in horses with PPID and surmised that m-calpains play an important role in PPID-associated muscle atrophy. However, this study did not evaluate horses with early-onset atrophy or posttranslational mechanisms, and requires further investigation.[57]

Carmalt and colleagues[58] investigated the differential expression of POMC and the prohormone convertase enzymes PC1 and PC2 from the pituitary gland of 10 horses with PPID and 6 control horses. The investigators also collected blood from the cavernous sinus to evaluate POMC protein expression in a separate cohort of 6 horses with PPID and 6 controls. The investigators determined that the expression of POMC, PC1, and PC2 messenger RNA (mRNA) were upregulated in horses with PPID, whereas there was no difference in POMC protein levels, amino acid sequences, or partial mRNA sequences of POMC and ACTH between groups. Thus, the investigators hypothesized that the lack of ACTH bioactivity in horses with PPID was not due to a genetic variant in the POMC or PC coding genes but a posttranslational modification or secretory defect. Notably, this study used whole pituitary gland extraction, which prevented evaluating the differential expression specifically in the par intermedia or pars distalis.[58]

PPID as a complex disease has not yet been proven and the next challenge will be to determine if/how much genetics is contributing to this disease. Accomplishing this goal will require the use of big data in well-phenotyped individuals. Initial steps, focusing on specific breeds, such as the Morgan horses and ponies, include (1) assessing the heritability to estimate how much of the phenotypic variation in PPID can be explained by genetics, (2) using whole-genome sequencing to assess candidate genes (for example, verified genes with causal variants for Parkinson disease), (3) performing GWA analyses using high-density SNP data, and (4) using a multi-omics approach including genomic and transcriptomic data to identify biological pathways responsible for PPID.

SUMMARY

Concrete evidence has supported the role of a genetic contribution to EMS. Heritability estimates of several biochemical measurements in 2 high-risk breeds were consistent with traits that were moderately to highly heritable, and GWA analyses has led to the identification of hundreds of regions of the genome contributing to EMS. Association analysis and fine-mapping has led to the proposal of *HMGA2* and *FAM174A* as candidate genes for EMS; although the allele in *FAM174A* was not verified in a replication study. PPID as a complex disease has not yet been proven, and initial studies have focused on using differential gene expression to identify pathways and potential genetic mechanisms contributing to PPID. The identification of the specific genetic risk factors for both EMS and PPID are in their infancy, but the continued research is crucial to gain a better understanding of the underlying pathophysiology of both diseases and allow for the development of a genetic test. As a complex disease, dozens to hundreds of risk alleles contribute to the genetic variation. Therefore, single-gene tests will not accurately determine a horse's risk of developing metabolic disease, but instead will require a genetic panel that represents both cross and within breed genetic risk variants. This information, in combination with environmental risk factors, will be essential for determining an individual's risk of either metabolic disease before they develop clinical signs or laminitis. Further, both EMS and PPID have been proposed to be naturally occurring models for human diseases, and identification of causal genetic variants has the potential to translate back to human health.

DISCLOSURE

The authors have nothing to disclose.

REFERENCES

1. Hall MA, Moore JH, Ritchie MD. Embracing complex associations in common traits: critical considerations for precision medicine. Trends Genet 2016;32(8):470–84.

2. Li YI, van de Geijn B, Raj A, et al. RNA splicing is a primary link between genetic variation and disease. Science 2016;352(6285):600–4.

3. Pickrell JK. Joint analysis of functional genomic data and genome-wide association studies of 18 human traits. Am J Hum Genet 2014;94(4):559–73.

4. Welter D, MacArthur J, Morales J, et al. The NHGRI GWAS Catalog, a curated resource of SNP-trait associations. Nucleic Acids Res 2014;42(Database issue):D1001–6.

5. Johnson PJ. The equine metabolic syndrome peripheral Cushing's syndrome. Vet Clin North Am Equine Pract 2002;18(2):271–93.

6. Alberti KG, Eckel RH, Grundy SM, et al. Harmonizing the metabolic syndrome: a joint interim statement of the International Diabetes Federation Task Force on Epidemiology and Prevention; National Heart, Lung, and Blood Institute; American Heart Association; World Heart Federation; International Atherosclerosis Society; and International Association for the Study of Obesity. Circulation 2009; 120(16):1640–5.

7. Durham AE, Frank N, McGowan CM, et al. ECEIM consensus statement on equine metabolic syndrome. J Vet Intern Med 2019;33(2):335–49.

8. Frank N. Equine metabolic syndrome. Vet Clin North Am Equine Pract 2011;27(1): 73–92.

9. Jeffcott LB, Field JR. Current concepts of hyperlipaemia in horses and ponies. Vet Rec 1985;116(17):461–6.

10. Jeffcott LB, Field JR, McLean JG, et al. Glucose tolerance and insulin sensitivity in ponies and standardbred horses. Equine Vet J 1986;18(2):97–101.

11. Robie SM, Janson CH, Smith SC, et al. Equine serum lipids: serum lipids and glucose in Morgan and thoroughbred horses and Shetland ponies. Am J Vet Res 1975;36(12):1705–8.

12. Bamford NJ, Potter SJ, Harris PA, et al. Breed differences in insulin sensitivity and insulinemic responses to oral glucose in horses and ponies of moderate body condition score. Domest Anim Endocrinol 2014;47:101–7.

13. Prentice AM. Early influences on human energy regulation: thrifty genotypes and thrifty phenotypes. Physiol Behav 2005;86(5):640–5.

14. Neel JV. Diabetes mellitus: a "thrifty" genotype rendered detrimental by "progress"? Am J Hum Genet 1962;14:353–62.

15. Stoger R. The thrifty epigenotype: an acquired and heritable predisposition for obesity and diabetes? Bioessays 2008;30(2):156–66.

16. Speakman JR. Thrifty genes for obesity, an attractive but flawed idea, and an alternative perspective: the 'drifty gene' hypothesis. Int J Obes (Lond) 2008; 32(11):1611–7.

17. Qasim A, Turcotte M, de Souza RJ, et al. On the origin of obesity: identifying the biological, environmental and cultural drivers of genetic risk among human populations. Obes Rev 2018;19(2):121–49.

18. Treiber KH, Kronfeld DS, Hess TM, et al. Evaluation of genetic and metabolic predispositions and nutritional risk factors for pasture-associated laminitis in ponies. J Am Vet Med Assoc 2006;228(10):1538–45.

19. Visscher PM, Hill WG, Wray NR. Heritability in the genomics era–concepts and misconceptions. Nat Rev Genet 2008;9(4):255–66.

20. Bayoumi RA, Al-Yahyaee SA, Albarwani SA, et al. Heritability of determinants of the metabolic syndrome among healthy Arabs of the Oman family study. Obesity (Silver Spring) 2007;15(3):551–6.

21. Henneman P, Aulchenko YS, Frants RR, et al. Prevalence and heritability of the metabolic syndrome and its individual components in a Dutch isolate: the Erasmus Rucphen Family study. J Med Genet 2008;45(9):572–7.

22. Khan RJ, Gebreab SY, Sims M, et al. Prevalence, associated factors and heritabilities of metabolic syndrome and its individual components in African Americans: the Jackson Heart Study. BMJ Open 2015;5(10):e008675.

23. Lin HF, Boden-Albala B, Juo SH, et al. Heritabilities of the metabolic syndrome and its components in the Northern Manhattan Family Study. Diabetologia 2005;48(10):2006–12.

24. Austin MA, Edwards KL, McNeely MJ, et al. Heritability of multivariate factors of the metabolic syndrome in nondiabetic Japanese Americans. Diabetes 2004; 53(4):1166–9.

25. Bellia A, Giardina E, Lauro D, et al. "The Linosa Study": epidemiological and heritability data of the metabolic syndrome in a Caucasian genetic isolate. Nutr Metab Cardiovasc Dis 2009;19(7):455–61.

26. Graziano F, Biino G, Bonati MT, et al. Estimation of metabolic syndrome heritability in three large populations including full pedigree and genomic information. Hum Genet 2019;138(7):739–48.

27. Henneman P, Aulchenko YS, Frants RR, et al. Genetic architecture of plasma adiponectin overlaps with the genetics of metabolic syndrome-related traits. Diabetes Care 2010;33(4):908–13.

28. Martin LJ, North KE, Dyer T, et al. Phenotypic, genetic, and genome-wide structure in the metabolic syndrome. BMC Genet 2003;4(Suppl 1):S95.

29. Mills GW, Avery PJ, McCarthy MI, et al. Heritability estimates for beta cell function and features of the insulin resistance syndrome in UK families with an increased susceptibility to type 2 diabetes. Diabetologia 2004;47(4):732–8.

30. Wu KD, Hsiao CF, Ho LT, et al. Clustering and heritability of insulin resistance in Chinese and Japanese hypertensive families: a Stanford-Asian Pacific Program in Hypertension and Insulin Resistance sibling study. Hypertens Res 2002; 25(4):529–36.

31. Zarkesh M, Daneshpour MS, Faam B, et al. Heritability of the metabolic syndrome and its components in the Tehran Lipid and Glucose Study (TLGS). Genet Res (Camb) 2012;94(6):331–7.

32. Musani SK, Martin LJ, Woo JG, et al. Heritability of the severity of the metabolic syndrome in whites and blacks in 3 large cohorts. Circ Cardiovasc Genet 2017; 10(2) [pii:e001621].

33. Lee C, Pollak EJ. Influence of sire misidentification on sire x year interaction variance and direct-maternal genetic covariance for weaning weight in beef cattle. J Anim Sci 1997;75(11):2858–63.

34. Yang J, Benyamin B, McEvoy BP, et al. Common SNPs explain a large proportion of the heritability for human height. Nat Genet 2010;42(7):565–9.

35. Vattikuti S, Guo J, Chow CC. Heritability and genetic correlations explained by common SNPs for metabolic syndrome traits. PLoS Genet 2012;8(3):e1002637.

36. Norton EM, Schultz NE, Rendahl AK, et al. Heritability of metabolic traits associated with equine metabolic syndrome in Welsh ponies and Morgan horses. Equine Vet J 2019;51(4):475–80.

37. Lee SH, DeCandia TR, Ripke S, et al. Estimating the proportion of variation in susceptibility to schizophrenia captured by common SNPs. Nat Genet 2012;44(3): 247–50.

38. Yang J, Lee SH, Goddard ME, et al. GCTA: a tool for genome-wide complex trait analysis. Am J Hum Genet 2011;88(1):76–82.

39. Lee SH, Wray NR, Goddard ME, et al. Estimating missing heritability for disease from genome-wide association studies. Am J Hum Genet 2011;88(3):294–305.

40. Manolio TA, Collins FS, Cox NJ, et al. Finding the missing heritability of complex diseases. Nature 2009;461(7265):747–53.

41. Norton E, Schultz N, Geor R, et al. Genome-wide association analyses of equine metabolic syndrome phenotypes in Welsh ponies and Morgan horses. Genes (Basel) 2019;10(11) [pii:E893].

42. Norton EM, Avila F, Schultz NE, et al. Evaluation of an HMGA2 variant for pleiotropic effects on height and metabolic traits in ponies. J Vet Intern Med 2019; 33(2):942–52.

43. Frischknecht M, Jagannathan V, Plattet P, et al. A non-synonymous HMGA2 variant decreases height in Shetland ponies and other small horses. PLoS One 2015;10(10):e0140749.

44. Lewis SL, Holl HM, Streeter C, et al. Genomewide association study reveals a risk locus for equine metabolic syndrome in the Arabian horse. J Anim Sci 2017;95(3): 1071–9.

45. Stefaniuk-Szmukier M, Ropla-Molik K, Bugno-Poniewierska M. Identyfikacja wariantu w rejonie genu FAM14A potencjalnie związanego z występowaniem syndromu metabolicznego (EMS) u koni czystej krwi arabskiej. Wiadomosci Zootechniczne 2017;5:46–8. Available at: https://www.google.com/url? sa=t&rct=j&q=&esrc=s&source=web&cd=1&cad=rja&uact=8&ved=2ahUK Ewjziq2Ap-boAhWGKs0KHfKxCKMQFjAAegQIAhAB&url=https%3A%2F%2Fw z.izoo.krakow.pl%2Ffiles%2FWZ_2017_5_art05.pdf&usg=AOvVaw3hg4jrAAQB kp3xsWidYYKN.

46. Roy M, Norton E, Rendahl, A, et al. Assessment of the FAM174A 11G allele as a risk allele for equine metabolic syndrome. Animal Genetics 2020.

47. McFarlane D. Advantages and limitations of the equine disease, pituitary pars intermedia dysfunction as a model of spontaneous dopaminergic neurodegenerative disease. Ageing Res Rev 2007;6(1):54–63.

48. Karikoski NP, Patterson-Kane JC, Singer ER, et al. Lamellar pathology in horses with pituitary pars intermedia dysfunction. Equine Vet J 2016;48(4):472–8.

49. Rommelfanger KS, Weinshenker D. Norepinephrine: The redheaded stepchild of Parkinson's disease. Biochem Pharmacol 2007;74(2):177–90.

50. Eriksen JL, Wszolek Z, Petrucelli L. Molecular pathogenesis of Parkinson disease. JAMA Neurol 2005;62(3):353–7.

51. Hamza TH, Payami H. The heritability of risk and age at onset of Parkinson's disease after accounting for known genetic risk factors. J Hum Genet 2010;55(4):241–3.

52. Keller MF, Saad M, Bras J, et al. Using genome-wide complex trait analysis to quantify 'missing heritability' in Parkinson's disease. Hum Mol Genet 2012; 21(22):4996–5009.

53. Klein C, Westenberger A. Genetics of Parkinson's disease. Cold Spring Harb Perspect Med 2012;2(1):a008888.

54. Alcalay RN, Caccappolo E, Mejia-Santana H, et al. Frequency of known mutations in early-onset Parkinson disease: implication for genetic counseling: the consortium on risk for early onset Parkinson disease study. Arch Neurol 2010; 67(9):1116–22.

55. Payami H, Zareparsi S, James D, et al. Familial aggregation of Parkinson disease: a comparative study of early-onset and late-onset disease. Arch Neurol 2002; 59(5):848–50.

56. Schott HC 2nd. Pituitary pars intermedia dysfunction: equine Cushing's disease. Vet Clin North Am Equine Pract 2002;18(2):237–70.

57. Aleman M, Nieto JE. Gene expression of proteolytic systems and growth regulators of skeletal muscle in horses with myopathy associated with pituitary pars intermedia dysfunction. Am J Vet Res 2010;71(6):664–70.

58. Carmalt JL, Mortazavi S, McOnie RC, et al. Profiles of pro-opiomelanocortin and encoded peptides, and their processing enzymes in equine pituitary pars intermedia dysfunction. PLoS One 2018;13(1):e0190796.

Genetics of Equine Muscle Disease

Stephanie J. Valberg, DVM, PhD

KEYWORDS

- Myopathy • Atrophy • Rhabdomyolysis • Tying up • Polysaccharide • Glycogen

KEY POINTS

- There are currently genetic tests for 5 equine myopathies that have been scientifically validated: hyperkalemic periodic paralysis (codominant), glycogen branching enzyme deficiency (recessive), type 1 polysaccharide storage myopathy (dominant), malignant hyperthermia (dominant), and myosin heavy chain myopathy (codominant).
- The breed, age, clinical signs shown, and mode of inheritance should all be considered when selecting the appropriate genetic test and interpreting the test for diagnostic or breeding purposes.
- With the exception of glycogen branching enzyme deficiency, the penetrance of clinical signs can be highly variable from individual to individual within a breed, and from breed to breed in the case of type 1 polysaccharide storage myopathy.

INTRODUCTION

For hundreds of years, horses have undergone genetic selection for muscular traits that promote athletic ability. A popular sire effect occurs in horses when a stud with desirable performance attributes is bred repeatedly, concentrating his genetics in the gene pool and perpetuating his traits.[1] Although this can enhance performance, it can also result in genetic disorders knowingly or unknowingly being passed along to thousands of offspring in subsequent generations. For example, hundreds of years ago when feed was scarce and horses worked for hours every day, the increased muscle glycogen storage that occurs with type 1 polysaccharide storage myopathy (PSSM1) had a selective advantage.[2] However, with modern high-quality feeds and periodic recreational use of horses, excessive muscle glycogen can disrupt energy metabolism causing muscle degeneration with intermittent exercise.[3] Thus, what was once a beneficial trait can now manifest as a detrimental trait. The 5 known single-gene mutations that cause muscle diseases in horses disrupt cell membrane electrical conduction, muscle energy metabolism, muscle contraction, and immunogenicity (**Fig. 1**).

Equine Sports Medicine, Department of Large Animal Clinical Sciences, College of Veterinary Medicine, Michigan State University, 736 Wilson Road, East Lansing, MI 48824, USA
E-mail address: valbergs@cvm.msu.edu

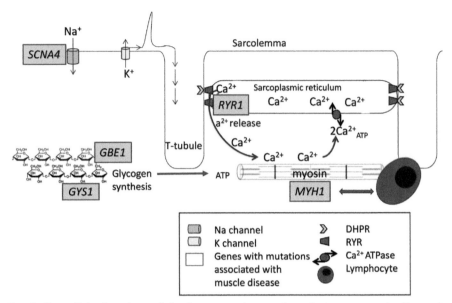

Fig. 1. The cellular locations of the 5 monogenic mutations that cause muscle disease in horses. The mutation causing hyperkalemic periodic paralysis (HYPP) occurs in the *SCNA4* gene encoding the sodium channel, the mutation causing glycogen branching enzyme disease (GBED) occurs in *GBE1* encoding glycogen branching enzyme, the mutation causing PSSM1 occurs in *GYS1* encoding glycogen synthase, the mutation causing malignant hyperthermia occurs in *RYR1*, and the mutation causing myosin heavy chain myopathies (MYHM) immune-mediated myositis and nonexertional rhabdomyolysis occurs in *MYH1* encoding the type 2X myofiber myosin heavy chain. DHPR, dihydropyridine receptor.

The muscle diseases included in this article have scientifically validated genetic tests that are recommended for use in the diagnosis of each disorder. Information on mode of inheritance, breeds affected, penetrance, age of onset, clinical signs, management, and prognosis are provided to assist veterinarians in making the best decisions for management and potential breeding (**Fig. 2**). The scientific validation that has been followed for the 5 genetic mutations comprise statistical association of the variant with the phenotype that was defined by the gold standard for diagnosis, high frequency of the variant in an affected population and low frequency in a healthy population, evidence that the variant changes the function or regulation of a protein, and peer-reviewed publication.

Genetic variants can be offered as commercial genetic tests without scientific validation to veterinarians and horse owners because there is no regulation of genetic testing in veterinary medicine. Validation steps are fundamentally important because genetic variants, including variants that change the amino acid sequence of a protein, are common in healthy horses, making them easy to discover and easy to falsely attribute to a disease. For example, our laboratory examined the sequence of genes expressed in skeletal muscle from 10 healthy thoroughbreds using RNA sequencing and found 20,710 sequence variants, 17,644 of which changed an amino acid sequence and 2750 of which were deemed potentially severe by the Ensembl variant effect predictor (Valberg, personal observation). These variants had no clinical effect in these healthy exercising horses. Because genetic variants with little clinical impact are common and testing is unregulated, the onus is on veterinarians to ensure that

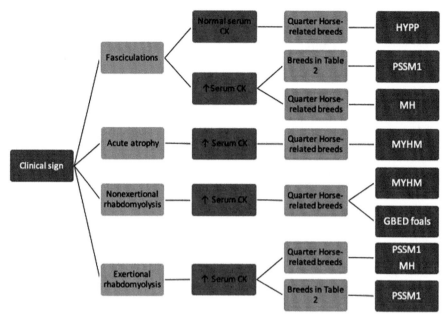

Fig. 2. Selection of the appropriate genetic test for horses with clinical signs of muscle disease. Decisions to use a genetic test for these myopathies should be based on the age, breed, clinical signs, and history of muscle degeneration as indicated by increased serum creatine kinase (CK) activity.

commercial genetic tests are scientifically validated before using them for diagnostic, prepurchase, or breeding decisions.

HYPERKALEMIC PERIODIC PARALYSIS

Hyperkalemic periodic paralysis (HYPP) was the first genetic disease in horses for which the molecular defect was determined.[4] This ground-breaking achievement resulted from an in-depth clinical investigation, strong parallels between equine and human cases of HYPP, and an available herd of horses segregating for the HYPP phenotype.[4–6]

Mutation

HYPP is caused by a phenylalanine to leucine substitution at codon 1416 (F1416L) in the alpha-subunit of the voltage-gated skeletal muscle sodium channel (SCN4A) (see **Fig. 1**).[4] Heterozygosity for the SCN4A mutation is sufficient to cause susceptibility to HYPP; however, a codominant mode of inheritance is apparent because clinical signs are more severe and more frequent in homozygous horses.[7] The common designation for genotypes is: heterozygous affected, N/H; homozygous affected, H/H; and homozygous normal, N/N.

Prevalence

HYPP affects quarter horses, American paint horses, Appaloosas, and quarter horse crossbred animals worldwide that are descendants of the stallion Impressive. Approximately 1.5% of the quarter horse breed and 4.5% of the American paint horse breed are affected (**Table 1**).[8] There seems to be selection for the heavily muscled

Table 1
Percentages of horses with a disease-causing variant within quarter horses and paint horse populations and within elite competitive quarter horse subgroups

| | Dominant | | | | Recessive | | |
| | | | | Horses with the Mutation (%) | | | |
Population	HYPP[8]	PSSM[8]	MH[a]	MYHM[64]	GBED[8]	HERDA[8]	OLWS[8]
QH	1.5	11.3	<1	7.4	11	3.5	0
APH	4.5	4.5	UN	UN	3.9	1.7	21.3
Halter	56.4	28.2	UN	16.0	5.1	0.8	0
Western Pleasure	1.1	8.6	UN	4.2	26.3	12.8	0
Cutting	0	6.7	UN	8.8	13.6	28.3	0
Reining	0	4.3	UN	24.3	3.1	9.3	0
Working Cow Horse	0	5.7	UN	17.0	9.5	11.5	0
Barrel Racing	1.2	1.4	UN	0	1.2	1.2	0
Racing	0	2	UN	0	0	0	0

Zero (0) indicates that the variant is not observed in the dataset evaluated.
Abbreviations: GBED, glycogen branching enzyme deficiency; HERDA, herditary regional dermal asthenia; MH, malignant hyperthermia; MYHM, myosin heavy chain myopathy; OWLS, overo lethal white syndrome; UN, unknown.
[a] Personal communication, Rebecca Bellone, University of California Davis, 2019.

phenotype associated with HYPP in the halter horse performance group, where 56% of horses possess the HYPP mutation (**Fig. 3**, see **Table 1**).[8,9] No change in prevalence of the HYPP mutation has occurred in quarter horses since the discovery of the genetic mutation in 1992, likely because preferential selection of halter horse breeding stock with the mutation has occurred because heavily muscled affected offspring are deemed superior halter horses in shows.[9]

Breed Standards

In 1996, the American Quarter Horse Association (AQHA) officially recognized HYPP as a genetic defect or undesirable trait and instituted mandatory HYPP testing for all foals descended from Impressive and that were born after January 1, 1998.[10] Results of genetic testing are recorded on the registration certificate. In 2004, the AQHA ruled that foals born in 2007 or later and that tested H/H would not be eligible for registration because of the severity of their clinical signs. Testing of breeding stallions for HYPP is required by the AQHA and American Paint Horse Association (APHA), with the results recorded on the horse's registration papers. Some Appaloosa registries also require genetic testing.

Clinical Signs

Clinical signs of HYPP occur with N/H and H/H genotypes and vary widely in N/H horses from asymptomatic to daily episodic muscle fasciculations and weakness.[5,11] Feeds high in potassium, starving, anesthesia, heavy sedation, trailer rides, and stress are common precipitators of an episode of HYPP.[5] Owners of affected horses should advise veterinarians of HYPP status before anesthesia or procedures requiring heavy sedation. Exercise does not seem to induce clinical signs and serum creatine kinase (CK) level is either normal or modestly increased during episodic fasciculations and weakness (see **Fig. 2**).[5,11]

Episodes of HYPP begin with a brief period of twitching or delayed relaxation of muscles and can include prolapse of the third eyelid.[10] Sweating and muscle

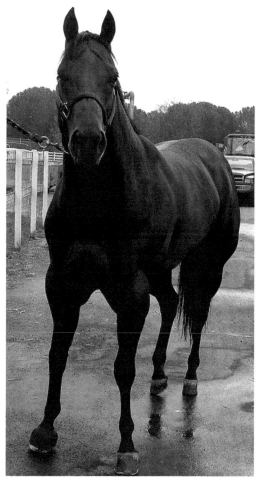

Fig. 3. Heavily muscled phenotype of a quarter horse with the HYPP mutation in *SCNA4*. (*Courtesy of* Dr. Gary Magdesian.)

fasciculations commonly occur in the flanks, neck, and shoulders. Stimulation and attempts to move can exacerbate muscle tremors, with some horses developing severe muscle cramping.[10] During mild episodes, horses remain standing. With more severe episodes, horses are often tachycardic and tachypneic, and fasciculations evolve into generalized weakness shown by swaying and dog-sitting, and progressing to lateral recumbency. Recumbent horses appear paralyzed but remain fully conscious. Episodes usually last for 15 to 60 minutes.[5] Respiratory distress caused by paralysis of upper respiratory muscles can occur in N/H and H/H horses during episodes and can require a tracheostomy to prevent death from anoxia.[7] After an episode of HYPP subsides, the horse appears normal.

Classically, by 2 to 3 years of age, most N/H horses have shown intermittent clinical signs once weaned, with no apparent abnormalities between episodes.[5] Foals homozygous for HYPP usually show clinical signs of disease in the first few days of life that include dysphagia, respiratory stridor, periodic obstruction of the upper respiratory tract, and respiratory distress.[7] Endoscopic findings include pharyngeal collapse and edema, laryngopalatal dislocation, and laryngeal paralysis.[7] Adults that are H/H usually have more frequent and severe episodes of HYPP compared with N/H horses and more severe signs of upper airway obstruction during an episode.[10] Homozygous affected horses also have a high-pitched whinny even between episodes.[10]

During episodes of muscle fasciculations, most horses have hyperkalemia (6–9 mEq/L), hemoconcentration, and mild hyponatremia with normal acid-base balance.[5] Serum potassium concentration returns to normal quickly after the cessation of clinical signs. Some affected horses have normal serum potassium concentrations during minor episodes of muscle fasciculations.[12] Electromyographic examination of asymptomatic HYPP horses between episodes reveals abnormal fibrillation potentials, complex repetitive discharges, with occasional myotonic potentials and trains of doublets.[5,13]

Pathophysiology

Sodium channels are normally briefly activated to allow transient sodium entry into muscle cells during the initial phase of the muscle action potential. Codon 1416 lies in a highly conserved segment of one of the 24 transmembrane domains of the SCN4A channel protein.[4] The F1416L HYPP mutation results in a failure of a subpopulation of sodium channels to inactivate when serum potassium concentrations are increased.[14] Inactivation seems to be more pronounced during times of increased extracellular potassium level, which can occur with diets high in potassium.[15] Failure of inactivation results in membrane depolarization, which manifests as muscle fasciculations and can eventually lead to depolarization block manifesting as muscular paresis or paralysis.[16]

Diagnosis

The definitive test to diagnose HYPP is demonstration of the C to G base-pair substitution in SCN4A, which causes an F1416L substitution.[4] This test clearly differentiates among H/H, N/H, and N/N.

Treatment

Mild episodes of HYPP can be aborted early on by feeding grain or corn syrup to stimulate insulin-mediated movement of potassium into cells and by initiating light exercise. Many horses spontaneously recover from episodes of paralysis and appear normal by the time a veterinarian arrives. Other acute treatment options include administration of epinephrine (3 mL of 1:1000/500 kg intramuscularly).[10] In severe cases, administration of calcium gluconate (0.2–0.4 mL/kg of a 23% solution diluted in 1 L of 5% dextrose, slowly) can produce immediate improvement.[10] An increase in extracellular calcium concentration increases the muscle-membrane threshold potential, which attenuates membrane hyperexcitability. Alternatively, to reduce serum potassium level, intravenous (IV) dextrose (6 mL/kg of a 5% solution) alone or combined with sodium bicarbonate (1–2 mEq/kg) can be used to enhance intracellular movement of potassium.[10] With severe dyspnea caused by laryngeal or pharyngeal obstruction, a tracheostomy can be necessary.

Management

Restricting dietary potassium is usually the most successful approach to managing HYPP.[15,17] Ideally, horses with recurrent episodes of HYPP should be fed a balanced diet containing between 0.6% and 1.1% total potassium concentration and meals containing less than 33 g of potassium.[15] The most common source of potassium is forage. Practical approaches include testing hay to ensure it has less than 1.1% potassium, and avoiding feeds high in molasses and supplements containing electrolytes and/or kelp. Pasture grazing need not be restricted because the gradual consumption of grasses, which have a high water content, prevents a spike in blood potassium concentrations.[10] Regular exercise and frequent turnout are beneficial.

In cases where dietary management is insufficient to control episodes of HYPP, drugs that increase renal losses of potassium are used. Acetazolamide (2–3 mg/kg every 8–12 hours by mouth) or hydrochlorothiazide (0.5–1 mg/kg every 12 hours by mouth) can be helpful. Owners should take note of restrictions on the use of these drugs during competitions.

Prognosis

HYPP is a manageable disorder in most cases. Recurrent bouts can occur in some horses and owners need to be aware that severe episodes can be fatal. Because HYPP is a dominant trait, breeding an N/H horse to a normal horse results in a 50% chance of producing a foal heterozygous for HYPP, whereas breeding an H/H horse to a normal horse results in a 100% chance of producing an N/H heterozygous affected horse. Horses descended from Impressive should be tested for HYPP during prepurchase examination.

GLYCOGEN BRANCHING ENZYME DEFICIENCY

Glycogen is a highly branched glucose polymer consisting of alpha-1,4 glycosidic linkages produced by glycogen synthase and numerous branching alpha-1,6 linkages formed by glycogen branching enzyme (GBE) (see **Fig. 1**). GBE deficiency (GBED) was discovered in 2001 through the observation of abnormal polysaccharide inclusions in tissues from neonatal foals that were either euthanized or died because of muscular weakness, respiratory failure, hypoglycemic seizures, or cardiac arrest (**Fig. 4**).[18,19]

Mutation

GBED is caused by a mutation in exon 1 of the *GBE1* gene that substitutes a tyrosine for a premature stop codon at amino acid 34 (Y34X), truncating the encoded GBE.[20] GBED is autosomal recessive with common designation for genotypes: heterozygous affected, Gb/N; homozygous affected, Gb/Gb; and normal horses, N/N. Heterozygous horses are clinically normal.

Prevalence

GBED occurs in quarter horse and paint horse breeds. Carrier frequency ranges from 8% to 11% in the quarter horse and 4% to 7% in the paint horse breeds (see **Table 1**).[8,21] The highest prevalence is seen in Western pleasure horses at 26% followed by cutting (14%) and working cow horses (10%) (see **Table 1**).[8]

Breed Standards

Genetic testing for GBED is mandatory for breeding stallions registered by the AQHA and APHA, with results recorded on the horse's registration papers. Some Appaloosa registries also require genetic testing.

Clinical Signs

Most foals homozygous for GBED seem to be aborted or stillborn based on the high prevalence of heterozygosity for GBED in the paint and quarter horse breeds and the

PAS   Amylase-PAS

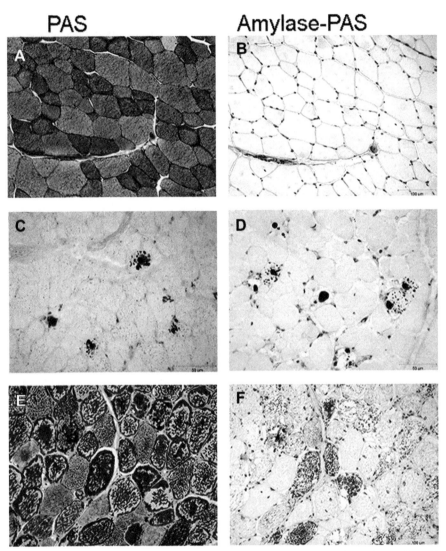

Fig. 4. (*A*) Glycogen in a cross section a skeletal muscle from a normal horse (periodic acid–Schiff [PAS], original magnification ×20). (*B*) Skeletal muscle from a normal horse showing complete digestion of glycogen in the muscle fibers (amylase PAS, original magnification ×20). (*C*) Muscle biopsy from a foal with GBED. Note the lack of normal PAS staining for the presence of glycogen and the accumulation of abnormal PAS-positive inclusions (*arrow*) (PAS, original magnification ×40). (*D*) Skeletal muscle from the same foal showing that the abnormal inclusions are amylase resistant (*arrow*) (amylase PAS, original magnification ×40). (*E*) Muscle biopsy from a horse with PSSM1. Note the dark stain indicating increased muscle glycogen concentrations and the presence of aggregates of PAS-positive material in many cells (PAS, original magnification ×20). (*F*) Skeletal muscle from the same horse showing that the abnormal aggregates are amylase resistant (amylase PAS, original magnification ×20).

low prevalence of live foals born with GBED.[21] Genotyping of 190 quarter horse foals that were aborted, stillborn, or died at full or near term of unknown causes found that approximately 4% were Gb/Gb, with most being aborted within the second trimester.[21] If foals survive to term, they usually appear weak and hypothermic at birth but, with support to nurse, can appear normal for the first weeks of life.[18] Early in life, affected foals usually have a slightly dull mentation and flexural limb deformities that are corrected by bandaging or tetracycline administration (**Fig. 5**). Hematologic and biochemical abnormalities include a leukopenia and moderate increases in serum CK, aspartate transaminase, and gamma glutamyl transferase activities.[18] Within weeks, GBED progresses to involve difficulty rising or respiratory failure or sudden death following hypoglycemic seizures or cardiac arrest. Regardless of the degree of intensive care provided, all affected foals studied to date have died or been euthanized by 18 weeks of age.[18,19,22]

Pathophysiology

The GBE provides an energy-dense structure through adding branching alpha-1,6 glycosidic linkages to the glycogen polymer (**see Fig. 1**). The stop codon introduced in *GBE1* results in no measurable GBE activity or immunodetectable GBE in tissues.[18] The production of straight chains of glycogen without branch points drastically decreases the number of nonreducing ends within the glycogen molecule, thereby limiting the rates of both synthesis and degradation.[23] As a result, cardiac and skeletal muscle, liver, and the brain cannot store or mobilize normally branched glycogen to maintain glucose homeostasis. Glucose-dependent tissues such as skeletal myocytes, cardiac myocytes, and cardiac Purkinje fibers are subject to catastrophic energy deficits in foals with GBED, creating weakness and cardiac dysfunction.[18]

Diagnosis

Definitive diagnosis of GBED requires genetic testing to identify foals homozygous for the C to A missense mutation in *GBE1*, which causes a Y34X amino acid change.[20] In the absence of tissue from the foal, parents can be genotyped for carrier status.

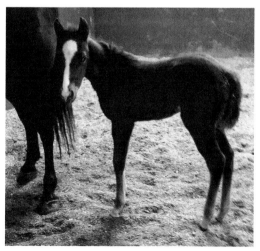

Fig. 5. Foal with GBED showing a slightly dull mentation and mild carpal flexural limb deformity. (*Courtesy of* Dr. Alicia Foley.)

Characteristic histopathologic findings in skeletal muscle, Purkinje fibers, or cardiac myocytes include basophilic globules and eosinophilic crystalline inclusions in hematoxylin and eosin stains and deeply magenta inclusions in periodic acid–Schiff (PAS) stains (see **Fig. 4**).[18,19] In contrast with polysaccharide storage myopathy (PSSM), cardiac and skeletal muscle tissues from GBED foals have little background staining for glycogen (see **Fig. 4**).

Management

Foals with GBED have survived for weeks in intensive care facilities; however, none of the foals have lived beyond 18 weeks of age. Euthanasia is recommended after identification of homozygous Gb/Gb foals to minimize unnecessary and futile expense.

Prognosis

GBED is invariably fatal by 18 weeks of age. Heterozygous horses show no clinical signs of disease. Breeding of 2 heterozygotes results in a 25% chance of producing an affected Gb/Gb foal.

TYPE 1 POLYSACCHARIDE STORAGE MYOPATHY
Mutation

PSSM1 is caused by a gain-of-function missense mutation in the glycogen synthase 1 gene (*GYS1*) that results in an arginine to histidine (R309H) substitution in the glycogen synthase enzyme (see **Fig. 1**).[2] It is inherited as an autosomal dominant disease. The common designation for genotypes is: heterozygous affected, P/N; homozygous affected, P/P; and normal horses, N/N.

Prevalence

More than 20 different breeds possess the *GYS1* mutation responsible for PSSM1 (**Table 2**).[24–28] The highest prevalence of the mutation occurs in continental European breeds derived from the Belgian draft (90% prevalence in), which also have a high prevalence of homozygous P/P horses (see **Table 2**).[24] North American Belgians and Percherons are derivatives of these European breeds and also have a high prevalence of PSSM1 at 36% and 54% of horses affected, respectively (see **Table 2**).[25] The prevalence of PSSM1 is very low in United Kingdom–derived breeds such as shires and Clydesdales, but the *GYS1* mutation is present in other United Kingdom–derived breeds such as Irish drafts, Irish sport horses, and cobs (see **Table 2**).[24,25] The *GYS1* mutation is present in Haflinger and gypsy Vanner breeds at about 18% to 20% prevalence and occurs at a low prevalence in some warmblood breeds (see **Table 2**).[24,27]

In quarter horses, the prevalence of *GYS1* mutation is 6% to 10% and in American paint and Appaloosa horses it is 6% to 8% (see **Table 1**).[8,25] The highest frequency of the mutation occurs in halter horses (28%) and the lowest frequency in barrel racing quarter horses (1.4%) (see **Table 1**).[8] The prevalence of *GYS1* mutation is very low to nonexistent in light horse breeds such as Arabians, Standardbreds, and thoroughbreds (see **Table 2**).[25,29]

Breed Standards

Testing of breeding stallions for PSSM1 is mandated by the AQHA and APHA, with results recorded on the horse's registration papers. Some Appaloosa registries also require genetic testing.

Table 2
The number of North American and European horses tested and the percentage of horses testing positive (heterozygous and homozygous) for the *GYS1* mutation in breeds sampled using random and nonrandom sampling

	Breed	No. Tested	Prevalence (%)
North America			
Random Sample[25]	Percheron	149	62
	Belgian	149	39
	Clydesdale	132	0
	Shire	195	0.5
	Quarter horse	335	7
	Paint	195	8
	Appaloosa	152	6
	Morgan	214	1
	Thoroughbred	96	0
	Arabian	100	0
	Norwegian fjord	46	0
	Icelandic horse	45	0
Europe			
Nonrandom Sample[24]	Belgian trekpaard	38	92
	Netherlands trekpaard	23	74
	Comtois	88	80
	Breton	51	63
	Swedish Ardennes	29	38
	Rhenish German coldblood	44	68
	South German coldblood	265	20
	Hanoverian	214	0
	Haflinger[27]	50	18
Additional Breeds			
Neuromuscular Diagnostic Laboratory[a]	Rocky Mountain horse	—	Present
	Tennessee walker	—	Present
	Mustang	—	Present
	Dutch warmblood	—	Present
	Hanoverian	—	Present
	Irish sport horse	—	Present
	Selle Français	—	Present
	Gypsy Vanner	—	Present
	Cobb	—	Present
	Suffolk punch	—	Present
	Normandy cob	—	Present
	American cream	—	Present

[a] Personal communication, Stephanie Valberg, Michigan State University.

Clinical Signs

On average, in light breed horses, clinical signs of PSSM1 may develop during or after light exercise around 5 years of age; however, this can range from 1 to 14 years of age. Acute clinical signs include tucking up of the abdomen, stretching out, fasciculations in the flank, muscle stiffness, sweating, reluctance to move forward, pawing, rolling, and overt firm muscle contractures (**Fig. 6**).[3,30] The hindquarters are frequently most affected, but epaxial muscles, abdomen, and forelimb muscles may also be involved. Signs of pain usually begin after 15 minutes of exercise and can last for more than

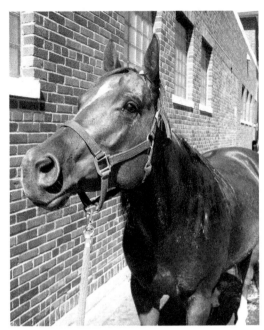

Fig. 6. A quarter horse with acute signs of rhabdomyolysis caused by PSSM1. Note the anxious expression, sweating, and muscle stiffness.

2 hours after exercise. Approximately 10% of cases are severe enough to cause temporary recumbency.[30] Severe coliclike pain and myoglobinuric renal failure are less common presenting complaints.[31] Acute episodes are usually associated with markedly increased serum CK activity of greater than 35,000 U/L and myoglobinuria.[30]

Draft horse and draft crosses

Many draft horses and Haflingers with the *GYS1* mutation are asymptomatic.[32–34] The average age of draft horses diagnosed with PSSM1 is 8 years of age.[35] Clinical signs occur most often in horses fed high-grain diets, exercised irregularly, with little turnout, or horses that undergo general anesthesia. When present, rhabdomyolysis can be severe and result in prolonged recumbency and possibly euthanasia.[31,36] Other signs of PSSM in draft horses, often homozygotes (P/P), include progressive weakness and muscle loss resulting in difficulty rising in horses with normal serum CK activity.[37] Although abnormal polysaccharide can be present in cardiac myocytes in P/P horses, there seems to be no clinical evidence of cardiac disease.[38,39]

Chronic signs in light breeds

Chronic signs of PSSM1 include a lack of energy when under saddle, reluctance to move forward, stopping and stretching out as if to urinate, and a sour attitude toward exercise.[3,30] PSSM1 may also present in dressage and show jumpers as chronic back pain, failure to round over fences, and fasciculations or pain on palpation of lumbar muscles.[40] Serum CK activities are often increased in unmanaged horses, even when horses are rested, or increase from normal values by 2-fold or more after 15 minutes of light exercise.[41]

Pathophysiology

The dominant gain-of-function mutation in the *GYS1* gene encoding glycogen synthase results in greater than 1.8-fold higher glycogen concentrations in skeletal muscle and accumulation of amylase-resistant polysaccharide in a small percentage of fast-twitch muscle fibers (see **Fig. 4**).[2,3,42] Ineffective regulation by phosphorylation of the glycogen synthase enzyme arising from the position of the *GYS1* mutation results in higher than normal activity of glycogen synthase in basal states and when activated by insulin and glucose-6-phosphate.[2,42] The formation of an abnormal polysaccharide is probably related to chronically enhanced glycogen synthase enzyme activity without the same relative activation of branching enzyme.[39] Over years, this leads to a less highly branched polysaccharide that becomes resistant to amylase digestion.[43]

The dysregulation of glycogen synthesis seems to alter energy generation in muscle fibers during exercise under certain dietary conditions that increase insulin levels.[44] One of the critical studies performed in horses with PSSM1 determined that high serum CK activity following 15 minutes of light aerobic exercise is associated with a deficit in energy metabolism (measured as high myofiber inosine monophosphate concentrations).[45] A potential scenario for an energy deficit in PSSM1 could be that myophosphorylase is inactive when glycogen synthase is active, resulting in minimal glycogen metabolism. Alternatively or in concert, dysregulation of glycogen concentrations could prevent nutrient switches (AMP [5'-adenosine monophosphate–activated protein] kinase) to fully activate enzymes such as pyruvate dehydrogenase during exercise, limiting adequate acetyl coenzyme A (CoA) for oxidative metabolism.[44] Thus, PSSM horses with maximal stimulation of glycogen synthase from high nonstructural carbohydrate (NSC) diets may be unable to generate enough acetyl CoA from either carbohydrate or fat metabolism to fuel muscle contraction. The common occurrence of clinical signs during the first 20 minutes of exercise may be because, at this stage of exercise, muscles rely heavily on glycogen/glucose for energy.[30]

Diagnosis

The gold standard for diagnosis of PSSM1 is identification of the G to A base substitution in exon 6 of the *GYS1*, which causes an R309H substitution in glycogen synthase.[2]

Muscle biopsy provides another means to diagnose PSSM1 in horses at 2 years of age.[3,43] The distinctive features of PSSM1 in muscle biopsy samples are numerous subsarcolemmal vacuoles and dense, crystalline PAS–positive, amylase-resistant inclusions in fast-twitch fibers (see **Fig. 4**).[3] A false-negative diagnosis of type 1 PSSM by muscle biopsy can occur if biopsy samples are small or if horses are less than 2 years of age.[43] A diagnosis of PSSM1 can be made irrespective of diet and proximity of sampling to recent episodes of rhabdomyolysis.

Note that, in draft horses of continental European origin, the very high prevalence of PSSM in essence means that there is a high chance that any clinical sign could be falsely associated with the disease PSSM1.[24] Thus, clinical judgment is required to determine whether the horse's clinical signs could reasonably be associated with a myopathy.

Acute Treatment

The objectives of treatment are to relieve anxiety and muscle pain, as well as to correct fluid deficits. The first line of treatment of horses with painful rhabdomyolysis should include acepromazine (0.04–0.07 mg/kg); xylazine (0.4–0.8 mg/kg); or, in more painful horses, detomidine (0.02–0.04 μg/kg) combined with butorphanol (0.01–0.04 mg/kg). In hydrated horses, nonsteroidal antiinflammatory drugs such as ketoprofen (2.2 mg/kg), phenylbutazone (2.2–4.4 mg/kg), or flunixin meglumine (1.1 mg/kg) can provide additional pain relief but the effect is not as immediately effective as tranquilization. Muscle relaxants such as methocarbamol (5–22 mg/kg, IV slowly) seem to produce variable results, possibly depending on the dosage used. Analgesic treatment is continued to effect, but most horses are relatively pain free within 18 to 24 hours. Hand-walking horses recovering from an episode of PSSM1 for more than 5 to 10 minutes at a time may trigger another episode of rhabdomyolysis. If possible, when a horse walks comfortably, stall confinement should be limited to 48 hours and turnout then provided in a small paddock.

For horses with extreme pain and distress, a constant rate infusion of detomidine (0.22 μg/kg IV followed by 0.1 μg/kg/min IV) or lidocaine (1.3 mg/kg IV followed by 0.05 mg/kg/min IV) or butorphanol (13 μg/kg/h) can make the difference between adequate time for recovery and euthanasia.

Dantrolene (2–4 mg/kg orally) repeated in intervals of 4 to 6 hours can be of value with severe rhabdomyolysis because it decreases the release of calcium from the sarcoplasmic reticulum, which provokes muscle contractures and necrosis.[46] Caution is advised when administering dantrolene to horses with concomitant PSSM1 and HYPP because it can increase serum potassium concentrations and precipitate an episode of HYPP.[47]

CHRONIC MANAGEMENT
Exercise

Prolonged rest should be avoided because serum CK activity and clinical signs of PSSM1 are more severe in horses without access to turnout.[43,48] If pastures are the available turnout areas, a grazing muzzle may be needed to reduce sugar intake when the grass is lush. Important principles to follow when starting exercise programs in horses with PSSM1 include (1) 2 weeks allowed for dietary adaptations before commencing exercise, (2) ensuring the program is gradually introduced and consistently performed, (3) regulating both the duration and the intensity of exercise, and (4) minimizing days without some form of exercise. Successive daily addition of 2-minute intervals of walk and trot in a round pen or on a lunge line beginning with only 4 minutes of exercise and working up to 30 minutes after 3 weeks is often recommended.[35] If horses had minor increases in 4 hours postexercise CK activity with the 15-minute exercise test, 15 minutes of exercise is a reasonable starting point. Advancing the horse too quickly often results in an episode of rhabdomyolysis and repeated frustration for the owner.[35] Work can usually begin under saddle after 3 weeks of ground work and can gradually be increased by adding 2-minute intervals of lope or canter to the initial relaxed warm-up period at a walk and trot. Unless a horse shows an episode of overt rhabdomyolysis during the initial 4 weeks of exercise, reevaluating serum CK activity is not helpful for the first month because serum CK activity can be increased but exercise needs to continue regardless. It is common to have subclinical increases in CK activity when exercise is reintroduced, and a return to normal levels often requires 4 to 6 weeks of gradual exercise.[49]

Diet

Horses with PSSM1 should be fed hay with less than 12% NSC in order to prevent an increase in serum insulin concentration, which stimulates the already overactive enzyme glycogen synthase.[50] The degree to which the NSC content of hay should be restricted to less than 12% depends on the caloric requirements of the horse.

Feeding a lower-NSC hay provides room to add additional fat to the diet of easy keepers without exceeding the daily caloric requirement. Some horses with PSSM1 do well on a low-NSC diet alone consisting of forage and a ration balancer that provides additional protein, vitamins, and minerals. Horses with PSSM1 requiring a higher caloric intake usually show the most improvement when a low-NSC diet is supplemented with at least 13% of daily digestible energy as fat.[49,51]

Fat can be added to the diet in the form of oils or solid fat, or a low starch (<15%) combined with high fat (>10% by weight) concentrate.[49,51,52] Long-chain fats found in corn oil and rice bran have been shown to decrease postexercise serum CK activity in horses with PSSM1 in controlled diet trials, whereas odd-chain fat (C7) is detrimental.[49,52,53] Whether there is any direct beneficial effect of providing energy in the form of omega-3 versus omega-6 fatty acids to horses with PSSM1 has yet to be determined. Vitamin E (1000–5000 U/d) should be fed to horses receiving high-oil diets because of the potential additional oxidant stress of fats.

In overweight horses with PSSM1, caloric intake can be reduced by using a grazing muzzle during turnout, feeding hay with a low NSC content at 1% to 1.5% of body weight, providing a low-calorie ration balancer, gradually introducing daily exercise, and fasting for 6 hours before exercise to increase plasma free fatty acids.[35] Fat can then be added to the diet if needed when a horse has achieved a normal body weight.

Prognosis

PSSM1 has a wide variety of presentations from asymptomatic to debilitating. Horses with the genetic mutation have an underlying predilection for muscle soreness.[3,32,35] With adherence to both diet and exercise recommendations, at least 70% of horses show notable improvement in clinical signs and many return to acceptable levels of performance.[30] Homozygous P/P horses have more severe clinical signs, as do horses with both the *GYS1* and *RYR1* mutations.[33,54] Because PSSM1 is a dominant trait, breeding a P/N horse to an N/N horse results in a 50% chance of producing a P/N foal, whereas breeding a P/P horse to an N/N horse results in a 100% chance of producing a P/N horse.

MALIGNANT HYPERTHERMIA
Mutation

In horses, malignant hyperthermia (MH) is caused by a mutation in exon 46 of the ryanodine receptor (*RYR1*), which causes an arginine to glycine (R2454 G) amino acid substitution in the skeletal muscle calcium release channel (ryanodine receptor) (see **Fig. 1**).[55,56] The disorder is autosomal dominant. Homozygosity seems to be lethal because no homozygous adults have been reported out of 24,000 horses tested (personal communication, R. Bellone, Veterinary Genetics Laboratory, University of California, Davis). The common designation for genotypes is: heterozygous affected, M/N; normal unaffected, N/N.

Prevalence

MH is rare, with less than 1% of 24,000 genetic tests for MH in quarter horses and paint horses being M/N (personal communication, R Bellone, Veterinary Genetics Laboratory, University of California, Davis, 2019). Halter and pleasure horse lines have the highest prevalence.[55]

Breed Standards

Testing of breeding stallions for MH is required by the AQHA and APHA breed associations, with the results recorded on the horse's registration papers. Some Appaloosa registries also require genetic testing.

Clinical Signs

Rhabdomyolysis may be induced by exercise and anesthesia but can be extremely intermittent.[55–57] Following exercise, horses intermittently develop signs of exertional rhabdomyolysis with the unusual feature of increased body temperature during episodes.[55] Some MH-affected horses have died suddenly after an episode of exertional rhabdomyolysis. Horses can possess both the *RYR1* mutation and the *GYS1* mutation for PSSM1.[54] Double *RYR1*, *GYS1* mutation–positive horses have more severe episodes of exertional rhabdomyolysis, higher serum CK activity after exercise, and a poorer response to the diet and exercise regimes recommended for PSSM1.[58]

During anesthesia, clinical signs of hyperthermia (41°C or 105°F), hypercapnea (partial pressure of carbon dioxide, 274 mm Hg), and acidosis (pH of 6.7) have been reported in horses with MH.[57] In 2 horses masked down with halothane in an experimental protocol, clinical signs occurred approximately 60 minutes after anesthesia began, death occurred from cardiopulmonary arrest, and profound rigor mortis was almost immediate.[56] Hematologic changes measured 2 minutes after death included hemoconcentration, hyperkalemia, hypercalcemia, hyperphosphatemia, hyperglycemia, and increased creatinine level. Serum CK activity was mildly increased at 843 U/L and myoglobin level was 10 times higher than the reference range in this horse.

Pathophysiology

A missense mutation in the *RYR1* gene decreases the activation and increases the deactivation threshold of the ryanodine receptor (calcium release channel) (see **Fig. 1**).[56] When triggered, the R2454G ryanodine receptor remains open, causing a drastic efflux of calcium from the sarcoplasmic reticulum and inducing a persistent muscle contracture.[56,57] The process of reuptake of myoplasmic calcium into the sarcoplasmic reticulum consumes large amounts of oxygen and ATP and generates carbon dioxide and excessive heat.[59] Myofibers are damaged by the depletion of ATP and possibly the high temperatures.

Diagnosis

A diagnosis of MH in quarter horse–related breeds is established by identifying the C to G base substitution in exon 46 of the *RYR1* gene, which causes an R2454G substitution in the ryanodine receptor.[55] Genetic testing is recommended in quarter horse and paint horses that have a severe or difficult-to-manage form of rhabdomyolysis and in horses of these breeds with a family history of postanesthetic complications.

Muscle biopsy is not particularly useful for diagnosing MH because samples often lack any histopathologic changes. Biopsies can contain mild myopathic changes, including increased variation in fiber sizes, centrally located nuclei, fiber necrosis, glycogen depletion, and ringbinden fibers.[55]

Treatment

Dantrolene binds to RYR1 and inhibits calcium release.[46] If horses with the *RYR1* mutation develop rhabdomyolysis, treatment with 4 mg/kg of dantrolene orally every 6 hours is advised until serum CK activity begins to decline. Caution should be used with repeated high doses because dantrolene at higher doses can cause muscle weakness.[60] There is no cost-effective means to deliver dantrolene to horses intravenously once an episode has begun under general anesthesia. Other means to address hyperthermia and acidosis include external application of alcohol, fans, chilled IV fluids with sodium bicarbonate, and mechanical ventilation. However, once a fulminant episode is underway under anesthesia, it is difficult to prevent cardiac arrest.

Prevention

Exertional rhabdomyolysis in horses with the *RYR1* mutation is so intermittent that it is hard to justify premedication with dantrolene before each exercise session.[55] The best means to try to prevent an episode of MH under anesthesia in horses with the *RYR1* mutation is pretreatment with oral dantrolene (4 mg/kg) 30 to 60 minutes before anesthesia. Because MH is a dominant trait, breeding an M/N horse to a normal horse results in a 50% chance of producing a foal heterozygous for MH.

MYOSIN HEAVY CHAIN MYOPATHIES

Myosin heavy chain myopathy (MYHM) is a new term that is used to describe 2 muscle diseases termed immune-mediated myositis and nonexertional rhabdomyolysis, which are now known to be caused by the same mutation.[58,61] The clinical presentation of MYHM can be either severe rhabdomyolysis or rapid muscle atrophy but it also can be sequential with muscle atrophy following rhabdomyolysis.

Mutation

MYHM is caused by a missense mutation in the myosin heavy chain 1 gene (*MYH1*) that results in a glutamic acid for glycine substitution in the myosin type 2X heavy chain.[61] This myosin heavy chain is present in the fastest contracting muscle fibers, type 2X (previous designation type 2B) (see **Fig. 1**). The common designation for genotypes is: heterozygous affected, My/N; homozygous affected, My/My; and normal unaffected, N/N. MYHM has an autosomal codominant mode of inheritance with variable penetrance. My/My homozygotes usually have more severe clinical signs and a recurrent presentation compared with heterozygotes.[58,61]

Prevalence

MYHM occurs in quarter horses, paint horses, Appaloosas, and related breeds.[62] The prevalence of the *MYH1* mutation in the general quarter horse population is estimated to be 7% (see **Table 1**). Prevalence has been evaluated in top quarter horse breeding stallions. The highest *MYH1* mutation prevalence was found in reining (24%), working cow (17%), and halter (16%) horse stallions (see **Table 1**).[62] To date, the mutation has not been observed in barrel and racing quarter horse stallions. The specific percentage of horses with the *MYH1* mutation that develop disease is not known at this time.

Breed Standards

The addition of MYHM to the quarter horse breed panel test has been proposed but not yet enacted.

CLINICAL SIGNS
Nonexertional Rhabdomyolysis

MYHM rhabdomyolysis is not induced by exercise and presents as muscle pain, stiffness, and potentially recumbency, frequently affecting young horses.[58] In some cases, horses have a concurrent *Streptococcus equi equi* infection. Episodes of stiffness, firm muscles, marked pain, weakness, and recumbency are often severe. Myoglobinuria is common with serum CK and aspartate transaminase (AST) activities often greater than 100,000 U/L.[58] Horses can recover from rhabdomyolysis with treatment, but 35% subsequently develop acute muscle atrophy typical of immune-mediated myositis.[58] The *MYH1* mutation is not associated with exertional rhabdomyolysis.[58]

Immune-Mediated Myositis

Immune-mediated myositis usually occurs in horses less than or equal to 8 years of age or greater than or equal to 17 years of age and is characterized by rapid symmetric atrophy of lumbar and gluteal muscles (**Fig. 7**).[63] The semimembranosus and semitendinosus muscles are relatively unaffected. The loss of 40% of muscle mass can occur within 48 hours and persist for months.[63] Triggering factors are reported in 39% of cases and include a history of being recently exposed to infectious diseases such as *S equi equi* or *Streptococcus zooepidemicus*; a respiratory virus; or vaccination with influenza, equine herpes virus 4, or *S equi equi*.[63,64] Muscle mass usually recovers gradually over months but can be hastened by corticosteroid treatment (see **Fig. 7**).[63,64] Horses homozygous for MYHM (My/My) have more severe and recurrent atrophy that does not always fully recovery.

Hematologic abnormalities associated with MYHM, such as a neutrophilia and increased fibrinogen level, are a result of a concurrent infectious process.[63–65] During the acute phase of muscle atrophy, serum CK and AST activities are moderately to markedly increased, but, during the later phase of chronic atrophy, serum CK and AST activities can be normal.

Systemic Calcinosis

A rare fatal syndrome of systemic dystrophic calcification called systemic calcinosis or calciphylaxis can occur in horses in association with clinical signs of immune-mediated myositis.[66,67] An early indicator of systemic calcinosis is the presence of ventral edema. Additional signs include malaise, mild fever, stiffness, muscle atrophy, and diverse organ failure (respiratory distress, colic, laminitis).[66] Horses with systemic calcinosis have characteristic mild leukocytosis, hyperfibrinogenemia, and hyperphosphatemia, with a product of total calcium level (mg/dL) multiplied by phosphorus level greater than 65 mg/dL (1 mg/dL of calcium = 0.25 mmol/L; 1 mg/dL of phosphorus = 3.1 mmol/L).

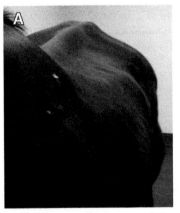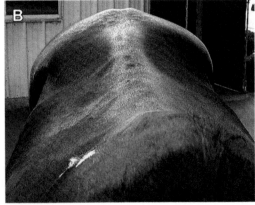

Fig. 7. (*A*) Rapid symmetric atrophy of the epaxial and gluteal muscles of a quarter horse with the *MYH1* mutation. (*B*) The same horse following treatment with corticosteroids for 1 month. Note the return of skeletal muscle mass. (*Courtesy of* Dr. Bonnie Rush.)

PATHOPHYSIOLOGY

Nonexertional Rhabdomyolysis

The *MYH1* mutation is located in the globular head of myosin near the ATP-binding pocket and it seems to affect the activity of the myosin ATPase enzyme of type 2X muscle fibers.[61] In 60% of horses, homozygous for the *MYH1* mutation myosin ATPase staining failed to clearly distinguish 2A and 2X, even though the 2A and 2X fibers were identified by immunofluorescent antibody staining.[58] The exact reason rhabdomyolysis develops is not known, but a role for abnormal actin/myosin interaction is postulated in a fashion similar to what occurs during an episode of hypercontraction during MH.[58] Lack of lymphocytic infiltrates in many muscle samples of horses with MYHM suggests that either the cell-mediated immune reaction in skeletal muscle was not captured in the muscles sampled or that an immune-mediated mechanism is not entirely responsible for rhabdomyolysis (**Fig. 8**A, B).[58]

Immune-Mediated Myositis

There seems to be a link between exposure to certain irritating vaccines or infectious agents and an immune-mediated response.[63,64,68] The innate immune response is suggested to be activated by release of the mutant form of myosin heavy chain from myofibers following muscle damage (trauma, vaccination). The loss of hydrogen bonds with the *MYH1* mutation is also postulated to lead to conformational changes in myosin that activate Toll-like receptors (TLRs) and autoimmunity.[61] The best-characterized link between myosin, inflammation, and muscle disease is immune-mediated myocarditis.[69] Fragments of cardiac myosin have been shown to activate TLR2, which strongly drives reactivity to self and subsequently determines the type of adaptive immune response (ie, T-helper [Th] 1, Th2) that occurs. Synergy between the activated innate immune response and the adaptive response of pathogenic T-cell epitopes seems to be important in the generation of chronic inflammation.[69] Similar to human myocarditis, the adaptive immune response could be triggered in immune-mediated myositis horses by shared epitopes between bacteria such as the M protein of *Streptococcus* sp and myosin.[61]

Systemic Calcinosis

Synergistic effects of cytokines released during inflammation, such as tumor necrosis factor-alpha and interleukin-6, on activation of the receptor activator of nuclear factor kappa B ligand (RANKL) have been reported that lead to enhanced bone resorption.[70] RANKL/RANK signaling regulates the formation of multinucleated osteoclasts from their precursors, as well as their activation and survival in normal bone remodeling. The combined impact of activation of RANKL is to increase resorption of bone, which may lead to hyperphosphatemia. In turn, hyperphosphatemia can induce dystrophic calcification through passive calcium phosphate deposition from phosphate supersaturation in the blood, an active process promoting the conversion of smooth muscle cells to osteogenic cell types, directly increasing parathyroid hormone secretion and transcription, and interference with renal production of 1,25-dihydroxyvitamin D levels.[66]

Diagnosis

MYHM is diagnosed by identifying the T to C substitution in *MYH1*, which produces an E321G amino acid change in the type 2X muscle fiber myosin heavy chain.[61]

Muscle biopsy samples from horses with nonexertional rhabdomyolysis are often normal, 30% show marked glycogen depletion, and less than 18% of muscle samples contain lymphocytic infiltrates (see **Fig. 8**A, B).[58] In contrast, during the acute phase of

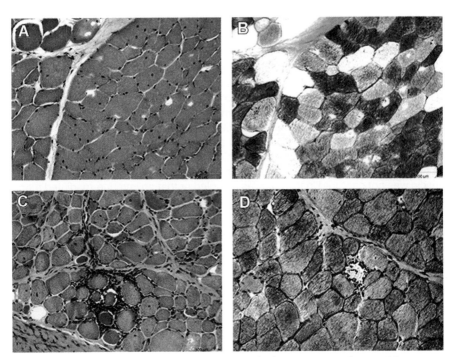

Fig. 8. (*A*) Cross section of semimembranosus muscle from a quarter horse with nonexertional rhabdomyolysis caused by a mutation in *MYH1*. Note the lack of inflammatory infiltrates (hematoxylin-eosin [HE], original magnification ×20). (*B*) PAS stain of the same muscle showing complete glycogen depletion in select muscle fibers, likely caused by increased glycolysis induced by hypercontracting myofibers (PAS, original magnification ×20). (*C*) Cross section of gluteal muscle from a horse with immune-mediated myositis caused by a mutation in *MYH1*. Note the presence of numerous lymphocytes surrounding and invading healthy myofibers caused by an immune reaction against myosin heavy chain in type 2X muscle fibers (*arrow*) (HE, original magnification ×20). (*D*) The same muscle showing normal background glycogen staining with minor glycogen depletion occurring only in the muscle fiber with lymphocytic infiltrates (PAS, original magnification ×20).

immune-mediated myositis, gluteal and epaxial muscles of horses have lymphocytic infiltrates in myofibers and surrounding small blood vessels without glycogen depletion (**Fig. 8**C, D).[58,61,64,68] Additional histopathologic findings in muscle samples from horses with systemic calcinosis include multinucleated giant cells and dystrophic calcification of muscle fibers.[66]

MANAGEMENT
Nonexertional Rhabdomyolysis

Acute management of nonexertional rhabdomyolysis is similar to that described for PSSM1 in this article. Dantrolene (2–4 mg/kg orally) repeated in hourly intervals until serum CK activity has declined significantly is recommended in order to prevent further muscle necrosis. Corticosteroids can be beneficial, but their use needs to be weighed against the severity of any ongoing infectious disease.[63,64] Antibiotic therapy for underlying infection can be combined with corticosteroids. A potential regime includes dexamethasone (0.05 mg/kg IV) for 3 days, followed by prednisolone (1 mg/kg by mouth) for 7 to 10 days tapered by 100 mg/wk over 1 month.[63]

Immune-Mediated Myositis

Antiinflammatory doses of corticosteroids for approximately 1 month (as described earlier), combined with antibiotics if infection is present, are often successful in halting muscle atrophy.

Prognosis

Horses with nonexertional rhabdomyolysis and immune-mediated myositis can make a full recovery. Muscle mass regenerates over weeks to months.[63] However, the *MYH1* mutation results in recurrent episodes in almost 50% of horses.[63] Horses homozygous My/My are more likely to have frequent episodes and more severe episodes with less return of normal muscle mass, which has led owners to contemplate euthanasia. Horses with systemic signs of calcinosis have a grave prognosis.[66]

Prevention

Minimizing exposure to infectious agents, using intranasal vaccines or intramuscular vaccines that cause the least muscle irritation, spreading out vaccines at 1-month intervals, and avoiding immunostimulants are advised.[63,64] Strangles vaccination is contraindicated in My/N and My/My horses. Breeding an My/N horse to an N/N horses has a 50% chance of producing a heterozygous affected offspring. Breeding an My/My horse to an N/N horse has a 100% chance of producing an MYHM susceptible horse. Breeding homozygous horses My/My or 2 My/N horses to each other should be discouraged.

MULTIPLE GENETIC MUTATIONS

The halter horse performance group of quarter horses has the highest prevalence of horses with multiple genetic mutations.[8] Out of 118 halter horses tested, 21 (18%) had 2 disease alleles (16 with HYPP/PSSM1, 2 with HYPP/GBED, 2 PSSM1/GBED), and 3 horses had 3 disease alleles (HYPP/PSSM/GBED).[8] Horses with HYPP and PSSM1 can have episodes of HYPP simultaneously with PSSM1-induced rhabdomyolysis resulting in horses being difficult to manage and prolonged recumbency. In addition, the *GYS1* mutation and the genetic mutation responsible for MH (*RYR1*) occur together in a small number of quarter horses and paint horses.[54] This condition results in particularly severe exertional rhabdomyolysis characterized by muscle pain; increased body temperature; a limited response to diet and exercise management; and, in some cases, sudden death.

SUMMARY

There are 5 single-gene mutations described to date that cause muscle disease in horses with the specific clinical signs depending on the pathway affected. HYPP causes muscle fasciculations without muscle fiber damage. GBED is fatal because of a lack of normal muscle glycogen synthesis, whereas muscle fiber degeneration and contracture occur with exercise in PSSM1 because of metabolic derangements related to excessive muscle glycogen synthesis. MH can have no evident clinical signs but occasionally causes fatal anesthetic hyperthermia or exertional rhabdomyolysis when the ryanodine receptor calcium release channel is triggered to delay closing. MYHM can cause severe muscle degeneration caused by an altered amino acid in myosin of fast-contracting type 2X muscle fibers or can cause atrophy triggered by an immune reaction to the altered myosin proteins. The likelihood that an animal with any of these mutations will show clinical signs depends on the mode of inheritance as well as environmental influences and interactions with other genes.

There are other muscle disorders in horses beyond those covered in this article that could potentially have a genetic basis. A variant in the highly conserved region of the chloride channel CLCN1 has been reported in a New Forest pony cross, and more information on this single case can be found in the published article.[71] Other myopathies with a potential inherited basis include type 2 PSSM,[35] myotonic dystrophy,[72,73] lipid storage myopathy,[74] centronuclear myopathy,[75] myofibrillar myopathy,[76,77] and recurrent exertional rhabdomyolysis.[78,79] A single-gene mutation has yet to be identified for these myopathies or the offered genetic tests have not been scientifically validated, as described earlier.

Selecting a genetic test for diagnostic purposes requires knowledge of clinical signs of disease as well as of the breeds that possess the genetic mutation. Variants in the genetic code occur commonly in horses and any of these can be offered as a commercial genetic test in an unregulated industry. Therefore, the onus is on veterinarians to ensure that there is adequate scientific validation for a genetic test before selecting it for use as a diagnostic test, prepurchase test, or consideration for breeding.

DISCLOSURE

Dr S Valberg has received Funding for research into genetic muscle diseases in horses was provided by The American Quarter Horse Association, the Morris Animal Foundation, the University of Minnesota Equine Center and the Mary Anne McPhail Endowment at Michigan State University.

REFERENCES

1. Petersen JL, Mickelson JR, Cothran EG, et al. Genetic diversity in the modern horse illustrated from genome-wide SNP data. PLoS One 2013;8:e54997.
2. McCue ME, Valberg SJ, Miller MB, et al. Glycogen synthase (GYS1) mutation causes a novel skeletal muscle glycogenosis. Genomics 2008;91:458–66.
3. Valberg SJ, Cardinet GH 3rd, Carlson GP, et al. Polysaccharide storage myopathy associated with recurrent exertional rhabdomyolysis in horses. Neuromuscul Disord 1992;2:351–9.
4. Rudolph JA, Spier SJ, Byrns G, et al. Periodic paralysis in quarter horses: a sodium channel mutation disseminated by selective breeding. Nat Genet 1992;2: 144–7.
5. Spier SJ, Carlson GP, Holliday TA, et al. Hyperkalemic periodic paralysis in horses. J Am Vet Med Assoc 1990;197:1009–17.
6. Rudolph JA, Spier SJ, Byrns G, et al. Linkage of hyperkalaemic periodic paralysis in quarter horses to the horse adult skeletal muscle sodium channel gene. Anim Genet 1992;23:241–50.
7. Carr EA, Spier SJ, Kortz GD, et al. Laryngeal and pharyngeal dysfunction in horses homozygous for hyperkalemic periodic paralysis. J Am Vet Med Assoc 1996; 209:798–803.
8. Tryon RC, Penedo MC, McCue ME, et al. Evaluation of allele frequencies of inherited disease genes in subgroups of American Quarter Horses. J Am Vet Med Assoc 2009;234:120–5.
9. Naylor JM. Selection of quarter horses affected with hyperkalemic periodic paralysis by show judges. J Am Vet Med Assoc 1994;204:926–8.

10. Finno CJ, Spier SJ, Valberg SJ. Equine diseases caused by known genetic mutations. Vet J 2009;179:336–47.

11. Naylor JM. Hyperkalemic periodic paralysis. Vet Clin North Am Equine Pract 1997;13:129–44.

12. Naylor JM. Equine hyperkalemic periodic paralysis: review and implications. Can Vet J 1994;35:279–85.

13. Robinson JA, Naylor JM, Crichlow EC. Use of electromyography for the diagnosis of equine hyperkalemic periodic paresis. Can J Vet Res 1990;54:495–500.

14. Zhou J, Spier SJ, Beech J, et al. Pathophysiology of sodium channelopathies: correlation of normal/mutant mRNA ratios with clinical phenotype in dominantly inherited periodic paralysis. Hum Mol Genet 1994;3:1599–603.

15. Reynolds JA, Potter GD, Greene LW. Genetic-diet interactions in the Hyperkalemic Periodic Paralysis syndrome in Quarter Horses fed varying amounts of potassium: III. The relationship between plasma potassium concentration and HYPP Symptoms. J Equine Vet Sci 1998;18:731–5.

16. Cannon SC, Hayward LJ, Beech J, et al. Sodium channel inactivation is impaired in equine hyperkalemic periodic paralysis. J Neurophysiol 1995;73:1892–9.

17. Reynolds AJ. Equine Hyperkalemic periodic paralysis (HYPP): overview & management strategies. Available at: https://www.admanimalnutrition.com/webcenter/content/conn/WCC1/uuid/dDocName%3AHYPP. Accessed September 15, 2019.

18. Valberg SJ, Ward TL, Rush B, et al. Glycogen branching enzyme deficiency in quarter horse foals. J Vet Intern Med 2001;15:572–80.

19. Render JA, Common RS, Kennedy FA, et al. Amylopectinosis in fetal and neonatal Quarter Horses. Vet Pathol 1999;36:157–60.

20. Ward TL, Valberg SJ, Adelson DL, et al. Glycogen branching enzyme (GBE1) mutation causing equine glycogen storage disease IV. Mamm Genome 2004;15: 570–7.

21. Wagner ML, Valberg SJ, Ames EG, et al. Allele frequency and likely impact of the glycogen branching enzyme deficiency gene in Quarter Horse and Paint Horse populations. J Vet Intern Med 2006;20:1207–11.

22. Sponseller BT, Valberg SJ, Ward TL, et al. Muscular weakness and recumbency in a Quarter Horse colt due to glycogen branching enzyme deficiency. Equine Vet Educ 2003;15:182–7.

23. Mickelson JR, Valberg SJ. The genetics of skeletal muscle disorders in horses. Annu Rev Anim Biosci 2015;3:197–217.

24. Baird JD, Valberg SJ, Anderson SM, et al. Presence of the glycogen synthase 1 (GYS1) mutation causing type 1 polysaccharide storage myopathy in continental European draught horse breeds. Vet Rec 2010;167:781–4.

25. McCue ME, Anderson SM, Valberg SJ, et al. Estimated prevalence of the type 1 polysaccharide storage myopathy mutation in selected North American and European breeds. Anim Genet 2010;41(Suppl 2):145–9.

26. Stanley RL, McCue ME, Valberg SJ, et al. A glycogen synthase 1 mutation associated with equine polysaccharide storage myopathy and exertional rhabdomyolysis occurs in a variety of UK breeds. Equine Vet J 2009;41:597–601.

27. Schwarz B, Ertl R, Zimmer S, et al. Estimated prevalence of the GYS-1 mutation in healthy Austrian Haflingers. Vet Rec 2011;169:583.

28. Herszberg B, McCue ME, Larcher T, et al. A GYS1 gene mutation is highly associated with polysaccharide storage myopathy in Cob Normand draught horses. Anim Genet 2009;40:94–6.

29. McKenzie EC, Eyrich LV, Payton ME, et al. Clinical, histopathological and metabolic responses following exercise in Arabian horses with a history of exertional rhabdomyolysis. Vet J 2016;216:196–201.

30. Firshman AM, Valberg SJ, Bender JB, et al. Epidemiologic characteristics and management of polysaccharide storage myopathy in Quarter Horses. Am J Vet Res 2003;64:1319–27.

31. Sprayberry KA, Madigan J, Lecouteur RA, et al. Renal failure, laminitis, and colitis following severe rhabdomyolysis in a draft horse-cross with polysaccharide storage myopathy. Can Vet J 1998;39:500–3.

32. Schroder U, Licka TF, Zsoldos R, et al. Effect of diet on haflinger horses with GYS1 mutation (polysaccharide storage myopathy type 1). J Equine Vet Sci 2015;35:598–605.

33. Naylor RJ, Livesey L, Schumacher J, et al. Allele copy number and underlying pathology are associated with subclinical severity in equine type 1 polysaccharide storage myopathy (PSSM1). PLoS One 2012;7:e42317.

34. Valentine BA, Habecker PL, Patterson JS, et al. Incidence of polysaccharide storage myopathy in draft horse-related breeds: a necropsy study of 37 horses and a mule. J Vet Diagn Invest 2001;13:63–8.

35. Valberg S. Muscling in on the cause of tying up. Proceedings of the 58th Annual Convention of the American Association of Equine Practitioners- AAEP - December 1-5, 2012. Anaheim, CA: American Assoc Equine Practitioners; 2012. p. 85–123.

36. Bloom BA, Valentine BA, Gleed RD, et al. Postanaesthetic recumbency in a Belgian filly with polysaccharide storage myopathy. Vet Rec 1999;144:73–5.

37. Valentine BA, Credille KM, Lavoie JP, et al. Severe polysaccharide storage myopathy in Belgian and Percheron draught horses. Equine Vet J 1997;29:220–5.

38. Naylor RJ, Luis-Fuentes V, Livesey L, et al. Evaluation of cardiac phenotype in horses with type 1 polysaccharide storage myopathy. J Vet Intern Med 2012; 26:1464–9.

39. Annandale EJ, Valberg SJ, Mickelson JR, et al. Insulin sensitivity and skeletal muscle glucose transport in horses with equine polysaccharide storage myopathy. Neuromuscul Disord 2004;14:666–74.

40. Quiroz-Rothe E, Novales M, Aguilera-Tejero E, et al. Polysaccharide storage myopathy in the M. longissimus lumborum of showjumpers and dressage horses with back pain. Equine Vet J 2002;34:171–6.

41. Valberg SJ, Mickelson JR, Gallant EM, et al. Exertional rhabdomyolysis in quarter horses and thoroughbreds: one syndrome, multiple aetiologies. Equine Vet J Suppl 1999;533–8.

42. Maile CA, Hingst JR, Mahalingan KK, et al. A highly prevalent equine glycogen storage disease is explained by constitutive activation of a mutant glycogen synthase. Biochim Biophys Acta 2017;1861:3388–98.

43. De La Corte FD, Valberg SJ, MacLeay JM, et al. Developmental onset of polysaccharide storage myopathy in 4 Quarter Horse foals. J Vet Intern Med 2002;16: 581–7.

44. Valberg SJ, McCue ME, Mickelson JR. The interplay of genetics, exercise, and nutrition in polysaccharide storage myopathy. J Equine Vet Sci 2011;31:205–10.

45. Annandale EJ, Valberg SJ, Essen-Gustavsson B. Effects of submaximal exercise on adenine nucleotide concentrations in skeletal muscle fibers of horses with polysaccharide storage myopathy. Am J Vet Res 2005;66:839–45.

46. Fruen BR, Mickelson JR, Louis CF. Dantrolene inhibition of sarcoplasmic reticulum Ca2+ release by direct and specific action at skeletal muscle ryanodine receptors. J Biol Chem 1997;272:26965–71.

47. McKenzie EC, Di Concetto S, Payton ME, et al. Effect of dantrolene premedication on various cardiovascular and biochemical variables and the recovery in healthy isoflurane-anesthetized horses. Am J Vet Res 2015;76:293–301.

48. De la Corte FD, Valberg SJ. Treatment of polysaccharide storage myopathy. Compend Contin Educ Vet 2000;22:782.

49. Ribeiro WP, Valberg SJ, Pagan JD, et al. The effect of varying dietary starch and fat content on serum creatine kinase activity and substrate availability in equine polysaccharide storage myopathy. J Vet Intern Med 2004;18:887–94.

50. Borgia L, Valberg S, McCue M, et al. Glycaemic and insulinaemic responses to feeding hay with different non-structural carbohydrate content in control and polysaccharide storage myopathy-affected horses. J Anim Physiol Anim Nutr (Berl) 2011;95:798–807.

51. Valentine BA, Van Saun RJ, Thompson KN, et al. Role of dietary carbohydrate and fat in horses with equine polysaccharide storage myopathy. J Am Vet Med Assoc 2001;219:1537–44.

52. Borgia L, Valberg SJ, Mcue M, et al. The effect of odd and even chain dietary fat on serum creatine kinase activity in horses with polysaccharide storage myopathy. J Vet Intern Med 2007;21:619.

53. Borgia LA, Valberg SJ, McCue ME, et al. Effect of dietary fats with odd or even numbers of carbon atoms on metabolic response and muscle damage with exercise in Quarter Horse-type horses with type 1 polysaccharide storage myopathy. Am J Vet Res 2010;71:326–36.

54. McCue ME, Valberg SJ, Jackson M, et al. Polysaccharide storage myopathy phenotype in quarter horse-related breeds is modified by the presence of an RYR1 mutation. Neuromuscul Disord 2009;19:37–43.

55. Aleman M, Nieto JE, Magdesian KG. Malignant hyperthermia associated with ryanodine receptor 1 (C7360G) mutation in Quarter Horses. J Vet Intern Med 2009;23:329–34.

56. Aleman M, Riehl J, Aldridge BM, et al. Association of a mutation in the ryanodine receptor 1 gene with equine malignant hyperthermia. Muscle Nerve 2004;30:356–65.

57. Aleman M, Brosnan RJ, Williams DC, et al. Malignant hyperthermia in a horse anesthetized with halothane. J Vet Intern Med 2005;19:363–6.

58. Valberg SJ, Henry ML, Perumbakkam S, et al. An E321G MYH1 mutation is strongly associated with nonexertional rhabdomyolysis in Quarter Horses. J Vet Intern Med 2018;32(5):1718–25.

59. Mickelson JR, Louis CF. Malignant hyperthermia: excitation-contraction coupling, Ca2+ release channel, and cell Ca2+ regulation defects. Physiol Rev 1996;76:537–92.

60. Valverde A, Boyd CJ, Dyson DH, et al. Prophylactic use of dantrolene associated with prolonged postanesthetic recumbency in a horse. J Am Vet Med Assoc 1990;197:1051–3.

61. Finno CJ, Gianino G, Perumbakkam S, et al. A missense mutation in MYH1 is associated with susceptibility to immune-mediated myositis in Quarter Horses. Skelet Muscle 2018;8:7.

62. Gianino GM, Valberg SJ, Perumbakkam S, et al. Prevalence of the E321G MYH1 variant for immune-mediated myositis and nonexertional rhabdomyolysis in

performance subgroups of American Quarter Horses. J Vet Intern Med 2019;33: 897–901.

63. Lewis SS, Valberg SJ, Nielsen IL. Suspected immune-mediated myositis in horses. J Vet Intern Med 2007;21:495–503.

64. Hunyadi L, Sundman EA, Kass PH, et al. Clinical implications and hospital outcome of immune-mediated myositis in horses. J Vet Intern Med 2017;31: 170–5.

65. Aulchenko YS, Hoppenbrouwers IA, Ramagopalan SV, et al. Genetic variation in the KIF1B locus influences susceptibility to multiple sclerosis. Nat Genet 2008;40: 1402–3.

66. Tan JY, Valberg SJ, Sebastian MM, et al. Suspected systemic calcinosis and calciphylaxis in 5 horses. Can Vet J 2010;51:993–9.

67. Fales-Williams A, Sponseller B, Flaherty H. Idiopathic arterial medial calcification of the thoracic arteries in an adult horse. J Vet Diagn Invest 2008;20:692–7.

68. Durward-Akhurst SA, Finno CJ, Barnes N, et al. Major histocompatibility Complex I and II expression and lymphocytic subtypes in muscle of horses with immune-mediated myositis. J Vet Intern Med 2016;30:1313–21.

69. Zhang P, Cox CJ, Alvarez KM, et al. Cutting edge: cardiac myosin activates innate immune responses through TLRs. J Immunol 2009;183:27–31.

70. Lam J, Takeshita S, Barker JE, et al. TNF-alpha induces osteoclastogenesis by direct stimulation of macrophages exposed to permissive levels of RANK ligand. J Clin Invest 2000;106:1481–8.

71. Montagna P, Liguori R, Monari L, et al. Equine muscular dystrophy with myotonia. Clin Neurophysiol 2001;112:294–9.

72. Hegreberg GA, Reed SM. Skeletal muscle changes associated with equine myotonic dystrophy. Acta Neuropathol 1990;80:426–31.

73. Reed SM, Hegreberg GA, Bayly WM, et al. Progressive myotonia in foals resembling human dystrophia myotonica. Muscle Nerve 1988;11:291–6.

74. Pinn TL, Divers TJ, Southard T, et al. Persistent hypoglycemia associated with lipid storage myopathy in a paint foal. J Vet Intern Med 2018;32:1442–6.

75. Polle F, Andrews FM, Gillon T, et al. Suspected congenital centronuclear myopathy in an Arabian-cross foal. J Vet Intern Med 2014;28:1886–91.

76. Valberg SJ, McKenzie EC, Eyrich LV, et al. Suspected myofibrillar myopathy in Arabian horses with a history of exertional rhabdomyolysis. Equine Vet J 2016; 48:548–56.

77. Valberg SJ, Nicholson AM, Lewis SS, et al. Clinical and histopathological features of myofibrillar myopathy in Warmblood horses. Equine Vet J 2017;49(6):739–45.

78. MacLeay JM, Valberg SJ, Sorum SA, et al. Heritability of recurrent exertional rhabdomyolysis in Thoroughbred racehorses. Am J Vet Res 1999;60:250–6.

79. Norton EM, Mickelson JR, Binns MM, et al. Heritability of recurrent exertional rhabdomyolysis in standardbred and thoroughbred racehorses derived from SNP genotyping data. J Hered 2016;107:537–43.

Genetics and Signaling Pathways of Laminitis

Hannah Galantino-Homer, VMD, PhD[a], Samantha A. Brooks, PhD[b],*

KEYWORDS

- Horse • Hoof equine • Founder • Proteostasis • Autoinflammatory disease
- Fibrosis

KEY POINTS

- Gene expression studies have examined many different induction models of the disease and a few sets of naturally occurring cases.
- Most mechanisms to initiate laminitis, whether experimental or naturally occurring, involve some aspects of cell stress, epidermal activation, and a sterile autoinflammatory cycle.
- Laminitis resembles many other types of organ failure, in which the wound healing response and fibrosis disrupt the ability to regenerate tissue function. In this case, the delicate structure of the secondary epidermal lamellae are affected.
- Genomics tools offer the potential to improve our understanding of the laminitis disease process.

INTRODUCTION

Laminitis, a common and crippling foot disease of equids and other ungulates, is associated with microanatomical and molecular lesions of the epidermal and dermal lamellae that can progress to structural failure of the suspensory apparatus of the distal phalanx (SADP) and dysplastic changes in the hoof and underlying tissues.[1–4] The 3 major types of laminitis are endocrinopathic laminitis (EL), sepsis-associated laminitis (SL), and laminitis in the limb contralateral to a reduced weight-bearing orthopedic condition, also called supporting limb laminitis (SLL). EL is the most common form of the disease,[5,6] occurring in horses and ponies with obesity, equine metabolic syndrome (EMS), and pituitary pars intermedia dysfunction, often in association with grazing pasture rich in nonstructural carbohydrate.[7–9] The major risk factor in these cases appears to be hyperinsulinemia (HI)[10] and the prolonged euglycemic-HI clamp is an established acute experimental model for EL.[11,12] The experimental models for SL include the oligofructose (OF), and carbohydrate overload (CHO), models and

[a] Department of Clinical Studies, New Bolton Center, School of Veterinary Medicine, University of Pennsylvania, Kennett Square, PA, USA; [b] Department of Animal Sciences, UF Genetics Institute, University of Florida, Gainesville, FL, USA
* Corresponding author.
E-mail address: samantha.brooks@ufl.edu

Vet Clin Equine 36 (2020) 379–394
https://doi.org/10.1016/j.cveq.2020.04.001
0749-0739/20/© 2020 Elsevier Inc. All rights reserved.
vetequine.theclinics.com

the black walnut extract (BWE) models.[13–15] An experimental model for SLL was recently developed by Gardner and colleagues.[16] The relevance of these models to naturally occurring disease is difficult to determine because of the relative lack of studies of these cases and differences in timing and disease stage at time of euthanasia.

Laminitis is an extremely complex disease that includes pathologies of multiple tissues of the foot and can more accurately be thought of as a disease of organ dysfunction or failure. Failure of the SADP is a primary and characteristic feature, with variable primary and secondary epidermal, dermal, vascular, and bone pathology at both acute and chronic stages.[4,17] Epidermal pathologies are grossly evident as the lamellar wedge, composed of the abnormal hyperplastic and acanthotic epidermal tissue that forms between the hoof wall and laminitic dermal-epidermal lamellar interface[3] and histologically as epidermal dysplasia, metaplasia, loss of cell-cell and cell-matrix adhesion, hyperplasia, apoptosis, and necrosis.[4] Dermal pathology is apparent histologically as dermal activation (enlarged myofibroblast nuclei), dermal fibrosis, and loss of dermal integrity (gaps and clefts) and biochemically as degradation of epithelial basement membrane and dermal connective tissues through matrix metalloproteinase (MMP)activity, probably secondary to inflammatory leukocyte infiltration and apparently a late event in HI-induced experimental laminitis.[18,19] With few exceptions, most of our knowledge of the molecular events of laminitis pathogenesis are derived from studies involving predetermined investigative targets based on disease processes in other tissues and species.

Among all equine diseases, laminitis presents the perfect storm of diverse etiologies, rapid and/or insidious progression, treatment resistance (lack of targeted treatment), and often irreversible damage. Genomics offers a suite of tools aimed at gene expression and trait mapping, as well as functional annotation key for enabling other approaches like proteomics and immunohistochemistry.[20] This article reviews the contributions of those studies to our understanding of signaling processes involved in laminitis pathogenesis and how broader discovery-mode approaches have been, or can be, applied to laminitis pathogenesis as a necessary basis for the development of improved laminitis diagnosis, treatment, and prevention.

Altered Proteostasis

Maintenance of the normal proteome, the set of expressed proteins in a cell or tissue necessary for its physical phenotype and physiologic function, involves cellular processes encompassing the initial synthesis of nascent proteins; the appropriate folding, transport, and secretion of mature proteins; and the degradation (and recycling) of damaged and redundant proteins within the cell. Lamellar proteins of particular interest for the maintenance of the SADP, due to their importance in epithelial and dermal tissue integrity, include cytoskeletal, adhesion complex, and extracellular matrix proteins. Termed proteostasis, this process is highly relevant to aging and disease. The following are cellular processes that maintain proteostasis and are associated with disease when they fail:

1. Endoplasmic reticulum (ER) stress-induced unfolded protein response (UPR)
2. The ubiquitin-proteasome system (UPS)
3. Autophagy

These functions are influenced by nutrient status, growth hormone, insulin/insulin-like growth factor (IGF)-1 and mammalian target of rapamycin (mTOR) (all pro-growth) signaling pathways, as well as inflammation. The footprint of these processes can be detected in the gene expression of lamellar tissues in crisis.

The most common trigger for naturally occurring laminitis is endocrinopathies that cause hyperinsulinemia, primarily EMS, but also pituitary pars intermedia dysfunction.[5,9,21] Administration of exogenous insulin, sufficient to induce acute hyperinsulinemia, will induce laminitis in experimental settings, suggesting that insulin itself can initiate laminitis pathogenesis.[11,12] Hyperinsulinemia is now well established as the primary risk factor for naturally occurring EL.[17,22–24] Anabolic signaling mechanisms and pro-growth pathways are likely triggered by hyperinsulinemia.[25] Yet, the underlying molecular connections between insulin-driven growth signaling and resulting lamellar pathologies are poorly understood.

Exposure to a diet high in nonstructural carbohydrates will drive up circulating insulin concentrations, especially in obese individuals, and concurrently increase the number of insulin receptor–bearing endothelial cells in the lamellae, but not in lamellae themselves.[8,9] Epithelial proliferation is one likely consequence of IGF-1R activation,[26] yet destabilization by excessive expansion of epithelium does not explain loss of integrity and lamellar damage observed in EL. In fact, the epidermal lamellae do not express the insulin receptor,[27,28] leading to the assumption that the insulin effect is mediated through IGF-1R. However, one study shows that the lamellar IGF-1R have a lower affinity for insulin and the insulin effect might therefore be indirect (eg, vascular effect) or through a direct effect on lamellar epidermal cells mediated through another receptor.[27] The lesions that contribute to failure of the SADP might be better explained by epidermal stress and activation in response to excessive anabolic stimulation or in response to damage and stress mediators originating from insulin-responsive tissues.[29,30]

The signaling pathway responsible for transmitting these anabolic triggers is not obvious, as there is significant overlap among downstream messengers for insulin resistance (IR), IGF-1R, and other growth factor and inflammatory mediators. The mitogen-activated protein kinase (*MAPK*) pathway seems a likely candidate, supported by increased activated ERK 1/2 and stress-activated protein kinase/Jun amino-terminal kinase (SAPK/JNK) following experimental induction of laminitis by the CHO model.[31] Yet this same study observed activation of this pathway to similar levels in the affected and unaffected (cryoprotected) limbs from the same horse following oligofructose induction of laminitis.

Evidence from the diet-induced and exogenously administered hyperinsulinemic HI experimental models[25] and the oligofructose overdose OF model[32] implicate *mTORC*. Cell stress, regardless of the initiator, activates interconnected stress response pathways such as ER stress/UPR, autophagy (*mTORC1* suppresses autophagy), apoptosis, and the antioxidant response.[33] Given the evidence supporting a role for *mTORC1* and *IGF-1R* in both experimental and naturally occurring laminitis, finding the remaining molecular connections between these 2 signaling pathways will be important to understand the earliest triggers of lamellar degradation.

The circulation of nutrients to the foot is of paramount importance to healthy function of the tissues within. Remarkably, even while at rest, the glucose consumption of the 4 hooves of the horse surpasses that of the head, and is presumably required to maintain the cytoskeletal, adhesion complex, and extracellular matrix proteins necessary for the integrity of a tissue subjected to high mechanical stress.[34] In the case of SLL, decreased cyclic loading negatively impacts lamellar capillary perfusion.[35] Mimicking this loss of perfusion by application of a shoe that reduces normal weight-bearing and cyclic loading decreases nutrient delivery to the contralateral foot.[16] Deprivation of glucose alone triggered the loss of lamellar adhesion in an in vitro cultured lamellar explant study.[36] Finally, glucose uptake in lamellae is likely mediated by the insulin-independent *GLUT1*, rather than the insulin-dependent

GLUT4, as the latter is undetectable in this tissue by quantitative polymerase chain reaction (qPCR).[37] Cellular starvation is a well-documented cause of ER stress and the UPR, which in turn triggers upregulation of ubiquitin/proteasome and autophagy pathways intended to recycle vital nutrients from organelles and proteins or, if it is prolonged and exceeds these compensatory responses, leads to apoptosis.[38]

Alternately, chronic overstimulation of anabolic pathways in lamellar tissue, as in EL, likely results in ER stress and activation of the UPR, contributing to the resulting tissue pathology, as it does in human metabolic diseases.[39] ER stress is triggered when the synthesis of new membrane and/or secreted proteins overwhelms the protein folding capacity within the ER lumen. Misfolded proteins are detected by 3 sensors in the ER membrane, which initiate the UPR signaling that results in increased synthesis of ER chaperones and other proteins required for protein folding in the ER and other mechanisms to restore proteostasis. Prolonged ER stress and UPR can lead to apoptosis if cell homeostasis is not restored.[38,40–42] It is also quite possible that the cell's attempts to restore proteostasis by decreasing protein synthesis and autophagic recycling weaken the mechanical integrity of lamellar tissue if these processes result in the loss of keratin cytoskeleton and adhesion complex proteins.

Gene expression changes support the involvement of ER stress/UPR in laminitis pathogenesis as following experimental induction by administration of BWE, key ER stress/UPR markers *XBP1*, *BiP*, and *Grp94* are all upregulated.[43] *Grp94* is also increased specifically within laminar basal epithelial cells postinduction of laminitis by CHO.[44] These gene expression changes are mirrored in the protein content of tissues from naturally occurring cases of laminitis. Cassimeris and colleagues[45] observed increased expression of the same 3 markers of ER stress (XBP1s, BiP/Grp78, and Grp94) in affected front limbs compared with either unaffected hind limbs from the same horses or feet from age-matched nonlaminitic controls. ER stress/UPR does not function independently of the larger signaling circuit that contributes to laminitis pathogenesis. As illustrated in **Fig. 1**, the UPR counters the protein anabolic signaling mediated by the mTORC1 pathway and ER stress can activate mTORC1 signaling via an ATF6α/PI3K/AKT pathway.[46] Crosstalk between these pathways maintains proteostasis but results in disease when they cannot restore this balance. Both mTORC1 and ER stress/UPR are affected by anabolic signaling through IGF-1R and other growth factor pathways and both can contribute to inflammation.[47,48] Crosstalk between mTORC1 and ER stress/UPR signaling also determines whether a cell undergoes the cannibalistic process of autophagy and activation of ER-associated protein degradation (ERAD)/UPS to replenish nutrients and survive or undergoes the programmed cell death process of apoptosis.[33] All of these processes could contribute to laminitis pathogenesis. Increased numbers of apoptotic cells or alive but compromised lamellar epidermal cells with decreased cytoskeletal and adhesion protein complexes can both reduce epithelial integrity.

In the epidermal lamellae, as in other epidermal-derived epithelia, keratin filaments interact with desmosomes and hemidesmosomes to integrate and provide mechanical stability to epithelial tissues.[49] Mouse keratin knockout studies have demonstrated that keratins are crucial for the maintenance of epithelial and cellular integrity in response to mechanical stress.[50] Equine hoof lamellae express novel keratin isoforms that may be particularly suited to this mechanical function.[51] Histopathological studies of lamellar tissue associates changes in lamellar cell size and shape with laminitis that would be the expected outcome of keratin degradation by autophagy and other cell stress responses during laminitis pathogenesis, although further study is needed to confirm this.[45,52,53] Disturbed proteostasis,

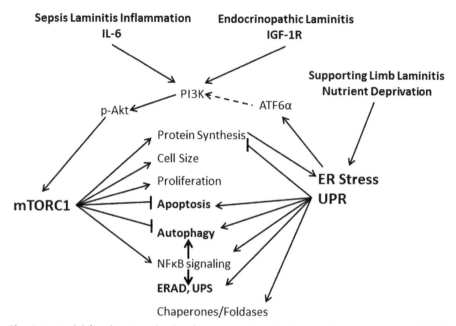

Fig. 1. A model for the central role of proteostasis in laminitis pathogenesis. The mTORC1 and ER stress/UPR pathways have opposing roles in the maintenance of proteostasis that could determine the function and survival of lamellar epidermal cells. Mechanisms that promote the degradation, recycling, and processing of excess misfolded proteins, the UPR, ERAD through the UPS, autophagy, and, ultimately, if these mechanisms chronically fail to restore proteostasis, apoptosis, are all activated by ER stress/UPR. In contrast, mTORC1 activates anabolic signals, protein synthesis, and cell growth and proliferation. Upregulation of protein synthesis by the mTORC1 pathway can exacerbate ER stress. ER stress/UPR can also activate mTORC1 through the ATF6α-PI3K-AKT pathway (p-Akt is the active, phosphorylated form of the Akt signaling factor). It has been proposed that mTORC1 signaling is activated in sepsis-associated laminitis via systemic IL-6 and activation of the PI3K-AKT pathway.[32] IGF-1R, potentially activated by the high insulin levels that are the primary risk factor for endocrinopathic laminitis, is also known to signal through this pathway.[25,109] We propose that supporting limb laminitis causes ER stress and activation of the UPR through the extrinsic effect on ER function in nutrient starvation due to poor lamellar perfusion. The UPR and mTORC1 pathways both contribute to nuclear factor (NF)-κB pathway activation, lipogenesis, and angiogenesis.[46] NF-κB signaling also upregulates ERAD and autophagy. The relative levels of these various pathways determine whether or not cells maintain proteostasis, including the cytoskeletal and adhesion complexes required for epithelial integrity, or undergo apoptosis. Arrows indicate stimulation and blunt-ended lines indicate inhibition.

particularly if it compromises the lamellar cytoskeletal, adhesion complex, and extracellular matrix structural proteins, weakens the SADP and lowers the threshold for tissue damage and loss of mechanical integrity.

Tissue Damage/Autoinflammatory Pathways

By the time laminitis has begun to damage tissue, the gene expression profile is profoundly dysregulated. The innate immune system turns from friend to foe, initiating autoinflammatory pathways that promote further destruction. Here, our best model is the body of work describing similar innate immune derailment in skin, causing release of antimicrobial peptides (AMPs), and effector molecules for cell migration, proliferation and differentiation, cytokine production, angiogenesis, and ultimately, wound healing.[54] Beneficial under most circumstances, within the inelastic capsule of the hoof, and under the feedback loop of inflammation causing injury that leads to more inflammation, these processes exacerbate disease.

Yet, equine lamellar keratinocytes, like skin keratinocytes from mice and humans, are not "innocent bystanders" to tissue injury and inflammation and are readily activated by stress stimuli to become inflammatory cells that produce large amounts of cytokines. These cytokines in turn amplify the original stimulus, driving keratinocytes to undergo functionally relevant changes in differentiation,.[29,44,55]

Epidermal activation in skin diseases and wounding causes keratinocytes to become inflammatory cells and to change their phenotype, shifting from epithelial to mesenchymal in morphology and adopting new expression patterns from keratin isoforms important for their mechanical function to the activated keratinocyte type II keratin (K) isoform, K17.[29] A hallmark of diverse (auto)-inflammatory skin diseases, the appearance of K17 expression correlates with epidermal hyperplasia and acanthosis in response to epidermal stress[30] and correlates with disease severity in human psoriasis.[56,57] Indeed, psoriasis is a surprisingly relevant model for the autoinflammatory feedback loop of laminitis. Sequence similarly between K17 peptide regions and streptococcal M6 protein could trigger a T-cell response once presented or released by damaged keratinocytes.[56] In turn, interleukin (IL)-22 and IL-17 from T cells upregulates K17 via the SOCS3/STAT3 pathway,[58] which is also activated in laminitic epidermal lamellae.[59]

Expression increases among numerous downstream targets of the inflammasome during both natural and experimentally induced laminitis. MMPs degrade proteins external to the cell and are important effectors of extracellular matrix dissolution.[60] Increased *MMP9* gene expression occurs in both the BWE and CHO experimental models of sepsis-related laminitis, as well as in clinical cases of the disease, and correlates with leukocyte infiltration.[61,62] Increased *MMP9* (and *MMP2*) enzymatic activity also occurs in naturally occurring laminitis, as well as in in vitro lamellar explants treated with MMP activators previously associated with lamellar detachment.[63–65]

In addition to MMPs, RNAs for inflammatory cytokines, like *IL-1β, IL-6,* and *IL-8,* increase during experimental induction.[62] Furthermore, in a more subtle "2-hit" model (mild systemic inflammation induced by endotoxin infusion followed by lower-dose oligofructose) gene expression changes are triggered in these same cytokines, but only among the horses that developed laminitis. Horses resistant to the experimental induction had less systemic inflammation, as evidenced by lower expression of genes for inflammatory cytokines in lung and liver tissues.[66] These findings remind us that the systemic proinflammatory components to this disease may pose a greater risk than those solely within the hoof.

In the CHO model, these changes are detected not just in the severely laminitic forelimbs, but also in the hindlimbs, and are joined by chemokine ligand genes (*CXCL1, CXCL6, CXCL8*) as early as the developmental time points.[67] Chemokines signal cellular migration in a number of settings. Notably, *CXCL1* induces expression of intercellular adhesion molecule-1 (*ICAM-1*).[68] More recent work observed many of these same changes in gene expression once lameness ensued post experimental induction, but not at the earlier developmental timepoints, when cell stress responses are likely the dominant processes.[59] *ICAM-1* and endothelial-leukocyte adhesion molecule-1 (*E-selectin*), both increased in the BWE model and others, promote leukocyte recruitment, adhesion, and translocation through the endothelium of the vascular wall.[62]

Expressed in both invading myeloid cells and secondary epidermal lamellae, calprotectin (dimer of *S100A8* and *S100A9*) appears in both models of sepsis-related laminitis where it likely contributes to cytokine secretion as well as leukocyte recruitment.[55,69,70] Early microarray studies examining the oligofructose model also detected increased expression of macrophage chemotactic protein, *CCL2*, a signaling molecule implicated in diverse inflammatory conditions for its role in orchestrating monocyte migration.[71] The reader is referred to Leise's[72] comprehensive recent review of the literature regarding leukocyte infiltration of lamellar tissue during laminitis for more information on this topic.

Inflammatory cytokines, produced either by infiltrating leukocytes or activated lamellar epidermal cells, also induce the prostaglandin manufacturing enzyme cyclooxygenase (*PTGS2*, formerly called *COX-2*). *COX-2* expression, as evaluated by quantitative reverse-transcriptase (qRT)-PCR, is increased in affected lamellae, likely contributing to the inflammatory response and degree of pain exhibited by laminitic horses.[62,67,73] However, *COX-2* upregulation occurs at both the RNA and protein levels in skin, secondary epidermal lamellae, endothelial, and vascular smooth muscle cells early during the BWE model, reflecting the systemic inflammatory nature of that experimental model of laminitis.[74] *COX-2* increases may precede other changes in lamellae, as they are detectable by qRT-PCR in response to feeding challenge in lean and obese ponies that did not induce laminitis.[75] *COX-2*, *MMP-9*, calprotectin, and other downstream effectors of inflammatory pathways are upregulated in lamellar tissue from SLL cases in comparison with controls, linking laminitis to other inflammatory diseases, such as human psoriasis and equine asthma.[76,77]

Inflammatory signaling pathways are clearly activated during laminitis pathogenesis, both within the foot, and more systemically, particularly in SL. Yet, what is just as fascinating is the key proinflammatory signaling genes that do not change in this setting, despite the severe tissue damage of laminitis. For the CHO and BWE SL models, no differences were detected at either the developmental or onset-of-lameness time points for cytokines *IL-2*, *IL-4*, and *IL-10*; tumor necrosis factor-α, a prominent proinflammatory product of macrophages/monocytes; *IFNG*, derived primarily from natural killer cells; and the gene encoding the prostaglandin synthase *COX-1*.[78] The immunomodulatory cytokine, IL-10, was elevated for the OF model.[67] In addition, there is a notable difference in the temporal pattern of inflammatory events between the BWE and CHO sepsis models, with most laminar inflammatory events appearing to occur at or near the onset of lameness in the CHO model, whereas many of these events peak earlier in the developmental stages in the BWE model.[78]

Wound healing/epithelial-mesenchymal transition

A third aspect of the disease, lamellar "wounding," results from programmed apoptosis/necrosis, the mechanical forces of weight-bearing on stressed and phenotypically abnormal cells under inflammatory insult and continuing onslaught from the initiating etiology, if unresolved.[16,35,79] Following injury, cellular responses initiate a transition from epithelial to mesenchymal morphology.[30] Inflammatory signals trigger invasion by leukocytes and activation of epidermal cells. This process leads to dermal activation with fibrosis, hyperplasia, a loss of cytoskeletal elements/adhesion complexes, and altered keratin isoform expression. In the skin, this response results in wound healing and scar formation, but, within the hoof capsule, it results in lamellar wedge formation and often a failure to regenerate a functioning SADP due to the inability to restore the delicate secondary epidermal lamellae (SEL) microanatomy. In many ways, this process is similar to other types of organ failure, such as liver failure, in which fibrosis prevents formation of functioning liver epithelium (anatomy and number of cells), in spite of the presence of progenitor cells capable of reforming the epithelium.[80,81]

Histologically, we observe evidence for these processes in laminitic tissues. Within the SEL, basal cells lose their normal morphology, becoming smaller and disorganized and suprabasal cells become elongated, undergo cornification, and become metaplastic and positive for periodic acid–Schiff stain. Hyperplasia and loss of adhesion to the basement membrane further contribute to loss of function.[4,12,17,45,52,53] Changes in K14 (a basal cell marker) detected by immunofluorescence are accompanied by decreased epithelial progenitor cell marker expression in horses with chronic laminitis and lamellar wedge formation.[82] Laminin-332, a trimeric protein responsible for anchoring the epidermis to the dermis, is lost from the basement membrane within 12 hours of experimental induction with oligofructose.[83] To illustrate the importance of this connection, loss of laminin-332 due to heritable defects either of 2 of the 3 chains results in junctional epidermolysis bullosa in horses,[84,85] a condition characterized by dramatic loss of large sections of skin and sloughing of the hooves due to exquisite congenital fragility.

Gene expression provides a further exploration of what is happening inside the cell. *MMP14* is secreted as a pro-protein and, once activated, is important in extracellular matrix remodeling.[60] Although its expression is increased during the acute phase of the oligofructose model, the protein itself is depleted from the basal cells, indicating that the products of that increased expression are quickly trafficked to the exterior of the cell.[86] In contrast, tissue inhibitor of metalloproteinases (TIMPs) balance the action of MMPs, helping to modulate these powerful enzymes.[60] As one might expect, the expression of TIMP2 is decreased following induction of laminitis by oligofructose.[86,87] Expression of *ADAMTS4*, an aggrecanase, also increases, likely contributing to degradation of the cartilage matrix concurrent with changes in the basement membrane.[87–89] Quantitative RT-PCR of lamellae from the BWE model, CHO model, and naturally occurring clinical cases often detected increases in *ADAMTS4*.[61] Yet, the timeline of remodeling of the extracellular matrix is not universal to all types of the disease. In the HI model, *MMP9* expression is increased, but no change occurs in *MMP2*, *MT1-MMP, TIMP3*, or *ADAMTS4* in either the developmental or acute phase.[19]

Immune response, tissue damage, and remodeling are linked processes. In the CHO experimental model, immune cell arrival within lamellar tissues correlates with increases in MMP9 concentration.[18,90] Cytochrome b-245 expression, tracked using the *CYBB* gene encoding the beta subunit, also increases 71 in these laminitic tissues. This proinflammatory product of neutrophils catalyzes generation of superoxide in the extracellular space, building oxidative stress within the tissue.[72]

The complex cascade of gene transcription necessary for wound reepithelialization is orchestrated by transcription factor signaling from the AP-1 family (heterodimers or homodimers of the Fos, Jun, and CREB/ATF protein families.) These AP-1 transcription factors regulate expression of many types of genes involved in wound healing, such as MMPs, integrins, and growth factors (reviewed in Ref.[91]). To date, only *Fos* was observed to increase in expression following induction by the oligofructose; however, as a master regulator, large-scale changes in gene expression are not needed to effect significant changes in their regulatory impact.[71]

Genetic predisposition

Anecdotal evidence has long supported different frequencies of laminitis among different breeds of horse. As breed formation is catalyzed by the action of selection on genes, this variation in the frequency of a phenotype across breeds is a valuable clue that a genetic component contributes to the trait. Selective pressure for survival in the challenging native environments of most pony breeds favored survival among those with a hardy, "easy-keeper" metabolism, as it does in people.[8,92] The only systematic across-breed study examining factors contributing to the onset of pasture-associated laminitis found that individuals from pony-type breeds were at a significantly higher risk of the disease.[93] However, this same selective pressure may fix genes for starvation resistance in ponies, reducing the variation in phenotype available for study and rendering pony breeds a less than ideal population for genetic studies. Adding difficulty to this task, there is considerable debate regarding the fundamental diagnostic definition of the primary underlying endocrinopathy for naturally occurring laminitis: EMS.[94] Yet, genomic calculations of heritability for diagnostic criteria indicative of EMS are moderate to high in these susceptible populations, indicating a strong genetic component to the disease.[95]

To date, only 2 studies have attempted to define loci contributing to this heritability for EMS. The first pilot study chose to sample the Arabian horse, a light horse breed with a moderate frequency of EMS.[96] Although the sample size was small, a genome-wide association to laminitis secondary to EMS pinpointed a single significant region on equine chromosome 14 bearing just one annotated gene: FAM174A. The function of FAM174A is unknown, although RNA interference knockdown studies with human cells suggest a role in cholesterol homeostasis for this transcript, validating a previous identification of this locus in a genome-wide study for blood lipid profiles in humans.[97] Both the SNP marker, and a homo-polymer polymorphism within the 3' end of the gene correlated with increased resting insulin levels, although no conclusive functional hypothesis could be tested.[96] Indeed, the causative genetic variation may lie anywhere within the associated 150k haplotype block, and further work is needed to narrow the candidate region and test haplotypes at this locus for association to similar phenotypes in other breeds. Still, as most studies of management or diet-based interventions target glucose-insulin hemostasis, this study highlights the need to further investigate the role of cholesterol/lipid control in the EMS horse.

A second study, focusing on a large sampling of Welsh ponies, identified a significant correlation between an SNP within the first exon of the HMGA2 gene and several diagnostic indicators of EMS (resting insulin, insulin after oral sugar test (OST), non-esterified fatty acids (NEFA), and triglycerides).[98] Strong signatures of selection across this locus suggest either recent breeder-driven selection for small height, or perhaps natural selection for resistance to starvation before the introduction of modern balanced diets and the end of use of most horses for transportation and agricultural labor. Notably, the allele correlated with larger body size and increases in diagnostic indicators for EMS is nearly fixed in most light horse breeds; therefore, this risk locus is unlikely to play a role in susceptibility to EMS in non-pony breeds.

High-mobility group A proteins serve to regulate inducible gene transcription by binding to promoter and enhancer regions of their target genes, and as such, can have broad action on the differentiation and expansion of cells.[99] Loss-of-function mutations in the mouse result in the relatively lean "pygmy" phenotype, in contrast to the horse, in which the small stature allele correlates with increases in diagnostics for obesity.[100] Diets were not quantified in this study, thus the interaction with environmental components, like the tendency for owners to overfeed smaller horses, cannot be ruled out. More work is needed to fully describe the biological action, and potential therapeutic implications, of this locus.

Aside from the predisposition to endocrinopathy, variation in systemic inflammatory responses to laminitis triggering stimuli and involvement of the innate immune system both suggest that we should be able to detect genetic variation contributing to laminitis resistance/susceptibility resulting from diverse etiology. Indeed, in most experimental induction models, horses develop laminitis at different timepoints and for some milder models, fail to develop clinical lameness.[16,66,75,101–103] There are many plausible explanations for this phenomenon, including gene-environment interaction. The interplay of genetic susceptibility with autoinflammatory diseases in humans is well established.[104] In one notable example, genome-wide association studies catalyzed new therapeutic strategies for psoriasis, a human autoinflammatory condition with strong potential as a model for laminitis. In a discovery-based, hypothesis-generating approach, associated regions from a population study highlighted a previously unknown role for activation of Th17 genes in psoriasis susceptibility.[105] With this knowledge, novel classes of biologic drugs targeting these pathways for other conditions were rapidly redeployed to treat psoriasis and are showing promising results in clinical trials.[106]

Examination of genetic predisposition offers promise for identification of individual horses with above-average susceptibility, enabling early targeted interventions though diet, management, and perhaps future pharmaceutical options to prevent this difficult-to-treat condition. In theory, these loci could be integrated into genomic selection programs to reduce the incidence of the disease in future generations. This is a promising field of study; however, it will require large sample sizes and significant investments in research funding to realize these benefits.

SUMMARY

None of the signaling processes described in this article are mutually exclusive and are likely all important to laminitis pathogenesis. The ultimate goal should be to determine their temporal and relative contributions to laminitis pathogenesis. The hoof is a unique and elegantly evolved biomechanical system for which there is no perfect substitute model. Yet, there are lessons to be learned from studies investigating diseases of the skin or other organs. If required, we can adjust our models, keeping in mind that the lamellar epithelium differs from skin in structure and in the content of the major keratins.

The constellation of gene expression patterns reflecting ongoing processes at the molecular level provide valuable clues to the biochemical puzzle. In particular, transcriptomics-level studies provide discovery-mode data and hypothesis-testable lines of investigation without a priori assumptions. Some of these targets provide candidate biomarkers for improved diagnosis and monitoring of the disease as well as signaling pathways that can be pharmacologically manipulated for laminitis prevention or treatment, as has been the case for human diseases.

Potential Interventions

A role for ER stress and autoinflammatory pathways is evidenced by the only empirically proven intervention for laminitis: digital hypothermia, which derails signaling and enzymatic processes across the board. Indeed, digital hypothermia prevents OF model-induced laminitis and decreases inflammatory markers detected by qRT-PCR.[67] Unfortunately, cryotherapy is not always feasible in the field, or applied early enough in the disease process.

With the help of novel hypothesis illuminated by gene expression studies, more sophisticated approaches are on the way. As discussed by Lane and colleagues,[25] rapamycin (an inhibitor of mTORC1) and other inhibitors acting on the mTORC1 pathway, are potential therapeutics for treatment and prevention of laminitis. Inhibitors of the mTORC1 pathway decrease ER stress by increasing autophagy and allowing cells to dispose of misfolded proteins. Although promising, rapamycin has shown toxicity in human trials,[107,108] and some investigators have suggested that rapamycin will be more effective in combination therapies.[107] The potential use of small molecules that either modulate protein function within the ER stress pathway or enhance the protein folding capacity within the ER lumen to relieve ER stress has been reviewed elsewhere.[45]

Still, by defining and connecting these critical pathways in the disease process with genomic tools, we can envision, for the first time, not just one novel therapeutic intervention but the possibility of several worthy of investigation in the near future. Just a decade or 2 ago, that would have seemed impossibly optimistic.

REFERENCES

1. Hood DM. The mechanisms and consequences of structural failure of the foot. Vet Clin North Am Equine Pract 1999;15(2):437–61.
2. Pollitt CC. The anatomy and physiology of the suspensory apparatus of the distal phalanx. Vet Clin North Am Equine Pract 2010;26(1):29–49.
3. Collins SN, van Eps AW, Pollitt CC, et al. The lamellar wedge. Vet Clin North Am Equine Pract 2010;26(1):179–95.
4. Engiles JB, Galantino-Homer HL, Boston R, et al. Osteopathology in the equine distal phalanx associated with the development and progression of laminitis. Vet Pathol 2015;52(5):928–44.
5. Donaldson MT, Jorgensen AJ, Beech J. Evaluation of suspected pituitary pars intermedia dysfunction in horses with laminitis. J Am Vet Med Assoc 2004; 224(7):1123–7.
6. Karikoski NP, Horn I, McGowan TW, et al. The prevalence of endocrinopathic laminitis among horses presented for laminitis at a first-opinion/referral equine hospital. Domest Anim Endocrinol 2011;41(3):111–7.
7. Carter RA, Geor RJ, Burton Staniar W, et al. Apparent adiposity assessed by standardised scoring systems and morphometric measurements in horses and ponies. Vet J 2009;179(2):204–10.
8. Treiber KH, Kronfeld DS, Hess TM, et al. Evaluation of genetic and metabolic predispositions and nutritional risk factors for pasture-associated laminitis in ponies. J Am Vet Med Assoc 2006;228(10):1538–45.
9. Carter R, Treiber K, Geor R, et al. Prediction of incipient pasture-associated laminitis from hyperinsulinaemia, hyperleptinaemia and generalised and localised obesity in a cohort of ponies. Equine Vet J 2009;41(2):171–8.
10. Johnson P, Messer N, Ganjam V. Cushing's syndromes, insulin resistance and endocrinopathic laminitis. Equine Vet J 2004;36(3):194–8.
11. Asplin KE, Sillence MN, Pollitt CC, et al. Induction of laminitis by prolonged hyperinsulinaemia in clinically normal ponies. Vet J 2007;174(3):530–5.
12. de Laat MA, McGowan CM, Sillence MN, et al. Equine laminitis: induced by 48 h hyperinsulinaemia in standardbred horses. Equine Vet J 2010;42(2):129–35.
13. van Eps AW, Pollitt CC. Equine laminitis induced with oligofructose. Equine Vet J 2006;38(3):203–8.
14. Pollitt CC, Visser MB. Carbohydrate alimentary overload laminitis. Vet Clin North Am Equine Pract 2010;26(1):65–78.
15. Galey F, Whiteley H, Goetz T, et al. Black walnut (*Juglans nigra*) toxicosis: a model for equine laminitis. J Comp Pathol 1991;104(3):313–26.
16. Gardner A, van Eps A, Watts M, et al. A novel model to assess lamellar signaling relevant to preferential weight bearing in the horse. Vet J 2017;221:62–7.

17. Karikoski N, McGowan C, Singer E, et al. Pathology of natural cases of equine endocrinopathic laminitis associated with hyperinsulinemia. Vet Pathol 2015; 52(5):945–56.

18. Black SJ. Extracellular matrix, leukocyte migration and laminitis. Vet Immunol Immunopathol 2009;129(3–4):161–3.

19. de Laat MA, Kyaw-Tanner MT, Nourian AR, et al. The developmental and acute phases of insulin-induced laminitis involve minimal metalloproteinase activity. Vet Immunol Immunopathol 2011;140(3–4):275–81.

20. Holl HM, Gao S, Fei Z, et al. Generation of a de novo transcriptome from equine lamellar tissue. BMC Genomics 2015;16(1):739.

21. Johnson PJ, Messer NT, Slight SH, et al. Endocrinopathic laminitis in the horse. Clin Tech Equine Pract 2004;3(1):45–56.

22. Menzies-Gow NJ, Harris PA, Elliott J. Prospective cohort study evaluating risk factors for the development of pasture-associated laminitis in the United Kingdom. Equine Vet J 2017;49(3):300–6.

23. Meier A, de Laat M, Reiche D, et al. The oral glucose test predicts laminitis risk in ponies fed a diet high in nonstructural carbohydrates. Domest Anim Endocrinol 2018;63:1–9.

24. Tadros EM, Fowlie JG, Refsal KR, et al. Association between hyperinsulinaemia and laminitis severity at the time of pituitary pars intermedia dysfunction diagnosis. Equine Vet J 2019;51(1):52–6.

25. Lane H, Burns T, Hegedus O, et al. Lamellar events related to insulin-like growth factor-1 receptor signalling in two models relevant to endocrinopathic laminitis. Equine Vet J 2017;49(5):643–54.

26. Hodak E, Gottlieb AB, Anzilotti M, et al. The insulin-like growth factor 1 receptor is expressed by epithelial cells with proliferative potential in human epidermis and skin appendages: correlation of increased expression with epidermal hyperplasia. J Invest Dermatol 1996;106(3):564–70.

27. Nanayakkara SN, Rahnama S, Harris PA, et al. Characterization of insulin and IGF-1 receptor binding in equine liver and lamellar tissue: implications for endocrinopathic laminitis. Domest Anim Endocrinol 2019;66:21–6.

28. Burns TA, Watts MR, Weber PS, et al. Distribution of insulin receptor and insulin-like growth factor-1 receptor in the digital laminae of mixed-breed ponies: an immunohistochemical study. Equine Vet J 2013;45(3):326–32.

29. Freedberg IM, Tomic-Canic M, Komine M, et al. Keratins and the keratinocyte activation cycle. J Invest Dermatol 2001;116(5):633–40.

30. Feldmeyer L, Werner S, French L, et al. Interleukin-1, inflammasomes and the skin. Eur J Cell Biol 2010;89(9):638–44.

31. Gardner A, Kelly C, van Eps A, et al. Mitogen-activated kinase pathway activation in epidermal lamellae in the acute stages of carbohydrate overload laminitis models and the effect of regional deep hypothermia on signalling pathways. Equine Vet J 2016;48(5):633–40.

32. Dern K, Burns TA, Watts MR, et al. Influence of digital hypothermia on lamellar events related to IL-6/gp130 signalling in equine sepsis-related laminitis. Equine Vet J 2019;52(3):441–8.

33. Sands WA, Page MM, Selman C. Proteostasis and ageing: insights from long-lived mutant mice. J Physiol 2017;595(20):6383–90.

34. Wattle O, Pollitt C. Lamellar metabolism. Clin Tech Equine Pract 2004;3(1):22–30.

35. Medina-Torres CE, Underwood C, Pollitt CC, et al. The effect of weightbearing and limb load cycling on equine lamellar perfusion and energy metabolism measured using tissue microdialysis. Equine Vet J 2016;48(1):114–9.
36. Pass MA, Pollitt S, Pollitt CC. Decreased glucose metabolism causes separation of hoof lamellae in vitro: a trigger for laminitis? Equine Vet J Suppl 1998;(26): 133–8.
37. Asplin K, Curlewis J, McGowan C, et al. Glucose transport in the equine hoof. Equine Vet J 2011;43(2):196–201.
38. Wang M, Kaufman R. Protein misfolding in the endoplasmic reticulum as a conduit to human disease. Nature 2016;529(7586):326–35.
39. Jung T, Choi K. Pharmacological modulators of endoplasmic reticulum stress in metabolic diseases. Int J Mol Sci 2016;17(2) [pii:E192].
40. Ozcan U, Cao Q, Yilmaz E, et al. Endoplasmic reticulum stress links obesity, insulin action, and type 2 diabetes. Science 2004;306(5695):457–61.
41. Salvadó L, Palomer X, Barroso E, et al. Targeting endoplasmic reticulum stress in insulin resistance. Trends Endocrinol Metab 2015;26(8):438–48.
42. Wang S, Kaufman RJ. The impact of the unfolded protein response on human disease. J Cell Biol 2012;197(7):857–67.
43. Noschka E, Vandenplas ML, Hurley DJ, et al. Temporal aspects of laminar gene expression during the developmental stages of equine laminitis. Vet Immunol Immunopathol 2009;129(3–4):242–53.
44. Leise BS, Watts M, Roy S, et al. Use of laser capture microdissection for the assessment of equine lamellar basal epithelial cell signalling in the early stages of laminitis. Equine Vet J 2014;47(4):478–88.
45. Cassimeris L, Engiles JB, Galantino-Homer H. Detection of endoplasmic reticulum stress and the unfolded protein response in naturally-occurring endocrinopathic equine laminitis. BMC Vet Res 2019;15(1):24.
46. Appenzeller-Herzog C, Hall MN. Bidirectional crosstalk between endoplasmic reticulum stress and mTOR signaling. Trends Cell Biol 2012;22(5):274–82.
47. Cai Q, Sheng ZH. Uncovering the role of Snapin in regulating autophagy-lysosomal function. Autophagy 2011;7(4):445–7.
48. Carmona-Gutierrez D, Hughes AL, Madeo F, et al. The crucial impact of lysosomes in aging and longevity. Ageing Res Rev 2016;32:2–12.
49. Moll R, Divo M, Langbein L. The human keratins: biology and pathology. Histochem Cell Biol 2008;129(6):705–33.
50. Ramms L, Fabris G, Windoffer R, et al. Keratins as the main component for the mechanical integrity of keratinocytes. Proc Natl Acad Sci U S A 2013;110(46): 18513–8.
51. Armstrong C, Cassimeris L, Da Silva Santos C, et al. The expression of equine keratins K42 and K124 is restricted to the hoof epidermal lamellae of *Equus caballus*. PLoS One 2019;14(9):e0219234.
52. Karikoski NP, Patterson-Kane JC, Asplin KE, et al. Morphological and cellular changes in secondary epidermal laminae of horses with insulin-induced laminitis. Am J Vet Res 2014;75(2):161–8.
53. Karikoski NP, Patterson-Kane JC, Singer ER, et al. Lamellar pathology in horses with pituitary pars intermedia dysfunction. Equine Vet J 2016;48(4):472–8.
54. Afshar M, Gallo R. Innate immune defense system of the skin. Vet Dermatol 2013;24(1):32–+.
55. Faleiros RR, Johnson PJ, Nuovo GJ, et al. Laminar leukocyte accumulation in horses with carbohydrate overload-induced laminitis. J Vet Intern Med 2011; 25(1):107–15.

56. Jin L, Wang G. Keratin 17: a critical player in the pathogenesis of psoriasis. Med Res Rev 2014;34(2):438–54.
57. Leigh IM, Navsaria H, Purkis PE, et al. Keratins (K16 and K17) as markers of keratinocyte hyperproliferation in psoriasis in vivo and in vitro. Br J Dermatol 1995; 133(4):501–11.
58. Zhang W, Dang E, Shi X, et al. The pro-inflammatory cytokine IL-22 up-regulates keratin 17 expression in keratinocytes via STAT3 and ERK1/2. PLoS One 2012; 7(7):e40797.
59. Leise BS, Watts M, Tanhoff E, et al. Laminar regulation of STAT1 and STAT3 in black walnut extract and carbohydrate overload induced models of laminitis. J Vet Intern Med 2012;26(4):996–1004.
60. Nissinen L, Kähäri VM. Matrix metalloproteinases in inflammation. Biochim Biophys Acta 2014;1840(8):2571–80.
61. Coyne MJ, Cousin H, Loftus JP, et al. Cloning and expression of ADAM-related metalloproteases in equine laminitis. Vet Immunol Immunopathol 2009;129(3–4): 231–41.
62. Loftus JP, Black SJ, Pettigrew A, et al. Early laminar events involving endothelial activation in horses with black walnut-induced laminitis. Am J Vet Res 2007; 68(11):1205–11.
63. Pollitt CC, Pass MA, Pollitt S. Batimastat (BB-94) inhibits matrix metalloproteinases of equine laminitis. Equine Vet J Suppl 1998;(26):119–24.
64. Mungall BA, Pollitt CC. Thermolysin activates equine lamellar hoof matrix metalloproteinases. J Comp Pathol 2002;126(1):9–16.
65. Visser MB, Pollitt CC. Lamellar leukocyte infiltration and involvement of IL-6 during oligofructose-induced equine laminitis development. Vet Immunol Immunopathol 2011;144(1–2):120–8.
66. Tadros EM, Frank N, Newkirk KM, et al. Effects of a "two-hit" model of organ damage on the systemic inflammatory response and development of laminitis in horses. Vet Immunol Immunopathol 2012;150(1–2):90–100.
67. van Eps A, Leise B, Watts M, et al. Digital hypothermia inhibits early lamellar inflammatory signalling in the oligofructose laminitis model. Equine Vet J 2012; 44(2):230–7.
68. Drechsler M, Duchene J, Soehnlein O. Chemokines control mobilization, recruitment, and fate of monocytes in atherosclerosis. Arterioscler Thromb Vasc Biol 2015;35(5):1050–5.
69. Faleiros R, Nuovo G, Belknap J. Calprotectin in myeloid and epithelial cells of laminae from horses with black walnut extract-induced laminitis. J Vet Intern Med 2009;23(1):174–81.
70. Wang S, Song R, Wang Z, et al. S100A8/A9 in inflammation. Front Immunol 2018;9:1298.
71. Budak MT, Orsini JA, Pollitt CC, et al. Gene expression in the lamellar dermis-epidermis during the developmental phase of carbohydrate overload-induced laminitis in the horse. Vet Immunol Immunopathol 2009;131(1–2):86–96.
72. Leise B. The role of neutrophils in equine laminitis. Cell Tissue Res 2018;371(3): 541–50.
73. Pawlak EA, Geor RJ, Watts MR, et al. Regulation of hypoxia-inducible factor-1α and related genes in equine digital lamellae and in cultured keratinocytes. Equine Vet J 2014;46(2):203–9.
74. Blikslager AT, Yin C, Cochran AM, et al. Cyclooxygenase expression in the early stages of equine laminitis: a cytologic study. J Vet Intern Med 2006;20(5): 1191–6.

75. Burns TA, Watts MR, Weber PS, et al. Effect of dietary nonstructural carbohy-drate content on activation of 5'-adenosine monophosphate-activated protein ki-nase in liver, skeletal muscle, and digital laminae of lean and obese ponies. J Vet Intern Med 2014;28(4):1280–8.

76. Korn A, Miller D, Dong L, et al. Differential gene expression profiles and selected cytokine protein analysis of mediastinal lymph nodes of horses with chronic recurrent airway obstruction (RAO) support an interleukin-17 immune response. PLoS One 2015;10(11):e0142622.

77. Albanesi C, Madonna S, Gisondi P, et al. The interplay between keratinocytes and immune cells in the pathogenesis of psoriasis. Front Immunol 2018;9:1549.

78. Leise BS, Faleiros RR, Watts M, et al. Laminar inflammatory gene expression in the carbohydrate overload model of equine laminitis. Equine Vet J 2011;43(1): 54–61.

79. Medina-Torres CE, Underwood C, Pollitt CC, et al. Microdialysis measurements of equine lamellar perfusion and energy metabolism in response to physical and pharmacological manipulations of blood flow. Equine Vet J 2016;48(6):756–64.

80. Novo E, di Bonzo LV, Cannito S, et al. Hepatic myofibroblasts: a heterogeneous population of multifunctional cells in liver fibrogenesis. Int J Biochem Cell Biol 2009;41(11):2089–93.

81. Oatmen KE, Cull E, Spinale FG. Heart failure as interstitial cancer: emergence of a malignant fibroblast phenotype. Nat Rev Cardiol 2019. https://doi.org/10. 1038/s41569-019-0286-y.

82. Carter RA, Engiles JB, Megee SO, et al. Decreased expression of p63, a regu-lator of epidermal stem cells, in the chronic laminitic equine hoof. Equine Vet J 2011;43(5):543–51.

83. Visser MB, Pollitt CC. The timeline of lamellar basement membrane changes during equine laminitis development. Equine Vet J 2011;43(4):471–7.

84. Milenkovic D, Chaffaux S, Taourit S, et al. A mutation in the LAMC2 gene causes the Herlitz junctional epidermolysis bullosa (H-JEB) in two French draft horse breeds. Genet Sel Evol 2003;35(2):249–56.

85. Graves KT, Henney PJ, Ennis RB. Partial deletion of the LAMA3 gene is respon-sible for hereditary junctional epidermolysis bullosa in the American Saddlebred Horse. Anim Genet 2009;40(1):35–41.

86. Kyaw-Tanner MT, Wattle O, van Eps AW, et al. Equine laminitis: membrane type matrix metalloproteinase-1 (MMP-14) is involved in acute phase onset. Equine Vet J 2008;40(5):482–7.

87. Visser MB, Pollitt CC. The timeline of metalloprotease events during oligofruc-tose induced equine laminitis development. Equine Vet J 2012;44(1):88–93.

88. Wang L, Pawlak E, Johnson PJ, et al. Effects of cleavage by a disintegrin and metalloproteinase with thrombospondin motifs-4 on gene expression and pro-tein content of versican and aggrecan in the digital laminae of horses with starch gruel-induced laminitis. Am J Vet Res 2012;73(7):1047–56.

89. Pawlak E, Wang L, Johnson PJ, et al. Distribution and processing of a disintegrin and metalloproteinase with thrombospondin motifs-4, aggrecan, versican, and hyaluronan in equine digital laminae. Am J Vet Res 2012;73(7):1035–46.

90. Loftus JP, Belknap JK, Black SJ. Matrix metalloproteinase-9 in laminae of black walnut extract treated horses correlates with neutrophil abundance. Vet Immu-nol Immunopathol 2006;113(3–4):267–76.

91. Schäfer M, Werner S. Transcriptional control of wound repair. Annu Rev Cell Dev Biol 2007;23:69–92.

92. Hales CN, Barker DJ. Type 2 (non-insulin-dependent) diabetes mellitus: the thrifty phenotype hypothesis. Diabetologia 1992;35(7):595–601.

93. Coleman MC, Belknap JK, Eades SC, et al. Case-control study of risk factors for pasture-and endocrinopathy-associated laminitis in North American horses. J Am Vet Med Assoc 2018;253(4):470–8.

94. Librado P, Der Sarkissian C, Ermini L, et al. Tracking the origins of Yakutian horses and the genetic basis for their fast adaptation to subarctic environments. Proc Natl Acad Sci U S A 2015;112(50):E6889–97.

95. Norton EM, Schultz NE, Rendahl AK, et al. Heritability of metabolic traits associated with equine metabolic syndrome in Welsh ponies and Morgan horses. Equine Vet J 2019;51(4):475–80.

96. Lewis SL, Holl H, Streeter C, et al. Genomewide association study reveals a risk locus for equine metabolic syndrome in the Arabian horse. J Anim Sci 2017; 95(3):1071–9.

97. Blattmann P, Schuberth C, Pepperkok R, et al. RNAi-based functional profiling of loci from blood lipid genome-wide association studies identifies genes with cholesterol-regulatory function. PLoS Genet 2013;9(2):e1003338.

98. Norton EM, Avila F, Schultz NE, et al. Evaluation of an HMGA2 variant for pleiotropic effects on height and metabolic traits in ponies. J Vet Intern Med 2019; 33(2):942–52.

99. Reeves R, Beckerbauer L. HMGI/Y proteins: flexible regulators of transcription and chromatin structure. Biochim Biophys Acta 2001;1519(1–2):13–29.

100. Xiang X, Benson KF, Chada K. Mini-mouse: disruption of the pygmy locus in a transgenic insertional mutant. Science 1990;247(4945):967–9.

101. Pollitt CC, Davies CT. Equine laminitis: its development coincides with increased sublamellar blood flow. Equine Vet J Suppl 1998;(26):125–32.

102. Milinovich GJ, Trott DJ, Burrell PC, et al. Fluorescence in situ hybridization analysis of hindgut bacteria associated with the development of equine laminitis. Environ Microbiol 2007;9(8):2090–100.

103. de Laat MA, Sillence MN, McGowan CM, et al. Continuous intravenous infusion of glucose induces endogenous hyperinsulinaemia and lamellar histopathology in standardbred horses. Vet J 2012;191(3):317–22.

104. Moghaddas F, Masters SL. The classification, genetic diagnosis and modelling of monogenic autoinflammatory disorders. Clin Sci (Lond) 2018;132(17): 1901–24.

105. Capon F. The genetic basis of psoriasis. Int J Mol Sci 2017;18(12):2526. https://doi.org/10.3390/ijms18122526.

106. Hawkes JE, Chan TC, Krueger JG. Psoriasis pathogenesis and the development of novel targeted immune therapies. J Allergy Clin Immunol 2017;140(3): 645–53.

107. Li J, Kim SG, Blenis J. Rapamycin: one drug, many effects. Cell Metab 2014; 19(3):373–9.

108. Kennedy BK, Lamming DW. The mechanistic target of rapamycin: the grand ConducTOR of metabolism and aging. Cell Metab 2016;23(6):990–1003.

109. Duan L, Maki CG. The IGF-1R/AKT pathway determines cell fate in response to p53. Transl Cancer Res 2016;5(6):664–75.

Genetics of Equine Reproductive Diseases

Terje Raudsepp, PhD

KEYWORDS

- Horse • Fertility • Sexual development • Chromosomes • Cryptorchidism
- Acrosome reaction • FKBP6 • Genetic testing

KEY POINTS

- Chromosome analysis remains the primary genetic test for reproductive disorders.
- No causative genes/mutations are known for reduced fertility or infertility in mares or stallions.
- The only available genetic test for stallion subfertility is based on a susceptibility gene, namely, *FKBP6*.
- A successful search for reproduction genes requires collection of many samples with accurate fertility records and clinical phenotypes.
- Progress in genetic testing for reproductive disorders requires teamwork of geneticists, clinicians, and breeders.

INTRODUCTION

Stallion and mare fertility are among the core components of the economy of the equine industry. Fertility and reproduction are complex traits influenced by environmental and genetic factors. The latter involve a network of thousands of genes, which undergo differential regulation during the development, and collectively govern a cascade of events from sex determination and sexual differentiation to sexual maturation and fertilization.[1,2] Although hundreds of candidate genes for male and female fertility have been identified using rodent models,[1,2] limited information is available for other species including the horse.[3–7]

Since sequencing the first horse genome a decade ago,[8] the progress of equine genomics has been unparalleled and marked by outstanding achievements in almost all fields, including the discovery of causative mutations for single-gene disorders and deciphering the genetic basis for several complex diseases.[6] However, compared with other complex traits, the genomics of equine reproduction has received relatively less attention, even though reproductive performance is of high economic importance for purebred horses and vital for survival in feral populations.[7,9] It is argued that

Department of Veterinary Integrative Biosciences, Molecular Cytogenetics Laboratory, Texas A&M University, College of Veterinary Medicine and Biomedical Sciences, Veterinary Research Building Room 306, 588 Raymond Stotzer Parkway, College Station, TX 77843-4458, USA
E-mail address: traudsepp@cvm.tamu.edu

Vet Clin Equine 36 (2020) 395–409
https://doi.org/10.1016/j.cveq.2020.03.013
0749-0739/20/© 2020 Elsevier Inc. All rights reserved.

vetequine.theclinics.com

breeding animals in the horse industry are selected on the basis of their pedigrees, athletic prowess, and appearance, but not for their reproductive potential. For example, stallions experience lower per-cycle conception rates compared with other livestock species.[10] Therefore, it is of particular importance to continue research on the genetic component of stallion and mare fertility for the discovery of genes and genomic regions responsible for various reproductive traits and disorders. Only this way we can develop genetics-based tests to evaluate breeding soundness of mares and stallions.

This article aims to provide a comprehensive overview about the current knowledge on genome mutations that are causative or associated with various equine reproductive diseases. We first describe the conditions that are caused by chromosome-level mutations, followed by reproductive disorders that are associated with sequence variants and candidate genes. Future prospective of developing genetic tests for equine reproductive disorders is discussed.

REPRODUCTIVE DISORDERS CAUSED BY CHROMOSOME MUTATIONS

In every cell, the genetic material, DNA, is packaged with diverse proteins into distinct structures—the chromosomes. The normal diploid chromosome number in the domestic horse (*Equus caballus*) is 64 and includes 31 pairs of autosomes and a pair of sex chromosomes—XX in females and XY in males. One-half of the chromosomes are inherited from the sire, and the other one-half from the dam. Changes in chromosome number or structure typically result in genomic imbalance and affect meiotic cell division, gametogenesis, and the viability of zygotes and embryos. Some chromosomal changes, such as translocations, may be genetically balanced and can be transmitted, causing fertility problems in subsequent generations. The association between numerical and structural chromosome abnormalities and reduced fertility in horses has been observed for decades and is well-reviewed.[11–23] These sections aim to succinctly outline the most commonly observed equine reproductive disorders that are caused by chromosomal rearrangements.

Infertile Mare with Gonadal Dysgenesis and 63,X Karyotype

Mares with normal external genitalia but with small ("pea-size") inactive ovaries, flaccid uterus and cervix, and in some cases small stature, may have X chromosome monosomy (63,X)—the equine equivalent of Turner's syndrome in humans. This chromosome abnormality is the most common one in female horses and is found in approximately 25% to 36% of mares with gonadal dysgenesis and primary infertility.[19,20,24] In contrast, the prevalence of pure X-monosomy in general female equine population is only about 0.4%.[25]

Cytogenetically, the condition is most commonly seen as complete absence of 1 X chromosome, but occasionally also as deletion of the short arm (p-arm) of 1 X chromosome,[19] or as an X chromosome, which is composed of 2 long arms (Xq), known as isochromosome Xq[26] (**Fig. 1**). All 3 forms result in the loss of Xp genetic material and genetic imbalance (haploinsufficiency) for genes that escape X chromosome inactivation. These genes must be expressed from both X chromosomes and are critical regulators during the development.[27] Underdevelopment of the female reproductive tract and sterility in X-monosomy is caused by haploinsufficiency for these genes, although the actual number and identity of these genes in horses is not known.[20]

Even though X-monosomy in horses is cytogenetically well-characterized, several aspects of the condition warrant more research. Only limited information is available for the parental origin of the retained X chromosome and whether or not this has

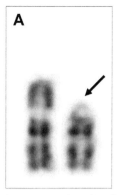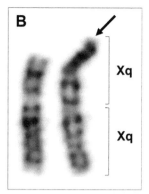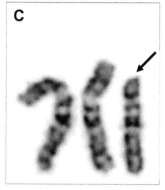

Fig. 1. Examples of X chromosome abnormalities and corresponding phenotypes found in infertile mares. (A) Deletion of Xp (arrow): small ovaries, no cycling, and no pregnancies. (B) Isochromosome Xq (arrow): small ovaries, short stature, and no pregnancies. (C) Trisomy of Xq: infantile uterus and ovaries.

any effect on the phenotype. For example, based on clinical reports, some 63,X mares have short stature, whereas others are of normal size and do not differ from their age and breed mates. Likewise, there are no systematic molecular data for the claim in the literature that a large percentage of mares with X-monosomy are mosaic for a normal 64,XX cell line.[19] There is also no information about the prevalence of X-monosomy among early or late equine abortions. In contrast, about 99% of human conceptions with nonmosaic X-monosomy do not survive gestation.[28]

Infertile Mare with Gonadal Dysgenesis and 65,XXX Karyotype

Some infertile mares with normal external genitalia but with very small ovaries, no cycling, and no pregnancies have 3 copies of the X chromosome and 65,XXX karyotype.[29–31] Compared with X-monosomy, the prevalence of X-trisomy among infertile mares is low.[24] For example, among the approximately 900 equine cytogenetic cases at Texas A&M Molecular Cytogenetics laboratory, only 4 were pure 65,XXX and 1 mare with infantile uterus and ovaries carried trisomy for Xq (see **Fig. 1**).

The equine data are contrasting that of humans, where X-trisomy is the most common chromosome abnormality in females, affects 1 in 1000 female live births, has a 99% fetal survival rate, and has a broad phenotype ranging from almost normal fertile females to those with premature ovarian failure.[32] Because infertility is usually the primary reason why horses are subjected to karyotyping, it may be that there are more 65,XXX mares in general population but have no reproductive problems or have not been used for breeding, and escape detection.[24] Genetic surveys in general equine populations do not support this idea; cytogenetic analysis of 500 young horses in Poland did not detect any 64,XXX individuals[25] and sex chromosome genotyping in 17,471 newborn foals in Japan found only 0.01% with X-trisomy.[33] It is possible that equine X-trisomy is not as viable it is in humans and additional surveys are needed to determine the actual prevalence of X-trisomy among female horses, as well as among embryonic and fetal losses.

Infertile Stallion

Compared with X chromosome aneuploidies in mares, there are no recurrent or prevalent cytogenetic conditions associated with stallion infertility. The majority of infertile stallions subjected for cytogenetic testing have normal 64,XY karyotype. The rare cases where an infertile stallion has chromosome abnormality are unique both clinically and cytogenetically.

Three cases of infertile stallions had nonmosaic or mosaic 65,XXY karyotype—the equine equivalent of Klinefelter's syndrome in humans. The first was a draft horse that had no scrotum but 2 small, soft, and flaccid palpable gonads; unusually large epididymides; and a normal penis and sheath.[34] The second was a French trotter that had relatively small, but normally descended, soft testes, a small penis, and a brownish azoospermic ejaculate.[35] The third case was an American Standardbred stallion with normal external genitalia but failure to produce pregnancy owing to azoospermia. This stallion had 60% 65,XXY cells and 40% normal 64,XY cells.[35] The overall incidence of XXY aneuploidy in horses is low (0.025%) as revealed by a large population survey.[33] In contrast, Klinefelter's syndrome is the most common form of aneuploidy in humans and affects 1 in 500 to 1 in 1000 males.[36]

A very recent case report describes a phenotypically normal 5-year-old Friesian stallion with normal external genitalia, normal erection, and ejaculation but no pregnancies owing to complete azoospermia.[37] Cytogenetic analysis revealed that the stallion carries a unique reciprocal translocation between the Y chromosome and chromosome 13. This case is the first of a phenotypically normal but sterile azoospermic stallion with a large rearrangement involving the Y chromosome and may be the first indication that, like in men and mice,[38] the Y chromosome is critical for normal spermatogenesis also in stallions.

Early Pregnancy Loss

Early pregnancy loss (EPL) between days 15 and 65 after breeding occurs in approximately 8% of equine pregnancies and has substantial economic and welfare implications.[39–41] The underlying pathology of the majority of cases is rarely identified and 80% remain without diagnosis.[41] A small fraction of EPL cases can be attributed to chromosomal mutations.

- *Recurrent EPL.* Normal mares and stallions whose conceptuses are repeatedly lost at early stages of pregnancy should be karyotyped to check for the presence of balanced translocations. Such translocations do not cause any gain or loss in the genetic material, do not have a noticeable effect on health or viability, and can easily remain unnoticed in carrier animals. However, translocations disturb meiosis and gametogenesis, resulting in the formation of both genetically balanced (1/3) and unbalanced (2/3) gametes.[22] The latter, if involved in fertilization, may result in EPL, whereas gametes with the balanced form of translocation will pass the defect to offspring. Therefore, to decrease the incidence of EPL, identification of translocation carriers is critical.

To date, 10 cases of recurrent EPL have been described where either the mare (7 cases) or the stallion (3 cases) is a carrier of a balanced autosomal translocations, whereas all translocations are different (**Table 1**). In 2 cases, where the stallion carried a translocation, samples for cytogenetic analysis were obtained from the offspring. As a proof of principle, in the first case, 8 out of 10 foals had the same chromosomal abnormality,[22] and in the other case, 5 out of 9 foals carried the same translocation as the sire (T. Raudsepp, unpublished data, 2018) (see **Table 1**). These findings further underscore the importance of cytogenetic testing to prevent propagating recurrent EPL.

- *EPL and mare age.* Balanced translocations explain only a small fraction of EPLs in horses and, in the majority of cases, both recurrent and spontaneous, the mare and the stallion are chromosomally normal. In the search for additional risk

Table 1
Cases of recurrent early embryonic loss caused by balanced autosomal translocations

Karyotype	Breed	Offspring Karyotypes	References
64,XX,t(1;3)	Thoroughbred	n/a	Power,[74] 1991
64,XY,t(1;30)	Thoroughbred	n/a	Long,[75] 1996
64,XX,t(1;16)	Thoroughbred	n/a	Lear et al,[76] 2002
64,XX,t(1;21)	Thoroughbred	n/a	Lear et al,[77] 2008
64,XX,t(16;22)	Thoroughbred	n/a	Lear et al,[77] 2008
64,XX,t(4;13)	Thoroughbred	n/a	Lear et al,[77] 2008
64,XY,t(5;16)+mar	Thoroughbred	8 with translocation; 2 normal	Durkin et al,[22] 2011
64,XX,t(2;13)	Thoroughbred	n/a	Lear et al,[78] 2014
64,XX,t(4;10)	Arabian	n/a	Ghosh et al,[79] 2016
64,XY;t(4;30)	Polo pony	5 with translocation; 4 normal	Raudsepp et al, 2018

Abbreviation: n/a, not applicable.

factors, the age of the mare has been identified as the most significant factor, with advancing age linked to increases in EPL.[39] It is thought that conceptuses of older mares have more chromosomal abnormalities and/or other large genomic structural rearrangements.[41] Because cytogenetic analysis of aborted dead embryos is difficult,[20] researchers use other genomics approaches. A deletion in the X chromosome involving the stromal antigen 2 gene (*STAG2*) was found in several male but not in female EPLs and was proposed as a candidate risk region for some cases.[41] Genomic studies on EPL are ongoing by whole genome sequencing the mares and their aborted conceptuses.

Infertility with Multiple Congenital Abnormalities

Infertile horses with multiple congenital defects should be karyotyped to determine whether they may have autosomal aneuploidy. To date, several cases have been described where congenital abnormalities are caused by autosomal trisomy, that is, the presence of 3 copies of a chromosome instead of the normal 2. All cases involve the smallest equine autosomes, namely, ECA23, 26, 27, 28, 30 and 31,[16,19,22,42] because genetic imbalance for larger chromosomes is not viable. In a case of a sterile stallion with azoospermia and trisomy ECA28, investigation of the behavior of the abnormal chromosome in meiosis confirmed that aneuploidy was the cause of meiotic arrest and azoospermia.[43]

Disorders of Sexual Development

Multiple forms of disorders of sexual development (DSDs) have been described in horses, all of which involve sterility. Genetic causes are known for only some DSDs, though a common feature of all is a discrepancy between chromosomal (genetic) sex and gonadal and/or phenotypic sex.[11,18,20,44]

- *Female or female-like horses with 64,XY karyotype and deletion of SRY (SRY-negative XY DSD).* Most of these horses have no somatic or behavioral abnormalities, although some may be small in size. They have normal female external genitalia, but are infertile owing to underdeveloped uterus and ovaries.[18,19,45] The overall phenotype is very similar to that of mares with X-monosomy, and the distinction between the 2 can be made only by karyotyping. Mares with *SRY*-negative DSD have XY sex chromosomes but the Y has lost the "maleness" gene *SRY*.[45] Therefore, in addition to karyotyping, it is necessary to test these animals for the presence or absence of *SRY* by polymerase chain reaction. *SRY*-negative XY DSD occurs in many breeds and, after X-monosomy, it is the most common sex chromosome abnormality in horses.[18,45]

- *Female-like horses with 64,XY karyotype and the SRY gene present (SRY-positive XY DSD)*. These are female-like horses with various degrees of masculinization and virilization. The genital tract is usually abnormal and the gonads can range from ovotestes to testicular feminization leading to male pseudohermaphroditism[11,18,45] (**Fig. 2**). Despite the female-like appearance, these horses are genetically male with an intact Y chromosome and a normal *SRY* gene. Genetic causes are known only for a few cases and are heterogeneous. In 3 families of different breeds, this DSD was associated with androgen insensitivity syndrome and different mutations in the androgen receptor gene (*AR*)[46–48] (**Table 2**). In 2 related Standardbred horses with male pseudohermaphroditism, a large (approximately 200 kb) homozygous deletion was found in ECA29.[49] The deletion involves genes that regulate sex hormone synthesis (aldo-keto reductase family 1 C; *AKR1C*) and may be causative for the DSD in these 2 horses. However, *AR* mutations or the ECA29 deletion are not present in other cases of *SRY*-positive XY DSDs (our unpublished data), suggesting that the molecular causes of the condition differ from case to case.

- *Intersexuality, hermaphroditism, and ambiguous sex.* Over the years, many cases have been described where it is difficult to decide about the gonadal and/or phenotypic sex of the horse. The external phenotype ranges from ambiguous genitalia to female-like or male-like genitalia. Most cases have an enlarged clitoris and an elongated fused vulva[18,19] (see **Fig. 2**). The majority of cases have normal female karyotype and are generally referred to as XX DSD. Causes of equine XX DSD are unknown.

Although all equine DSDs are a dead end from the perspective of reproduction, it is important to continue their clinical and genomic research to develop genetics-based tools for diagnostics and improve the very limited knowledge about the genes regulating sexual development in horses.

Stallion Subfertility and Sperm Aneuploidies

In cases where the stallion is phenotypically and chromosomally normal but constitutively subfertile, cytogenetic evaluation can be extended to chromosomes in sperm by a method known as sperm-fluorescence in situ hybridization (FISH).[20,50] Sperm-FISH is used to determine the percentage of sperm carrying sex chromosome aneuploidies. In normal fertile stallions, this ranges from 0.32% to 1.14%, but increases significantly[50,51] in older stallions. The latter have more sperm with disomies XY, XX, YY, and trisomy XXY.[51] Similar positive correlation between male age and the rate of sperm aneuploidies has been reported for men.[52] The rate of sex chromosome aneuploidies may also be higher in subfertile stallions. For example, sperm-FISH in subfertile Sorraia stallions revealed a more than 10 times higher rate (11%) of sex chromosome aneuploidies.[53] Sperm-FISH is too laborious for routine testing, but can be a useful additional method for genetic evaluation of some stallions.

MOLECULAR GENETICS OF REPRODUCTIVE DISORDERS

The findings of clinical cytogenetics indicate that only a fraction of equine reproductive problems is confined to chromosomal abnormalities, suggesting that genetic

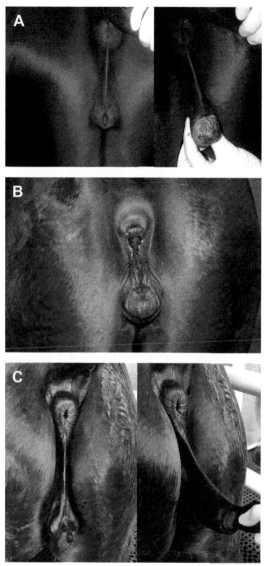

Fig. 2. Examples of equine DSDs. (*A*) Male pseudohermaphrodite with a female-like appearance, fused vulva and penis-like structure protruding from vulva, abdominal rudimentary testes, and *SRY*-positive 64,XY karyotype. (*B*) Intersex with penis growing from vagina, ovary-like abdominal gonads, no tubular structures and 64,XX karyotype. (*C*) Male pseudohermaphrodite with fused vulva and protruding penis, inguinal testes, no female structures by ultrasound examination, and a 64,XX karyotype.

causes of the majority of cases lie at the DNA sequence level. Despite of the recent progress in deciphering the genetic basis of equine single-gene and complex diseases,[6] reproduction has been given relatively less attention. To date, only a few reproductive phenotypes have been associated with candidate or susceptibility genes (see **Table 2**), but without actual knowledge about the genetic cause and mechanism.

Table 2
Summary data about causative and candidate genes for equine reproductive disorders

Reproductive Phenotype	Gene/Candidate Gene	Type of Variant	Horse Chromosome(s) (ECA)	Breed	References
64,XY SRY-negative DSD	SRY	Various size deletions in Y, all including SRY	Y	Multiple	Raudsepp et al,[45] 2010
64,XY SRY-positive DSD; male pseudohermaphroditism	AKR1C gene cluster	Candidate risk CNV; 200 kb homozygous deletion	29	Standardbred	Ghosh et al,[49] 2014
AIS; 64,XY SRY-positive DSD	AR	Regulatory	X	American Quarter Horse family	Révay et al,[46] 2012
AIS; 64,XY SRY-positive DSD	AR	Missense	X	Thoroughbred family	Bolzon et al,[47] 2016
AIS; 64,XY SRY-positive DSD	AR	Deletion 25 bp	X	Warmblood	Welsford et al,[48] 2017
CO	AKR1C gene cluster	Candidate risk CNV; 200 kb homozygous deletion	29	Multiple	Ghosh et al,[68] 2016; Ghosh et al,[80] 2014
EPL	STAG2	Candidate risk CNV for male embryos	X	Thoroughbred	Smart et al,[41] 2018
Stallion fertility	CFTR, OVGP1, FBXO43, TSSK6, PKD1, FOXP1, TCP11, SPATA31E1, NOTCH1	Candidate genes with high impact variants	4, 5, 9, 21, 13, 16, 20, 25	19 European breeds	Schrimpf et al,[69] 2016
Stallion fertility—paternal component for pregnancy rate per estrus	CRISP3	Candidate gene	20	Hanoverian	Hamann et al,[81] 2007

Stallion fertility—paternal component for pregnancy rate per estrus	PRLR	Candidate gene	21	Hanoverian	Giesecke et al,[82] 2010
Stallion fertility—paternal component for pregnancy rate per estrus	SPATA1	Candidate gene	5	Hanoverian	Giesecke et al,[83] 2009
Stallion fertility—paternal component for pregnancy rate per estrus	INHBA	Candidate gene	4	Hanoverian	Giesecke et al,[5] 2010
Stallion fertility—sperm-egg fusion	CRISP1	Candidate gene	20	Multiple	Giese et al,[84] 2002
Stallion fertility- reorganization of sperm chromatin during spermiogenesis	STK31	Candidate gene	4	Not determined	Sabeur et al,[85] 2008
Stallion fertility; increased conception rate	FKBP6	Candidate gene	13	Hanoverian	Schrimpf et al,[60] 2015
Stallion subfertility owing to impaired acrosome reaction	FKBP6	Susceptibility gene	13	Thoroughbred	Raudsepp et al,[59] 2012

Abbreviations: AIS, androgen insensitivity syndrome; ECA, Equus caballus.

Genetic Test for Stallion Subfertility Owing to Impaired Acrosome Reaction

Acrosome is a single secretory granule in sperm head and secretion of this granule, known as acrosomal reaction (AR), is necessary for natural fertilization. Impaired acrosome reaction (IAR) leads to subfertility or infertility.[54,55] The stallions with IAR have normal physical and semen characteristics and typically pass a breeding soundness evaluation, because AR test is not part of routine semen analysis.[54,56,57] The problem is noticed later as consistently low pregnancy rates because the failure of AR affects about 97% of the sperm, although the remaining 3% can perform normal AR for fertilization.[58]

So far, IAR has been confirmed as a cause of subfertility only in Thoroughbred breeding stallions.[58] Genome-wide association study identified *FKBP6* as a strong candidate gene.[59] The gene encodes for FK506 binding protein 6 (FKBP6) and is involved in sperm development and functions. The association is most significant between IAR and a homozygous A/A–A/A haplotype for 2 single nucleotide polymorphisms in *FKBP6* exon 5. Because neither of the 2 variants change protein function, the cause for the association is not known and *FKBP6* is considered only as a susceptibility gene.[59] *FKBP6* genotyping is currently the only genetic test for stallion subfertility, although it is informative only for Thoroughbreds because the susceptibility genotype is rarely found in other horse breeds.[53]

The *FKBP6* gene may have even broader interest with regard to stallion fertility because it shows contrasting associations in different breeds: in Thoroughbreds it is significantly associated with subfertility,[59] whereas homozygous A/A genotype in one of the single nucleotide polymorphisms is associated with higher conception rates in Hanoverians stallions.[60]

Cryptorchidism

Cryptorchidism (CO) is the most common nonlethal equine developmental defect affecting 2% to 8% of full-term male live births, and is more frequent in ponies and draft horses.[61] CO can occur as a single defect or as a part of complex congenital abnormalities and is manifested as the failure of 1 (unilateral) or both (bilateral) testes to descend into the scrotum. In all cases, CO affects normal testicular functions and can result in reduced fertility or infertility. Although stallions with unilateral CO generally produce sufficient normal sperm to yield acceptable pregnancy rates, surgical removal of a retained testis might be indicated because the undescended testis increases the risk for testicular tumors.[62–64] Also, the undescended testes continue testosterone production, owing to which males with bilateral CO show the same behavioral characteristics as normal stallions. Surgical removal of an undescended testis may be challenging and further increases the health risk,[63,65] as well as the financial costs for the owner.

The etiology of CO is complex and involves the interaction of environmental and genetic factors.[66] An indication about genetic predisposition is that some breeds, like Percherons, American Saddlebreds, American Quarter Horses, Friesians, and ponies, are more prone to have CO than, for example, Thoroughbreds.[61,67] Preliminary genomic studies show that about 9% of CO horses have the same approximately 200-kb deletion around *AKR1C* genes in ECA29 as was found in the 2 male pseudohermaphrodites with *SRY*-positive XY DSD (described elsewhere in this article).[49,68] The region is considered as a putative risk factor for CO, though more research is warranted to confirm this. No genetic tests are available for CO.

Candidate Genes for Stallion Fertility

Genomic search for stallion fertility genes has been ongoing for decades, but has so far given just a handful of candidate genes, the majority of which are associated with the paternal component of pregnancy rate in Hanoverian stallions (see **Table 2** for details). Further evaluation of 9 candidate genes in 337 fertile stallions across 19 breeds confirmed their high impact on stallion fertility.[69] This is a good start for the development of genetic tests for stallion evaluation in the future.

Mare Subfertility

After EPL and gonadal dysgenesis (described elsewhere in this article), the most common subfertile phenotype in mares is the failure to become pregnant.[70] Genetic causes of pregnancy failure are not known. Currently, there are no genetics tests for mare subfertility.

Reproductive Success and Inbreeding

Inbreeding in general has a negative effect on fertility because of the accumulation of deleterious recessive alleles in the population.[6] Therefore, fertility problems are more pronounced in high inbred closed breeds. Of particular effect on reproductive success may have the genetic similarity/dissimilarity of the major histocompatibility complex (MHC). For example, Friesians have high incidence (54%) of retained placenta, which is attributed to inbreeding and too similar MHC antigens between mare and foal.[71] Also, mares are more likely to become pregnant if exposed to a stallion with more dissimilar MHC[72] and stallion semen quality improves when exposed to an MHC-dissimilar mare.[73]

SUMMARY

Reproductive disorders are genetically heterogeneous and complex, and the available genetic tests are limited to chromosome analysis and a few candidate genes. Chromosome analysis should be the first test for horses with decreased fertility, infertility, early embryonic loss, and various DSDs. Cytogenetic testing is necessary to confirm or rule out the presence of chromosomal abnormalities and inform about the prognosis or help with management decisions. To date, no genes are known for decreased fertility or infertility in mares. For stallions, a few candidate genes have been proposed and genetic testing is available for one (FKBP6). Although it is anticipated that the ongoing progress in equine genomics will improve the poor status of genetic testing for reproductive disorders, there are inherent difficulties. Subfertility and infertility do not facilitate the collection of large numbers of samples or pedigrees for genetic studies. Difficulties are encountered in the precise clinical characterization of reproductive disorders because in most cases the causes remain unknown. Therefore, constructive cross-talk between the geneticists, clinicians, breeders, and owners remains the critical backbone for any further progress.

ACKNOWLEDGMENTS

The author was supported by grants from American Quarter Horse Foundation, Morris Animal Foundation (D19EQ-051), and USDA-NIFA (2019-67015-29322).

DISCLOSURE

The author has nothing to disclose.

REFERENCES

1. Matzuk MM, Lamb DJ. Genetic dissection of mammalian fertility pathways. Nat Cell Biol 2002;4(Suppl):s41–9.

2. Matzuk MM, Lamb DJ. The biology of infertility: research advances and clinical challenges. Nat Med 2008;14:1197–213.
3. Leeb T, Sieme H, Topfer-Petersen E. Genetic markers for stallion fertility–lessons from humans and mice. Anim Reprod Sci 2005;89:21–9.
4. Leeb T. The horse genome project–sequence based insights into male reproductive mechanisms. Reprod Domest Anim 2007;42(Suppl 2):45–50.
5. Giesecke K, Sieme H, Distl O. Infertility and candidate gene markers for fertility in stallions: a review. Vet J 2010;185:265–71.
6. Raudsepp T, Finno CJ, Bellone RR, et al. Ten years of the horse reference genome: insights into equine biology, domestication and population dynamics in the post-genome era. Anim Genet 2019;50(6):569–97.
7. Raudsepp T, Das PJ, Chowdhary BP. Genomics of reproduction and fertility. In: Chowdhary BP, editor. Equine genomics. John Wiley & Sons; 2013. p. 199–216.
8. Wade CM, Giulotto E, Sigurdsson S, et al. Genome sequence, comparative analysis, and population genetics of the domestic horse. Science 2009;326:865–7.
9. Metzger J, Karwath M, Tonda R, et al. Runs of homozygosity reveal signatures of positive selection for reproduction traits in breed and non-breed horses. BMC Genomics 2015;16:764.
10. Griffin RA, Baker M, Aitken RJ, et al. What makes a fertile sperm? Unique molecular attributes of stallion fertility. Reproduction 2019;158(4):R125–37.
11. Villagomez DA, Parma P, Radi O, et al. Classical and molecular cytogenetics of disorders of sex development in domestic animals. Cytogenet Genome Res 2009;126:110–31.
12. Villagomez DA, Pinton A. Chromosomal abnormalities, meiotic behavior and fertility in domestic animals. Cytogenet Genome Res 2008;120:69–80.
13. King WA. Chromosome variation in the embryos of domestic animals. Cytogenet Genome Res 2008;120:81–90.
14. Ducos A, Revay T, Kovacs A, et al. Cytogenetic screening of livestock populations in Europe: an overview. Cytogenet Genome Res 2008;120:26–41.
15. Chowdhary BP, Raudsepp T. Cytogenetics and physical gene maps. In: Bowling AT, Ruvinsky A, editors. The genetics of the horse. Wallingford (England): CABI; 2000. p. 171–242.
16. Lear TL, Bailey E. Equine clinical cytogenetics: the past and future. Cytogenet Genome Res 2008;120:42–9.
17. Lear TL. Chromosomal analysis. In: McCue JDAP, editor. Equine reproductive procedures. John Wiley & Sons, Inc; 2014. p. 77–82.
18. Lear TL, McGee RB. Disorders of sexual development in the domestic horse, Equus caballus. Sex Dev 2012;6:61–71.
19. Lear TL, Villagomez DAF. Cytogenetic evaluation of mares and foals. In: McKinnon AO, Squires EL, Vaala WE, et al, editors. Equine reproduction. Blackwell Publishing Ltd.; 2011. p. 1951–62.
20. Raudsepp T, Chowdhary BP. Chromosome aberrations and fertility disorders in domestic animals. Annu Rev Anim Biosci 2016;4:15–43.
21. Szczerbal I, Switonski M. Chromosome abnormalities in domestic animals as causes of disorders of sex development or impaired fertility. INTECH; 2016. p. 207–25.
22. Durkin K, Raudsepp T, Chowdhary B. Cytogenetic evaluation of the stallion. In: McKinnon AO, Squires EL, Vaala WE, et al, editors. Equine reproduction. Wiley Blackwell; 2011. p. 1462–8.

23. Raudsepp T, Das PJ. Genomics of reproduction & fertility. In: Chowdhary BP, editor. Equine genomics. Oxford (United Kingdom): John Wiley & Sons, Inc., Wiley-Blackwell; 2013. p. 199–216.
24. Raudsepp T, Das PJ, Avila F, et al. The pseudoautosomal region and sex chromosome aneuploidies in domestic species. Sex Dev 2012;6:72–83.
25. Bugno M, Slota E, Koscielny M. Karyotype evaluation among young horse populations in Poland. Schweiz Arch Tierheilkd 2007;149:227–32.
26. Mäkela O, Gustavsson I, Hollmen T. A 64,X,i(Xq) karyotype in a standardbred filly. Equine Vet J 1994;26:251–4.
27. Bellott DW, Hughes JF, Skaletsky H, et al. Mammalian Y chromosomes retain widely expressed dosage-sensitive regulators. Nature 2014;508:494–9.
28. Hook EB, Warburton D. Turner syndrome revisited: review of new data supports the hypothesis that all viable 45,X cases are cryptic mosaics with a rescue cell line, implying an origin by mitotic loss. Hum Genet 2014;133:417–24.
29. de Lorenzi L, Molteni L, Zannotti M, et al. X trisomy in a sterile mare. Equine Vet J 2010;42:469–70.
30. Mäkinen A, Hasegawa T, Mäkila M, et al. Infertility in two mares with XY and XXX sex chromosomes. Equine Vet J 1999;31:346–9.
31. Bugno M, Slota E, Wieczorek M, et al. Nonmosaic X trisomy, detected by chromosome painting, in an infertile mare. Equine Vet J 2003;35:209–10.
32. Tartaglia NR, Howell S, Sutherland A, et al. A review of trisomy X (47,XXX). Orphanet J Rare Dis 2010;5:8.
33. Kakoi H, Hirota K, Gawahara H, et al. Genetic diagnosis of sex chromosome aberrations in horses based on parentage test by microsatellite DNA and analysis of X- and Y-linked markers. Equine Vet J 2005;37:143–7.
34. Kubien EM, Pozor MA, Tischner M. Clinical, cytogenetic and endocrine evaluation of a horse with a 65,XXY karyotype. Equine Vet J 1993;25:333–5.
35. Mäkinen A, Katila T, Andersson M, et al. Two sterile stallions with XXY-syndrome. Equine Vet J 2000;32:358–60.
36. Los E, Ford GA. Klinefelter syndrome. In: StatPearls. 2019. Treasure Island (FL).
37. Ruiz AJ, Castaneda C, Raudsepp T, et al. Azoospermia and Y chromosome-autosome translocation in a Friesian stallion. J Equine Vet Sci 2019;82:102781.
38. Hughes JF, Page DC. The biology and evolution of mammalian Y chromosomes. Annu Rev Genet 2015;49:507–27.
39. de Mestre AM, Rose BV, Chang YM, et al. Multivariable analysis to determine risk factors associated with early pregnancy loss in thoroughbred broodmares. Theriogenology 2019;124:18–23.
40. Rose BV, Firth M, Morris B, et al. Descriptive study of current therapeutic practices, clinical reproductive findings and incidence of pregnancy loss in intensively managed thoroughbred mares. Anim Reprod Sci 2018;188:74–84.
41. Smart H, Rose BV, Baldwin G, et al. Profiling of aneuploidies and structural genomic variants in placentae from mares that suffer early pregnancy loss. J Equine Vet Sci 2018;66:234.
42. Brito LFC, Sertich PL, Durkin K, et al. Autosomic 27 trisomy in a standardbred colt. J Equine Vet Sci 2008;28(7):431–6.
43. Power MM, Gustavsson I, Switonski M, et al. Synaptonemal complex analysis of an autosomal trisomy in the horse. Cytogenet Cell Genet 1992;61:202–7.
44. Villagomez DA, Lear TL, Chenier T, et al. Equine disorders of sexual development in 17 mares including XX, SRY-negative, XY, SRY-negative and XY, SRY-positive genotypes. Sex Dev 2011;5:16–25.

45. Raudsepp T, Durkin K, Lear TL, et al. Molecular heterogeneity of XY sex reversal in horses. Anim Genet 2010;41(Suppl 2):41–52.
46. Révay T, Villagomez DA, Brewer D, et al. GTG mutation in the start codon of the androgen receptor gene in a family of horses with 64,XY disorder of sex development. Sex Dev 2012;6:108–16.
47. Bolzon C, Joone CJ, Schulman ML, et al. Missense mutation in the ligand-binding domain of the horse androgen receptor gene in a thoroughbred family with inherited 64,XY (SRY+) disorder of sex development. Sex Dev 2016;10:37–44.
48. Welsford GE, Munk R, Villagomez DA, et al. Androgen insensitivity syndrome in a family of warmblood horses caused by a 25-bp deletion of the DNA-binding domain of the androgen receptor gene. Sex Dev 2017;11:40–5.
49. Ghosh S, Qu Z, Das PJ, et al. Copy number variation in the horse genome. PLoS Genet 2014;10:e1004712.
50. Bugno M, Jablonska Z, Tischner M, et al. Detection of sex chromosome aneuploidy in equine spermatozoa using fluorescence in situ hybridization. Reprod Domest Anim 2010;45:1015–9.
51. Bugno-Poniewierska M, Kozub D, Pawlina K, et al. Determination of the correlation between stallion's age and number of sex chromosome aberrations in spermatozoa. Reprod Domest Anim 2011;46:787–92.
52. Templado C, Vidal F, Estop A. Aneuploidy in human spermatozoa. Cytogenet Genome Res 2011;133:91–9.
53. Kjöllerström HJ, do Mar Oom M, Chowdhary BP, et al. Fertility assessment in Sorraia stallions by sperm-fish and Fkbp6 genotyping. Reprod Domest Anim 2016; 51:351–9.
54. Varner DD, Johnson L. From a sperm's eye view - revisiting our perception of this intriguing cell. AAEP Proceedings 2007;53:104–77.
55. Mayorga LS, Tomes CN, Belmonte SA. Acrosomal exocytosis, a special type of regulated secretion. IUBMB Life 2007;59:286–92.
56. Bosard T, Love C, Brinsko S, et al. Evaluation and diagnosis of acrosome function/dysfunction in the stallion. Anim Reprod Sci 2005;89:215–7.
57. Varner DD. Developments in stallion semen evaluation. Theriogenology 2008;70: 448–62.
58. Brinsko SP, Love CC, Bauer JE, et al. Cholesterol-to-phospholipid ratio in whole sperm and seminal plasma from fertile stallions and stallions with unexplained subfertility. Anim Reprod Sci 2007;99:65–71.
59. Raudsepp T, McCue ME, Das PJ, et al. Genome-wide association study implicates testis-sperm specific FKBP6 as a susceptibility locus for impaired acrosome reaction in stallions. PLoS Genet 2012;8:e1003139.
60. Schrimpf R, Metzger J, Martinsson G, et al. Implication of FKBP6 for male fertility in horses. Reprod Domest Anim 2015;50:195–9.
61. Hayes HM. Epidemiological features of 5009 cases of equine cryptorchism. Equine Vet J 1986;18:467–71.
62. Pratt SM, Stacy BA, Whitcomb MB, et al. Malignant Sertoli cell tumor in the retained abdominal testis of a unilaterally cryptorchid horse. J Am Vet Med Assoc 2003;222:486–90, 450.
63. Arighi M. Testicular descent. In: McKinnon AO, Squires EL, Vaala WE, et al, editors. Equine reproduction, Vol. 1. New Delhi (India): Wiley-Blackwell; 2011. p. 1099–112.
64. Foster RA, Ladds PW. Male genital system. In: Maxie MG, editor. Pathology of domestic animals. Philadelphia: Elsevier Saunders; 2007. p. 564–619.

65. Russell TM, Pollock PJ. Cryptorchid castration. In: McKinnon AO, Squires EL, Vaala WE, et al, editors. Equine reproduction, Vol. 1. New Delhi (India): Wiley-Blackwell; 2011. p. 1531–9.
66. Barthold JS. Undescended testis: current theories of etiology. Curr Opin Urol 2008;18:395–400.
67. Stout TAE. Can and should we do more to reduce the incidence of cryptorchidism? Equine Vet J 2013;45:531–2.
68. Ghosh S, Arnold C, Wade C, et al. AKR1C genes as candidate loci for equine cryptorchidism. J Equine Vet Sci 2016;43:S56–82.
69. Schrimpf R, Gottschalk M, Metzger J, et al. Screening of whole genome sequences identified high-impact variants for stallion fertility. BMC Genomics 2016;17:288.
70. Coutinho da Silva MA. When should a mare go for assisted reproduction? Theriogenology 2008;70:441–4.
71. Sevinga M, Vrijenhoek T, Hesselinks JW, et al. Effect of inbreeding on the incidence of retained placenta in Friesian horses. J Anim Sci 2004;82:982–6.
72. Burger D, Thomas S, Aepli H, et al. Major histocompatibility complex-linked social signalling affects female fertility. Proc Biol Sci 2017;284 [pii:20171824].
73. Jeannerat E, Marti E, Berney C, et al. Stallion semen quality depends on major histocompatibility complex matching to teaser mare. Mol Ecol 2018;27:1025–35.
74. Power MM. The first description of a balanced reciprocal translocation [t(1q;3q)] and its clinical effects in a mare. Equine Vet J 1991;23:146–9.
75. Long SE. Tandem 1;30 translocation: a new structural abnormality in the horse (Equus caballus). Cytogenet Cell Genet 1996;72:162–3.
76. Lear TL, Layton G. Use of zoo-FISH to characterise a reciprocal translocation in a thoroughbred mare: t(1;1 6)(q16;q21.3). Equine Vet J 2002;34:207–9.
77. Lear TL, Lundquist J, Zent WW, et al. Three autosomal chromosome translocations associated with repeated early embryonic loss (REEL) in the domestic horse (Equus caballus). Cytogenet Genome Res 2008;120:117–22.
78. Lear TL, Raudsepp T, Lundquist JM, et al. Repeated early embryonic loss in a thoroughbred mare with a chromosomal translocation [64,XX,t(2;13)]. J Equine Vet Sci 2014;34:805–9.
79. Ghosh S, Das PJ, Avila F, et al. A non-reciprocal autosomal translocation 64,XX, t(4;10)(q21;p15) in an Arabian mare with repeated early embryonic loss. Reprod Domest Anim 2016;51:171–4.
80. Ghosh S, Das PJ, Arnold C, et al. Contribution of DNA copy number variants to equine cryptorchidism. J Equine Vet Sci 2014;34:29.
81. Hamann H, Jude R, Sieme H, et al. A polymorphism within the equine CRISP3 gene is associated with stallion fertility in Hanoverian warmblood horses. Anim Genet 2007;38:259–64.
82. Giesecke K, Hamann H, Sieme H, et al. Evaluation of prolactin receptor (PRLR) as candidate gene for male fertility in Hanoverian warmblood horses. Reprod Domest Anim 2010;45:e124–30.
83. Giesecke K, Hamann H, Stock KF, et al. Evaluation of SPATA1-associated markers for stallion fertility. Anim Genet 2009;40:359–65.
84. Giese A, Jude R, Kuiper H, et al. Molecular characterization of the equine AEG1 locus. Gene 2002;292:65–72.
85. Sabeur K, Ball BA, Corbin CJ, et al. Characterization of a novel, testis-specific equine serine/threonine kinase. Mol Reprod Dev 2008;75:867–73.

Genetics of Equine Behavioral Traits

Carissa Wickens, PhD[a], Samantha A. Brooks, PhD[b],*

KEYWORDS

- Equine • Behavior • Genetics • Heritability • Personality • Neurotransmitters
- Startle • Stereotypies

KEY POINTS

- Behavior is a valuable quantitative trait in the horse because of its impact on performance, work, recreation, and prerequisite close interactions with humans.
- Heritability studies have relied on traditional pedigree-derived estimates of relatedness, versus more accurate genomic estimation approaches enabled by high-throughput genotyping arrays.
- Extensive research on behavioral traits in laboratory species has revealed examples of the impact of genetic polymorphism on highly conserved pathways controlling aspects of temperament.
- Previous research supports a genetic basis for stereotypic behavior, although stereotypies in horses are most likely the result of genetics and environment.

INTRODUCTION

Behavior is a valuable quantitative trait in all domesticated livestock species. No production system can operate effectively when excessive fear, aggression or abnormal behavior jeopardizes the safety and well-being of the animals and their human caretakers. This is especially true for the horse, because of their value as a performance, working, and recreational animal and subsequent close interactions with humans. Behavior and cognitive traits are so fundamental to the domestication process that selection acts on them swiftly. Paleogenomic studies comparing modern horses with their predomestication counterparts highlighted regions of the genome with reduced nucleotide diversity characteristic of the action of selection. Modern-day horses possess several of these signatures of selection across chromosome regions harboring an enrichment of genes important for cognitive development and behavior.[1]

With the availability of the tools of modern genomics, reference genomes, single-nucleotide polymorphism (SNP) genotyping arrays, and next-generation sequencing,

[a] Department of Animal Sciences, University of Florida, Gainesville, FL, USA; [b] Department of Animal Sciences, UF Genetics Institute, University of Florida, 2250 Shealy Drive, Gainesville, FL 32611-0910, USA
* Corresponding author.
E-mail address: samantha.brooks@ufl.edu

Vet Clin Equine 36 (2020) 411–424
https://doi.org/10.1016/j.cveq.2020.03.014
0749-0739/20/© 2020 Elsevier Inc. All rights reserved.

there is now the scientific power to dissect the complex interplay between genetics and the environment. Here, we review the current field of genetics and behavior in the horse, management considerations for breeders or clinicians, and discuss the potential for future research studies aimed at identifying genetic correlates of specific behavioral traits. Ultimately, these studies enhance the understanding of the biology of behavior in the horse, improve handler and rider safety, and benefit horse welfare.

HOW MUCH OF HORSE BEHAVIOR IS HERITABLE?

Even in the absence of outright aggression, qualities of temperament still rank highly among the most important economic qualities in the horse because it influences much of the reaction to human handlers. From a scientific perspective, temperament governs an animal's reaction to a situation and is a stable component of personality over time. Among those reactions, fear plays a key role in survival because the ability to identify and escape danger frequently draws the line between life and death in the wild. In domesticated settings, predation is largely eliminated, yet because of the intrinsic nature of this most basic instinct, some aspect of the fear response remains even in the most docile pets.[2] A complex emotive reaction, fear itself presents a particularly challenging trait to quantify experimentally. Thus, most work aimed at identifying aspects of behavior under genetic control in any species breaks the behavior down into simpler, more measurable endophenotypes within the context of specific experimental procedures.

In the horse, as in other livestock and laboratory species, the novel arena, novel object, and startle test methods assess fear in absence of a handler (**Fig. 1**). The approach test, forced approach test, and restraint tests integrate a human with or without involuntary interaction.[2] During these experiments, diverse variables assess aspects of fearfulness including behavioral frequencies quantified by an ethogram; physical proximity measured by distance or time to approach; and physiologic

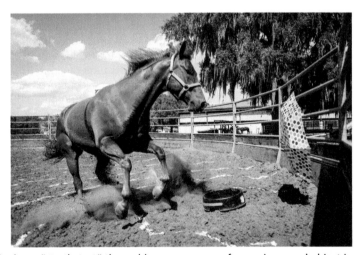

Fig. 1. During a "startle test" the sudden appearance of a moving novel object is presented to the horse and the degree of response measured using behavioral and physiologic variables. Triggered initially by the startle reflex and then carried on to outward behaviors by fearfulness, this trait is stable over time, and an important economic trait in the horse given the risk to handlers potentially caught in the path of an unwanted flight response. (*Courtesy of* Camila Guillen, IFAS Communications, UF).

parameters, most notably heart rate. In the search for genetic components of variation in response, variables that are stable over time and maturity, and therefore more likely intrinsic to the horse and not an effect of the environment, offer the most tractable targets. In the horse, this type of repeatability within horse is documented within novel object and startle tests for measures of physical proximity to the fear-inducing stimulus.[3] Even for these fairly stable measures of fearfulness, specific experimental introduction of enrichment stimuli (eg, social interactions and new foods) can alter the response to novel stimuli.[4] Yet, the positive benefits of an enriched environment may emerge in part through the action of genetic predispositions and epigenetics modifications because the effect of enrichment are clearly observed in the alteration of gene expression.[4]

Either as a direct result of selection, or as a coincidence of a population bottleneck occurring at breed formation, genetic divergence results from differentiation of breeds over time. Thus, allele frequencies at functional and nonfunctional loci differ between breeds. Variation in a trait that correlates with breed, and that is reproducibly observed across breeds even when they are maintained in a similar environment, likely has a strong genetic component.

There are significant differences across breeds for diverse aspects of personality, generally considered to the be sum resulting from temperament and life experiences. These are inexpensively detected using owner responses to a questionnaire, and were observed in European[5] and American populations.[6] Breed also strongly influences temperament-driven responses to novel object and learning tests among riding school horses, but this effect was modulated by the type of housing in which the horse was kept (stall vs pasture).[7] In a large sampling of 702 horses, Hausberger and colleagues[8] attributed 30% of the variation in a novel-object driven component to the breed, and 27.8% to the type of housing. Even within breed, changes in the response to a novel object test are observed between the dressage and show-jumping subtypes,[9] two groups valued for slightly different performance related behaviors and diverging genetically.[10] Even the influence of a particular sire or dam was detected for a learning test administered to semiferal ponies.[11]

Unfortunately, few studies have sought to objectively quantify the heritability evidenced by these trends. Just 17% of the variation in an observational behavior study conducted during breed inspection proceedings could be attributed to genetics, even in a large population of 323 Danish Warmblood horses.[12] In a massive examination of 4453 Thoroughbred horses, a similar effect size of 0.23 was attributed to genetic factors when assessing the need for restraint during a routine veterinary examination.[13] However, both studies are limited by the use of these opportunistic and accessible but environmentally complex "reactivity during presentation/examination" traits. Estimates were somewhat higher, 0.2 to 0.5, for behavioral responses to experimental measures within a large sampling across breeds.[8] However, each of these studies has used the traditional pedigree-derived estimates of relatedness, rather than more accurate genomic estimation approaches enabled by high-throughput genotyping arrays for the horse.

MOLECULAR GENETICS OF HORSE BEHAVIOR

Given the difficulties associated with large-scale genome-wide approaches, most progress in the understanding of the genetics of behavior in the horse has come from candidate gene studies. Extensive research on behavioral traits in laboratory species has revealed many examples of the impact of genetic polymorphism on highly conserved pathways controlling the startle response, and other aspects of temperament.[14–17] Among these, neurotransmitter-related genes yielded some of the most profound findings, and led to logical hypotheses regarding the cause of the associated phenotypes.[18]

Monoamine neurotransmitters bridge the gap of the synapse as they are released by one neuron and captured in the corresponding receptor on the opposing axon (**Fig. 2**, reviewed in Ref.[18]). Extensively studied dopaminergic pathways have yielded multiple genetic associations with startle, fear-driven, and thrill-seeking behavior in multiple diverse species. Multiple mutations in Dopamine Receptor D4 (*DRD4*) increase the likelihood of certain personality traits in humans including drug abuse, novelty-seeking behavior, and stranger fear in young children,[19–21] whereas studies in mice, dogs, and birds have all demonstrated impacts on startle, fear, and aggression.[14,17,22,23]

Although well-known for its relationship with the reward system, dopamine pathways are better described as balancing motivation and satisfaction. Dopamine itself can have either an excitatory or inhibitory effect, dependent on the subtype and receptor expression pattern of the individual neuron.[24] The dopamine coding sequence possesses a highly polymorphic region of tandem repeats in exon three.[25] The repeat structure and number of units differs across diverse mammalian species, including the horse, where it comprises an 18-bp motif tandemly recurring between 8 and 10 times.[26,27] However, the nine-repeat allele is fixed in most light horse breeds.[26] Several amino acid–altering SNPs also occur in the horse and are more useful for study because they are highly polymorphic in the popular Thoroughbred breed.[26]

Two studies identified significant associations between the *A292 G* nonsynonymous SNP in *DRD4* and behavioral phenotypes in the horse. The first compared survey reports from grooms and handlers familiar with the horses' daily routine on the racetrack.[28] This survey used questions structured around specific situations (ie, during grooming, or loading on a trailer) and qualitative assessments (on a score of 1–5, how nervous is the horse) and correlated well with changes in heart rate observed in a controlled novel object test of the same horses.[28] The survey phenotypes yielded a strong statistical association between the *A292 G* polymorphism and questions

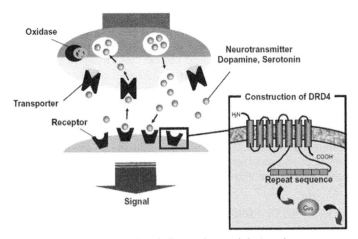

Fig. 2. Neurotransmitter pathways alter behavior by modulating the transport, oxidation, and receptor binding properties of the signaling cascade. Each gene product in the pathway is a potential candidate gene for behavioral phenotypes. Polymorphism in the *DRD4* coding sequence, especially the repetitive region of exon 3 (*inset*), alters temperament in several species, including the horse. (*From* Inoue-Murayama M. Genetic polymorphism as a background of animal behavior. *Anim Sci J.* Apr 2009;80(2):113-120; with permission.)

aimed at "curiosity" and "vigilance" components of temperament.[29,30] A second study of just 21 stabled horses also detected significant increases in frustration behaviors at feeding time in individuals with the *G/G* rather than the *G/A* or *A/A* genotypes at this same SNP.[31]

Known colloquially as the "worrier or warrior" locus in humans, catechol-O-methyltransferase (the *COMT* gene), is responsible for degradation of dopamine in the brain.[32] Early work suggests an association between postrace stress levels in Spanish Trotting Horses and a polymorphism upstream of the coding sequence.[33] These authors used a unique physiologic measure of stress, noninvasive detection of eye temperature by infrared thermography. This phenotype is advantageous for use in the field given the portability of the equipment and ability to take measurements without potentially stress-inducing restraint or procedures on the animal.[34] Yet, how the horse outwardly expresses the perception of this stress may differ based on yet other environmental variables and genetic loci. A nonsynonymous mutation (*G217 A*) in *COMT* was identified in a group of Mongolian horses, presumed to be a "landrace" with characteristics similar to the native horses present around the time of early domestication.[35] The *G217 A* variant supported a trend for association with a "competitiveness" trait in this breed.[35]

Dopamine β-hydroxylase, encoded by the *DBH* gene, converts dopamine to noradrenaline[36] and in humans, possesses several coding polymorphisms that alter enzyme levels so profoundly that the differences are detected in plasma.[37] Several neurologic and psychiatric conditions are associated with these polymorphisms, although most of these studies lack validation.[37] A leucine to glutamine change in the coding sequence exists in the Mongolian horse, and showed some statistical association with acceptance of novel situations (eg, swimming), tolerance, and affection to other horses.[35] More work is needed to examine the frequency, and possible phenotypes, of this allele in other populations.

The serotonin pathway is also a strong candidate for behavioral phenotypes based on findings from other species (reviewed in Ref.[24]). No association was detected between the caretaker survey variables in the Thoroughbred and sequence polymorphism in the *SLC6A4* gene for the serotonin transporter.[38] However, postperformance physiologic stress in harness racers and dressage horses differed by genotypes at a distant 3′ polymorphism for this locus.[33] Mongolian horses possess a *SLC6A4* coding sequence variant (*T1362 C*) associated with various traits described as "independence," "nervousness," and "reaction to harness."[35] At a different point in the pathway, investigation of the sequence for the Serotonin Receptor 1A (*HTR1A*) identified a nonsynonymous mutation associated with several components of a survey designed to detect anxiety during early training activities, especially in fillies.[39]

Targeted exome sequencing in a small set of aggressive and docile Thoroughbreds identified interesting polymorphisms in two candidate genes *AR* (for the androgen receptor) and *MAOA* (encoding monoamine oxidase A).[40] *MAOA* is particularly notable because it specifically recycles dopamine.[40] Alleles at this locus generate a variety of startling neuropsychiatric phenotypes in humans including panic disorder; delinquent behavior; and the most severe alleles, the violent and aggressive Brunner syndrome.[41–43] These two functional candidate polymorphisms will be interesting to follow in future population studies.

Aside from the action of neurotransmitters, the way an individual perceives stimuli can alter their behavioral response. The Agouti (*ASIP*)-Melanocortin Receptor 1 (*MC1R*) signaling pathway controls variation in base coat color in the horse. A frame-shift deletion within *ASIP* modifies the wild-type distribution of black pigment at the points to black pigment production evenly across the body (black allele, *a/a* genotype).[44] A loss of function mutation in the *MC1R* receptor abolishes signaling capacity, even when bound to the *ASIP* ligand, leading to a loss of black pigment production observed as the chestnut coat color phenotype.[45] In addition to the well-documented pigmentation phenotypes, these loci generate pleiotropic traits of obesity and pain response.[46] In humans, individuals with a similar loss-of-function mutation in *MC1R* have reduced tolerance to thermal pain and reduced relief of pain by analgesic drugs.[47]

Using an owner survey Finn and colleagues[48] did not detect an association with unwanted behaviors among chestnut horses of a variety of breeds, as expected based on common horsemen's mythology, but did see increases in willingness to approach novel objects. However, the investigators did not genotype each horse for the coat color variants, leaving significant room for error in color designation, and no option to assess associations by genotype. Within Tennessee Walking Horse mares an association was detected between the *ASIP* genotype and a survey-measured component of independence.[49]

Altered perception likely also played a role in another study observing increased responses to a startle test. Icelandic horses with the *Silver* dilution are more wary to approach an experimental test ring, although their responses to a startle type test are similar to their non-*Silver* compatriots.[50] There is no known neurophysiologic interaction for the *PMEL17* gene responsible for the *Silver* allele, although horses with this variant do contract several progressive ocular anomalies impairing vision, especially in older individuals.[51] Thus, altered vision may make *Silver* horses more fearful of unfamiliar surroundings.

STEREOTYPIC BEHAVIORS: ARE THEY GENETIC OR ARE THEY LEARNED?

Stereotypies are defined as repetitive, invariant patterns of behavior with no apparent goal or function.[52] It has been suggested that stereotypic behavior may serve as a coping mechanism, functioning to reduce stress or to provide the animal with some form of control over its environment.[52,53] The presence of stereotypies has been used as an indicator of poor welfare,[54,55] although whether the welfare is currently poor or has simply been poor in the past is more difficult to determine. Stereotypic behavior is not known to occur in feral, free-ranging horses, but is observed in domestic[56,57] and captive wild horses (eg, Przewalski horse).[58] It is widely reported in the literature that crib-biting (**Fig. 3**), and other stereotypic behaviors, are viewed by owners as being problematic and undesirable[59]

Despite researchers' significant efforts to elucidate the cause of stereotypic behaviors in horses, uncertainty and debate remains concerning stereotypic behavior development. Specifically, it has been difficult to determine whether environment or genetics are primarily involved or if stereotypies are the result of a combination of genetics and environment. There are well established environmental risk factors that increase the likelihood of stereotypies (eg, impeded foraging opportunities and limited social contact, provision of high concentrate diets, and abrupt weaning), yet even when horses are managed under similar, stressful or suboptimal conditions, not all individuals exhibit stereotypic behavior. A long-held belief within the equine community is that horses "learn" to perform stereotypic behavior through observation of another horse engaging in the behavior. However, to date, there is little scientific evidence to support the view that stereotypic behaviors develop through observational learning.

Previous research has demonstrated certain breeds are more likely to exhibit stereotypic behavior, including crib-biting. In a survey of stereotypic behavior in Swiss horses, Bachmann and colleagues[60] found Warmbloods and Thoroughbreds were

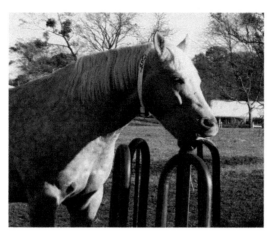

Fig. 3. A horse crib-biting on a metal hay feeder. Horses that exhibit crib-biting behavior set their incisor teeth on a fixed object, arch the neck, pull backward, and emit an audible grunting noise as air is drawn into the proximal esophagus and then expelled. This is a repetitive, seemingly functionless behavior that individual horses perform in much the same way and often even in a preferred location within the stall or paddock each time the behavior is performed. Some horses spend up to 15% to 20% of their day engaged in this behavior. The horse shown here is wearing an identification collar, not an anticribbing collar. (*Courtesy of* Dr. Carissa Wickens).

at 1.8 and 3.1 times greater risk of performing stereotypic behavior, respectively, compared with other breeds. Albright and colleagues[61] found that among US horses, Thoroughbreds were three times more likely to exhibit crib-biting behavior than Quarter Horses and five times more likely than Arabians. Vecchiotti and Galanti[62] suggested the involvement of a genetic component in the performance of stereotypic behavior, as evidenced by the finding that one or more relatives in eight families of Thoroughbreds exhibited crib-biting behavior. Luescher and colleagues[63] found a higher prevalence of crib-biting in geldings and stallions compared with mares, and a greater risk of crib-biting among Thoroughbred horses. Horses used for competitive disciplines, such as racing, eventing, show-jumping, and dressage, are often kept individually with limited free movement and social contact, and Thoroughbreds and Warmbloods are frequently engaged in these sports. Stallions also are frequently housed in individual enclosures to prevent accidental breeding and aggression.

Specific investigations into the cause of stereotypic behavior in horses using molecular genetics and genomics are limited. Cabib and colleagues[64] found that stress induces significant changes in dopamine receptor densities within the mesoaccumbens and nigrostriatal systems in mice. In inbred strains of mice, these stress-induced changes in dopamine neurophysiology have been associated with the development of stereotypic behavior.[65] McBride and Hemmings[66] reported significantly lower dopamine D_1-like receptor subtypes in the caudate nucleus (dorsomedial striatum) and significantly higher dopamine D_1-like and D_2-like receptor subtypes in the nucleus accumbens (ventral striatum) of crib-biting horses. Wickens and colleagues[67] conducted a study to examine the integrity and function of gastric mucosa in mature horses with a history of crib-biting behavior but found no differences in the number or severity of squamous mucosal lesions between crib-biting and normal horses maintained on pasture. However, serum gastrin response to concentrate feeding was shown to be higher in crib-biting horses compared with control animals, providing some additional evidence that gastrointestinal physiology may be altered in horses exhibiting crib-biting behavior. It was suggested that gastrin-stimulated acid secretion may be enhanced in crib-biting horses because of greater G cell numbers or increased secretory capacity of the existing G cells, but this idea can only be confirmed through further investigation involving molecular genetic techniques. It would be interesting to discover whether pathways involved in gastric acid secretion are upregulated and/or if gastric mucosal protective pathways are downregulated in crib-biting horses.

Hemmann and colleagues[68] tested associations of known or suspected stereotypic genes (Ghrelin [GHRL], Ghrelin receptor [GHS-RIA], Leptin [Lep], Dopamine receptor [DRD1], μ-opioid receptor [OPRM1], N-cadherin [CDH2], Serotonin receptor [HTR1B], and Semaphorin [SEMA6]) with equine crib-biting. In this candidate gene study with a case-control design (98 crib-biting and 135 control horses of two breeds, Finnhorses and Finnhorse crosses), detailed phenotypic information on crib-biting behavior was surveyed through an owner-completed questionnaire. SNPs flanking the candidate genes were genotyped using either Sanger sequencing or TaqMan assays. Comparison of allele frequencies between the cases and control animals for each breed separately did not provide evidence of an association at any of the tested loci. Although the results suggest previously known stereotypic genes are not associated with crib-biting behavior in horses, other candidate genes important in the development of stereotypy in mice including dopamine D_3 receptor gene (DRD3), GABA A-receptor beta-3 gene (GABRB3), serotonin receptor 2C gene (HTR2C or 5HT2C), and the disk large-associated protein-3 gene (DAP-3 or SAP90/PSD-95-associated protein 3 or SAPAP3) were not investigated and may be of interest in future studies.[69] Hemmann and colleagues[68] recommended pursuit of genome-wide association approaches in a larger population of horses. In a parallel study, Hemmann and colleagues[70] generated a heritability estimate of 0.68 for crib-biting in Finnhorses, a remarkably high heritability, although the authors cautioned readers to critically consider the results given the small study population and the inability to estimate possible effects of housing.

A genetic basis for stereotypic behavior is further supported through studies demonstrating the transmission of locomotor stereotypy from parents to offspring. In a study conducted by Jones and colleagues,[71] stereotypy prevalence in striped mice was five times greater in the offspring of stereotypic than nonstereotypic females, regardless of stereotypic status of the sire, and three times greater in offspring of stereotypic males paired with nonstereotypic females than in offspring from nonstereotypic parents. Surprisingly, offspring with two stereotypic parents were not at a greater risk of developing stereotypy than offspring with only a stereotypic mother. A finding of further interest was that pairings where the mother was stereotypic produced nearly twice the number of offspring compared with other pairings (nonstereotypic female with stereotypic male and both nonstereotypic parents). The finding that maternal stereotypy was a better predictor of stereotypic behavior in the offspring indicates, however, that nongenetic mechanisms are also at play. Although a previous study using a cross-foster experimental design helped refute social facilitation in the transmission of stereotypy from mother to offspring,[72] Jones and colleagues[71] and Mostard[69] suggested the influence of epigenetic factors, specifically gestational effects between conception and birth (eg, prenatal stress) that might predispose offspring to a stereotypic phenotype.

Interconnections between genetic and environmental factors, specifically interactions between breed and management, or gender and management, almost certainly play a role in the development of stereotypic behavior, and these relationships warrant further consideration in future experimental and epidemiologic studies. Nonetheless, there is some evidence for a genetic predisposition in the display of the behavior and additional studies aimed at identification of specific genes responsible for stereotypic behavior in horses through pedigree analysis and association mapping are warranted.

Concerning the question whether horses learn to perform stereotypic behavior by watching stereotypic stable or pasture mates, Albright and colleagues[61] reported that only 1% of horses surveyed started to crib-bite after being exposed to another crib-biting horse. Most (86%) horses were turned out in the same pasture with other horses and extent of contact with conspecifics was not statistically related to risk, although nearly 50% of owners surveyed believed crib-biting is learned by observation. The current authors' experience with situations where nonstereotypic horses have been housed with stereotypic horses in the same or adjacent pastures with fence-line contact has been that these behaviors are not "transmitted" between horses. However, Nagy and colleagues[73] found an increased risk of stereotypic behavior (crib-biting and weaving) in horses exposed to stereotypic neighbors. It was the presence of a weaving neighbor that increased the risk of crib-biting.

It has been suggested,[74,75] and more recently demonstrated,[76] that familiarity with other horses and dominance hierarchies between horses may be important factors in the ability of horses to learn or copy a particular behavior by observation, but this hypothesis has not been empirically tested with respect to stereotypic behaviors. Perhaps those horses with a genetic predisposition for stereotypic behavior are at greater risk when exposed to inciting management factors that include stereotypic conspecifics. At present, when multiple horses at a facility are observed performing stereotypic behavior, these horses may be exposed to common stressors or inciting environmental factors or alternatively, the presence of several horses with established history of stereotypic behavior may largely be coincidental (eg, greater number of stereotypic horses because of nonexclusion). Misconceptions within the equine industry on this topic lead to negative bias toward stereotypic horses. Such bias presents challenges for owners of stereotypic horses and can reduce the welfare of horses (eg, when horses with stereotypic behavior are isolated from other horses). Subsequent empirical and epidemiologic investigation is needed before reaching a definitive conclusion about the ability of horses to imitate stereotypic behavior through observation.

SUMMARY

Behavioral traits are among some of the most complex attributes under selection in animal agriculture. Influenced by heritable predispositions, epigenetics, and environment, then altered by learning and life experience, they are literally a moving target. Yet, the neurophysiologic changes initiated at domestication and still in progress today are witnessed as signatures and polymorphisms in the horse genome. Several behavioral traits have substantial heritable components worthy of expanded research.

Genomic tools are not limited to the study of heritable variations. Circadian and circannual behaviors influence several important economic traits, such as reproductive seasonality, feeding, and athletic performance.[77,78] Gene expression provides a valuable tool for tracking changes in physiologic processes, and the signaling pathways responsible for entraining them.[77] Novel gene variants altering patterns of activity, especially those contributing to circannual reproductive behavior, could be fruitful areas for future research because several successful examples are found in humans and other livestock species.[79,80]

Molecular studies have identified many novel polymorphisms in key candidate genes. These new polymorphisms, especially those implicated in multiple studies, such as the *A292 G DRD4* variation, could be used in informing selection of breeding and training stock, although the value of these markers is not currently well communicated to the horse industry. Most require further validation, and investigation of the allele frequencies and action on the genetic background of other breeds, before one can fully interpret their impact on gene function and the resulting phenotype.

Stereotypical behaviors impact the welfare and market value of the horses exhibiting them. Given the difficulty in controlling or modifying these behaviors, horse professionals have sought several explanations for the development of stereotypy and are quick to blame affected horses as setting a bad example for others in the barn. Yet, there is little evidence that stereotypies are learned, and, whereas they may be triggered by stressful management conditions, not all horses in these environments develop a stereotypical coping mechanism. Based on animal models it seems likely that genetics plays a strong role in stereotypy in horses, although large-scale genomics studies in this area are required. Certainly, quantification of genes involved in fear, aggression, and abnormal behaviors, including stereotypic behaviors, will allow owners to identify predisposed individuals, which may enhance the ability to proactively manage, handle, and train horses for more successful outcomes.

REFERENCES

1. Librado P, Gamba C, Gaunitz C, et al. Ancient genomic changes associated with domestication of the horse. Science 2017;356(6336):442–5.
2. Forkman B, Boissy A, Meunier-Salauen M, et al. A critical review of fear tests used on cattle, pigs, sheep, poultry and horses. Physiol Behav 2007;92(3):340–74.
3. Lansade L, Bouissou M, Erhard H. Fearfulness in horses: a temperament trait stable across time and situations. Appl Anim Behav Sci 2008;115(3–4):182–200.
4. Lansade L, Valenchon M, Foury A, et al. Behavioral and transcriptomic fingerprints of an enriched environment in horses (Equus caballus). PLoS One 2014; 9(12):e114384.
5. Lloyd A, Martin J, Bornett-Gauci H, et al. Horse personality: variation between breeds. Appl Anim Behav Sci 2008;112(3–4):369–83.
6. Sackman J, Houpt K. Equine personality: association with breed, use, and husbandry factors. J Equine Vet Sci 2019;72:47–55.
7. Lesimple C, Fureix C, LeScolan N, et al. Housing conditions and breed are associated with emotionality and cognitive abilities in riding school horses. Appl Anim Behav Sci 2011;129(2–4):92–9.
8. Hausberger M, Bruderer U, Le Scolan N, et al. Interplay between environmental and genetic factors in temperament/personality traits in horses (Equus caballus). J Comp Psychol 2004;118(4):434–46.
9. von Borstel U, Duncan I, Lundin M, et al. Fear reactions in trained and untrained horses from dressage and show-jumping breeding lines. Appl Anim Behav Sci 2010;125(3–4):124–31.
10. Rovere G, Ducro BJ, van Arendonk JA, et al. Genetic correlations between dressage, show jumping and studbook-entry inspection traits in a process of specialization in Dutch Warmblood horses. J Anim Breed Genet 2017;134(2):162–71.
11. Bonnell M, McDonnell S. Evidence for sire, dam, and family influence on operant learning in horses. J Equine Vet Sci 2016;36:69–76.
12. Rothmann J, Christensen O, Sondergaard E, et al. A note on the heritability of reactivity assessed at field tests for Danish Warmblood horses. J Equine Vet Sci 2014;34(2):341–3.

13. Oki H, Kusunose R, Nakaoka H, et al. Estimation of heritability and genetic correlation for behavioural responses by Gibbs sampling in the Thoroughbred racehorse. J Anim Breed Genet 2007;124(4):185–91.
14. Ralph RJ, Paulus MP, Fumagalli F, et al. Prepulse inhibition deficits and perseverative motor patterns in dopamine transporter knock-out mice: differential effects of D1 and D2 receptor antagonists. J Neurosci 2001;21(1):305–13.
15. Powell SB, Zhou X, Geyer MA. Prepulse inhibition and genetic mouse models of schizophrenia. Behav Brain Res 2009;204(2):282–94.
16. Wan M, Hejjas K, Ronai Z, et al. DRD4 and TH gene polymorphisms are associated with activity, impulsivity and inattention in Siberian Husky dogs. Anim Genet 2013;44(6):717–27.
17. Våge J, Wade C, Biagi T, et al. Association of dopamine- and serotonin-related genes with canine aggression. Genes Brain Behav 2010;9(4):372–8.
18. Inoue-Murayama M. Genetic polymorphism as a background of animal behavior. Anim Sci J 2009;80(2):113–20.
19. Lansade L, Bertrand M, Boivin X, et al. Effects of handling at weaning on manageability and reactivity of foals. Appl Anim Behav Sci 2004;87(1–2):131–49.
20. Fureix C, Pagès M, Bon R, et al. A preliminary study of the effects of handling type on horses' emotional reactivity and the human-horse relationship. Behav Process 2009;82(2):202–10.
21. Konig von Borstel U, Euent S, Graf P, et al. Equine behavior and heart rate in temperament tests with or without rider or handler. Physiol Behav 2011;104:454–63.
22. Nicol C. Equine learning: progress and suggestions for future research. Appl Anim Behav Sci 2002;78(2–4):193–208.
23. Fidler A, van Oers K, Drent P, et al. Drd4 gene polymorphisms are associated with personality variation in a passerine bird. Proc Soc Biol Sci 2007;274(1619):1685–91.
24. McBride S, Parker M, Roberts K, et al. Applied neurophysiology of the horse; implications for training, husbandry and welfare. Appl Anim Behav Sci 2017;190: 90–101.
25. Larsen SA, Mogensen L, Dietz R, et al. Identification and characterization of tandem repeats in exon III of dopamine receptor D4 (DRD4) genes from different mammalian species. DNA Cell Biol 2005;24(12):795–804.
26. Hori Y, Ozaki T, Yamada Y, et al. Breed differences in dopamine receptor D4 gene (DRD4) in horses. J Equine Sci 2013;24(3):31–6.
27. Hasegawa T, Sato F, Ishida N. Determination and variability of nucleotide sequences for D4 dopamine receptor genes (DRD4) in genus Equus. J equine Sci 2002;13(2):57–62.
28. Momozawa Y, Ono T, Sato F, et al. Assessment of equine temperament by a questionnaire survey to caretakers and evaluation of its reliability by simultaneous behavior test. Appl Anim Behav Sci 2003;84(2):127–38.
29. Momozawa Y, Takeuchi Y, Kusunose R, et al. Association between equine temperament and polymorphisms in dopamine D4 receptor gene. Mamm Genome 2005; 16(7):538–44.
30. Momozawa Y, Takeuchi Y, Tozaki T, et al. SNP detection and radiation hybrid mapping in horses of nine candidate genes for temperament. Anim Genet 2007; 38(1):81–3.
31. Ninomiya S, Anjiki A, Nishide Y, et al. Polymorphisms of the dopamine D4 receptor gene in stabled horses are related to differences in behavioral response to frustration. Animals (Basel) 2013;3(3):663–9.
32. Stein DJ, Newman TK, Savitz J, et al. Warriors versus worriers: the role of COMT gene variants. CNS Spectr 2006;11(10):745–8.

33. Negro S, Sánchez-Guerrero M, Bartolomé E, et al. Evidence for the effect of serotoninergic and dopaminergic gene variants on stress levels in horses participating in dressage and harness racing. Anim Prod Sci 2019;59(12):2206–11. https://doi.org/10.1071/AN18358.

34. Hall C, Burton K, Maycock E, et al. A preliminary study into the use of infrared thermography as a means of assessing the horse's response to different training methods. J Vet Behav Clin Appl Res 2011;6(5):291–2. https://doi.org/10.1016/j.jveb.2011.05.005.

35. Ren X, Yang H, Zhao Y, et al. Association analysis between major temperament traits and diversification of the candidate gene in Mongolian horse (Equus caballus). J Agric Biotechnol 2017;25(3):405–14.

36. Kim CH, Zabetian CP, Cubells JF, et al. Mutations in the dopamine beta-hydroxylase gene are associated with human norepinephrine deficiency. Am J Med Genet 2002;108(2):140–7.

37. Tunbridge EM, Narajos M, Harrison CH, et al. Which dopamine polymorphisms are functional? Systematic review and meta-analysis of COMT, DAT, DBH, DDC, DRD1-5, MAOA, MAOB, TH, VMAT1, and VMAT2. Biol Psychiatry 2019; 86(8):608–20.

38. Momozawa Y, Takeuchi Y, Tozaki T, et al. Polymorphism identification, RH mapping, and association analysis with the anxiety trait of the equine serotonin transporter (SLC6A4) gene. J Vet Med Sci 2006;68(6):619–21.

39. Hori Y, Tozaki T, Nambo Y, et al. Evidence for the effect of serotonin receptor 1A gene (HTR1A) polymorphism on tractability in Thoroughbred horses. Anim Genet 2016;47(1):62–7.

40. Song S, Oh D, Cho G, et al. Targeted next-generation sequencing for identifying genes related to horse temperament. Genes Genomics 2017;39(12):1325–33.

41. Guo G, Ou XM, Roettger M, et al. The VNTR 2 repeat in MAOA and delinquent behavior in adolescence and young adulthood: associations and MAOA promoter activity. Eur J Hum Genet 2008;16(5):626–34.

42. Deckert J, Catalano M, Syagailo YV, et al. Excess of high activity monoamine oxidase A gene promoter alleles in female patients with panic disorder. Hum Mol Genet 1999;8(4):621–4.

43. Brunner HG, Nelen M, Breakefield XO, et al. Abnormal behavior associated with a point mutation in the structural gene for monoamine oxidase A. Science 1993; 262(5133):578–80.

44. Rieder S, Taourit S, Mariat D, et al. Mutations in the agouti (ASIP), the extension (MC1R), and the brown (TYRP1) loci and their association to coat color phenotypes in horses (Equus caballus). Mamm Genome 2001;12(6):450–5.

45. Marklund L, Moller MJ, Sandberg K, et al. A missense mutation in the gene for melanocyte-stimulating hormone receptor (MC1R) is associated with the chestnut coat color in horses. Mamm Genome 1996;7(12):895–9.

46. Harris RB, Zhou J, Shi M, et al. Overexpression of agouti protein and stress responsiveness in mice. Physiol Behav 2001;73(4):599–608.

47. Liem EB, Joiner TV, Tsueda K, et al. Increased sensitivity to thermal pain and reduced subcutaneous lidocaine efficacy in redheads. Anesthesiology 2005; 102(3):509–14.

48. Finn J, Haase B, Willet C, et al. The relationship between coat colour phenotype and equine behaviour: A pilot study. Appl Anim Behav Sci 2016;174:66–9.

49. Jacobs LN, Staiger EA, Albright JD, et al. The MC1R and ASIP coat color loci may impact behavior in the horse. J Hered 2016;107(3):214–9.

50. Brunberg E, Andersson L, Cothran G, et al. A missense mutation in PMEL17 is associated with the silver coat color in the horse. BMC Genet 2006;7:46.
51. Johansson MK, Jäderkvist Fegraeus K, Lindgren G, et al. The refractive state of the eye in Icelandic horses with the silver mutation. BMC Vet Res 2017;13(1):153.
52. Mason G. Stereotypies: a critical-review. Anim Behav 1991;41:1015–37.
53. Cooper J, Albentosa M. Behavioural adaptation in the domestic horse: potential role of apparently abnormal responses including stereotypic behaviour. Livestock Prod Sci 2005;92(2):177–82.
54. Broom DM. Stereotypies as animal welfare indicators. In: Schmidt D, editor. Indicators relevant to farm animal welfare. The Hague (the Netherlands): Martinus Nijhoff; 1983. p. 81–7.
55. Mason G, Latham N. Can't stop, won't stop: is stereotypy a reliable animal welfare indicator? Anim Welfare 2004;13:S57–69.
56. Houpt K, Mcdonnell S. Equine stereotypies. Compend Contin Educ Vet 1993; 15(9):1265–72.
57. Mills D. Recent advances in the treatment of equine stereotypic behavior [Serial online]. Animal Behavior Cognition and Welfare Group; 2002.
58. Boyd L. Behavior problems of equids in zoos. Vet Clin North Am Equine Pract 1986;2(3):653–64.
59. Wickens C, Heleski C. Crib-biting behavior in horses: a review. Appl Anim Behav Sci 2010;128(1–4):1–9.
60. Bachmann I, Audige L, Stauffacher M. Risk factors associated with behavioural disorders of crib-biting, weaving and box-walking in Swiss horses. Equine Vet J 2003;35(2):158–63.
61. Albright J, Mohammed H, Heleski C, et al. Crib-biting in US horses: breed predispositions and owner perceptions of aetiology. Equine Vet J 2009;41(5):455–8.
62. Vecchiotti G, Galanti R. Evidence of heredity of cribbing, weaving and stall-walking in thoroughbred horses. Livestock Prod Sci 1986;14(1):91–5.
63. Luescher U, McKeown D, Dean H. A cross-sectional study on compulsive behaviour (stable vices) in horses. Equine Vet J 1998;30(S27):14–8.
64. Cabib S, Giardino L, Calza L, et al. Stress promotes major changes in dopamine receptor densities within the mesoaccumbens and nigrostriatal systems. Neuroscience 1998;84(1):193–200.
65. Cabib S, Bonaventura N. Parallel strain-dependent susceptibility to environmentally-induced stereotypies and stress-induced behavioral sensitization in mice. Physiol Behav 1997;61(4):499–506.
66. McBride S, Hemmings A. Altered mesoaccumbens and nigro-striatal dopamine physiology is associated with stereotypy development in a non-rodent species. Behav Brain Res 2005;159(1):113–8.
67. Wickens CL, McCall CA, Bursian S, et al. Assessment of gastric ulceration and gastrin response in horses with history of crib-biting. J equine Vet Sci 2013; 33(9):739–45.
68. Hemmann K, Ahonen S, Raekallio M, et al. Exploration of known stereotypic behaviour-related candidate genes in equine crib-biting. Animal 2014;8(3):347–53.
69. Mostard K. General understanding, neuro-endocrinologic and (epi) genetic factors of stereotypy. Nijmegen: Radboud University of Nijmegen; 2011.
70. Hemmann K, Raekallio M, Vainio O, et al. Crib-biting and its heritability in Finnhorses. Appl Anim Behav Sci 2014;156:37–43.
71. Jones M, van Lierop M, Pillay N. All a mother's fault? Transmission of stereotypy in striped mice Rhabdomys. Appl Anim Behav Sci 2008;115(1–2):82–9.

72. Schwaibold U, Pillay N. Stereotypic behaviour is genetically transmitted in the African striped mouse Rhabdomys pumilio. Appl Anim Behav Sci 2001;74(4): 273–80.

73. Nagy K, Schrott A, Kabai P. Possible influence of neighbours on stereotypic behaviour in horses. Appl Anim Behav Sci 2008;111(3–4):321–8.

74. Murphy J, Arkins S. Equine learning behaviour. Behav Process 2007;76(1):1–13.

75. Ninomiya S. Social leaning and stereotypy in horses. Behav Process. 2007;76(1): 22–3 [discussion: 57–60].

76. Krueger K, Heinze J. Horse sense: social status of horses (Equus caballus) affects their likelihood of copying other horses' behavior. Anim Cogn 2008; 11(3):431–9.

77. Martin AM, Elliott JA, Duffy P, et al. Circadian regulation of locomotor activity and skeletal muscle gene expression in the horse. J Appl Physiol (1985) 2010;109(5): 1328–36.

78. Murphy B. Circadian and circannual regulation in the horse: internal timing in an elite athlete. J Equine Vet Sci 2019;76:14–24.

79. Jones SE, Lane JM, Wood AR, et al. Genome-wide association analyses of chronotype in 697,828 individuals provides insights into circadian rhythms. Nat Commun 2019;10(1):343.

80. Posbergh CJ, Thonney ML, Huson HJ. Genomic approaches identify novel gene associations with out of season lambing in sheep. J Hered 2019;110(5):577–86.

Moving?

Make sure your subscription moves with you!

To notify us of your new address, find your **Clinics Account Number** (located on your mailing label above your name), and contact customer service at:

Email: journalscustomerservice-usa@elsevier.com

800-654-2452 (subscribers in the U.S. & Canada)
314-447-8871 (subscribers outside of the U.S. & Canada)

Fax number: 314-447-8029

Elsevier Health Sciences Division
Subscription Customer Service
3251 Riverport Lane
Maryland Heights, MO 63043

*To ensure uninterrupted delivery of your subscription, please notify us at least 4 weeks in advance of move.

Printed and bound by CPI Group (UK) Ltd, Croydon, CR0 4YY

03/10/2024

01040403-0002